Yamada's Handbook of Gastroenterology

Yamada's Handbook of Gastroenterology

EDITOR

Tadataka Yamada, MD

Board Member
Chief Medical and Scientific Officer
Executive Vice-President
Takeda Pharmaceutical Corporation
Tokyo, Japan

Adjunct Professor
Department of Internal Medicine
Division of Gastroenterology
University of Michigan Medical School
Ann Arbor, MI, USA

ASSOCIATE EDITOR

John M. Inadomi, MD

Cyrus E. Rubin Professor of Medicine
Head, Division of Gastroenterology
University of Washington
Seattle, WA, USA

CONTRIBUTING AUTHORS

Renuka Bhattacharya, MD

Clinical Associate Professor, Division of Gastroenterology
Chief of Clinical Hepatology
Medical Director for Liver Transplantation
University of Washington
Seattle, WA, USA

Jason A. Dominitz, MD, MHS

National Program Director, Gastroenterology
Veterans Health Administration
Professor, Division of Gastroenterology
University of Washington
Seattle, WA, USA

Joo Ha Hwang, MD, PhD

Associate Professor, Division of Gastroenterology
Director of Endoscopic Research
University of Washington
Seattle, WA, USA

THIRD EDITION

WILEY-BLACKWELL

A John Wiley & Sons, Ltd., Publication

Contents

Foreword

From its inception, the *Textbook of Gastroenterology* was intended to provide an encyclopedic reference to the rapidly evolving science and practice of gastroenterology to practitioners who encountered patients with digestive and liver diseases and to researchers in the field. Recognizing the need to provide access to the essential elements of the *Textbook* in a more concise format that was optimized to provide information of particular usefulness to medical students, house officers and fellows, we undertook the editing of *Yamada's Handbook of Gastroenterology*. The success of the first two editions of the *Handbook* has provided evidence of its utility not only as a guide to those in training but also as a resource for practicing physicians.

Dr. John Inadomi, the Associate Editor, has carried forward the best elements of past editions and improved on them in the third edition of *Yamada's Handbook of Gastroenterology*, with important additions such as key practice points, case studies, management algorithms and questions and answers, all within fewer pages. Moreover, this edition is available in electronic format to make it more compatible with the needs of practicing physicians.

I am indebted to Dr. Inadomi and his contributing authors Drs. Renuka Bhattacharya, Jason Dominitz and Joo Ha Hwang for the enormous time and effort they put into making this edition so clear and complete and hope that these qualities provided to the reader will help them to deliver the best possible care to their patients.

Tadataka Yamada
2013

Preface

On behalf of my co-authors, Drs. Bhattacharya, Dominitz and Hwang, I am pleased to introduce the third edition of *Yamada's Handbook of Gastroenterology*. *Yamada's Handbook* is based on the *Textbook of Gastroenterology* and *Principles of Clinical Gastroenterology* by Tadataka Yamada, and is divided into two major sections: symptom-based evaluation chapters and disease-based management chapters. In addition to updating the content for this version of *Yamada's Handbook*, Dr. Yamada challenged us to change the format for this version by incorporating pedagogical features that would enhance the learning experience for the reader. For this reason this version differs from previous editions of *Yamada's Handbook* by providing Key Practice Points, easily identified in "call-out boxes" in each chapter, which highlight the most important factors that guide clinical care. The case scenarios created for each chapter in Part 1: "Approach to Patients with Gastrointestinal Symptoms" are accompanied by discussions that we hope will provide the context necessary to translate medical knowledge to clinical practice. Finally, we have written a series of questions, with detailed answers located in the back of *Yamada's Handbook*, that should provide a means to test and solidify the reader's knowledge base.

We hope *Yamada's Handbook of Gastroenterology* is a useful companion to the Yamada *Textbook of Gastroenterology* and *Principles of Clinical Gastroenterology*, especially for readers interested in a condensed reference guiding the care of patients with gastrointestinal and liver diseases. In addition, we expect that trainees of all levels will benefit from *Yamada's Handbook* by providing a solid foundation upon which they may build a comprehensive understanding of this exciting and rapidly evolving field of medicine.

John M. Inadomi
2013

List of Abbreviations

5-ASA	5-aminosalicylate
6-MMP	6-methylmercaptopurine
6-MP	6-mercaptopurine
6-TG	6-thioguanine
ACCR	amylase-to-creatinine clearance ratio
ACE	angiotensin-converting enzyme
ADH	alcohol dehydrogenase
AFP	α-fetoprotein (AFP
AIDS	acquired immunodeficiency syndrome
AIH	autoimmune hepatitis
ALD	alcoholic liver disease
ALDH	acetaldehyde dehydrogenase
ALT	alanine aminotransferase
AMA	antimitochondrial antibody
ANA	antinuclear antibody
APC	adenomatous polyposis coli; argon plasma coagulation
ASCA	anti-*Saccharomyces cerevisiae* antibody
ASMA	anti-smooth muscle antibody
AST	aspartate aminotransferase
BRIC	benign recurrent intrahepatic cholestasis
BUN	blood urea nitrogen
CBC	complete blood count
CC	chronic constipation
CCK	cholecystokinin
CDC	Centers for Disease Control and Prevention
CEA	carcinoembryonic antigen
CHRPE	congenital hypertrophy of the retinal pigment epithelium
CREST	calcinosis, Raynaud phenomenon, esophageal dysmotility, sclerodactyly, and telangiectasia
CRP	C-reactive protein
CT	computed tomography
CTC	computed tomography colonography
DES	diffuse esophageal spasm
DS	double strength

EAC	esophageal adenocarcinoma
ECG	electrocardiogram
EGD	esophagogastroduodenoscopy
EGG	electrogastrography
EHEC	enterohemorrhagic *Escherichia coli*
EIEC	enteroinvasive *Escherichia coli*
ELISA	enzyme-linked immunosorbent assay
EMR	endoscopic mucosal resection
EPEC	enteropathogenic *Escherichia coli*
ERCP	endoscopic retrograde cholangiopancreatography
ERP	endoscopic retrograde pancreatography
ESD	endoscopic submucosal dissection
ESR	erythrocyte sedimentation rate
ETEC	enterotoxigenic *Escherichia coli*
EUS	endoscopic ultrasound
FAP	familial adenomatous polyposis
FIT	fecal immunochemical test
FNA	fine needle aspiration
FOBT	fecal occult blood test
GABA	γ-aminobutyric acid
GAVE	gastric arteriovenous ectasia, gastric antral vascular ectasia
GERD	gastroesophageal reflux disease
GGT	γ-glutamyl-transferase
GI	gastrointestinal
GIST	gastrointestinal stromal tumor
HAART	highly active antiretroviral therapy
HAV	hepatitis A virus
HBIG	hepatitis B immune globulin
HBV	hepatitis B virus
HCC	hepatocellular carcinoma
HCT	hematocrit
HCV	hepatitis C virus
HDV	hepatitis D virus
HE	hepatic encephalopathy
HEV	hepatitis E virus
HGD	high-grade dysplasia
HHC	hereditary hemochromatosis
HIAA	hydroxyindoleacetic acid
HII	hepatic iron index
HIV	human immunodeficiency virus
HNPCC	hereditary nonpolyposis colorectal cancer
HPF	high-power field
HVPG	hepatic venous pressure gradient

IBD	inflammatory bowel disease
IBS	irritable bowel syndrome
IBS-C	irritable bowel syndrome – constipation predominant
ICU	intensive care unit
Ig	immunoglobulin
IGF	insulin-like growth factor
IHC	immunohistochemistry
IL	interleukin
IM	intramuscular
I-MIBG	I-labeled metaiodobenzylguanidine
INR	international normalized ratio
IPMN	intraductal papillary mucinous neoplasm
IPSID	immunoproliferative small intestinal disease
IU	international unit
IV	intravenous
LAP	leucine aminopeptidase
LDH	lactate dehydrogenase
LES	lower esophageal sphincter
MALT	mucosa-associated lymphoid tissue
MCV	mean corpuscular volume
MELD	Model for End-Stage Liver Disease
MEN	multiple endocrine neoplasia
MRCP	magnetic resonance cholangiopancreatography
MRI	magnetic resonance imaging
NADH	nicotinamide adenine dinucleotide
NAFLD	nonalcoholic fatty liver disease
NASH	nonalcoholic steatohepatitis
NCCN	National Comprehensive Cancer Network
NG	nasogastric
NSAID	nonsteroidal anti-inflammatory drug
OLT	orthotopic liver transplantation
pANCA	perinuclear antineutrophil cytoplasmic antibody
PAS	periodic acid-Schiff
PBC	primary biliary cirrhosis
PCNA	proliferating cell nuclear antigen
PCR	polymerase chain reaction
PDGFR	platelet-derived growth factor receptor
PEG	polyethylene glycol
PEI	percutaneous ethanol injection
PET	positron emission tomography
PFIC	progressive familial intrahepatic cholestasis
PICC	peripherally inserted central catheter
PJS	Peutz–Jeghers syndrome

po	*per os*
PPI	proton pump inhibitor
PPN	peripheral parenteral nutrition
PSBL	primary small bowel lymphoma
PSC	primary sclerosing cholangitis
PTC	percutaneous transhepatic cholangiography
PUD	peptic ulcer disease
qid	*quater in die*
RFA	radiofrequency ablation
RUQ	right upper quadrant
SAAG	serum-ascites albumin gradient
SBP	spontaneous bacterial peritonitis
SCC	squamous cell carcinoma
SGOT	serum glutamic oxaloacetic transaminase
SGPT	serum glutamic pyruvic transaminase
SLA	soluble liver antigen
SO	sphincter of Oddi
SOD	sphincter of Oddi dysfunction
SVR	sustained virological response
TACE	transarterial chemoembolization
TARE	transaterial radioembolization
TCA	tricyclic antidepressant
TGF	transforming growth factor
TIBC	total iron-binding capacity
TIPS	transjugular intrahepatic portosystemic shunt
TLESR	transient lower esophageal sphincter relaxation
TNF	tumor necrosis factor
TPMT	thiopurine methyltransferase
TPN	total parenteral nutrition
TSH	thyroid-stimulating hormone
tTG	tissue transglutaminase
TTS	through-the-scope
UES	upper esophageal sphincter
UGT	uridine diphosphate glucuronosyltransferase
VCE	video capsule endoscopy
VEGF	vascular endothelial growth factor
VIP	vasoactive intestinal peptide
WBC	white blood count
WDHA	watery diarrhea, hypokalemia, and achlorhydria
ZES	Zollinger–Ellison syndrome

PART 1
Approach to Patients with Gastrointestinal Symptoms

CHAPTER 1

Approach to the Patient with Dysphagia or Odynophagia

Dysphagia is the sensation of food hindered in its passage from the mouth to the stomach. Dysphagia is differentiated from odynophagia (pain on swallowing) and from globus sensation (perception of a lump, tightness, or fullness in the throat that is temporarily relieved by swallowing). The act of swallowing has four phases: the oral preparation phase, the oral transfer phase, the pharyngeal phase, and the esophageal phase. An abnormality of any of the phases can produce dysphagia. Dysphagia is usually divided into two categories: (1) oropharyngeal: disorders of the oral preparation, oral transfer, or pharyngeal phases of swallowing; and (2) esophageal: dysfunction of the esophageal phase of swallowing (Table 1.1).

Clinical presentation

History

The patient's symptoms help define whether dysphagia or odynophagia is oropharyngeal or esophageal in location and structural or neuromuscular in origin. If dysphagia occurs within 1 sec of swallowing or is associated with drooling, choking, coughing, aspiration, or nasal regurgitation, an oropharyngeal process is likely. Conversely, an esophageal cause is probable if dysphagia occurs more than 1 sec after swallowing, if there is retrosternal pain or if there is regurgitation of unchanged food. Dysphagia perceived in the retrosternal or subxiphoid area is nearly always diagnostic of an esophageal source. Dysphagia perceived in the cervical area may result from either oropharyngeal or esophageal disease. Structural esophageal disorders generally produce solid food dysphagia with progression to liquid dysphagia only if lumenal narrowing becomes severe. Patients with neuromuscular disorders of the esophagus usually report both liquid and solid dysphagia from the onset of symptoms. Both structural and neuromuscular oropharyngeal disorders produce early liquid dysphagia.

Yamada's Handbook of Gastroenterology, Third Edition. Edited by Tadataka Yamada and John M. Inadomi.

Table 1.1 Differential diagnosis of dysphagia and odynophagia

Oropharyngeal dysphagia
Neuromuscular diseases
Cerebrovascular accident
Parkinson disease
Amyotrophic lateral sclerosis
Brainstem tumors
Bulbar poliomyelitis
Myasthenia gravis
Muscular dystrophies
Polymyositis
Metabolic myopathy
Amyloidosis
Systemic lupus erythematosus

Local mechanical lesions
Inflammation (pharyngitis, abscess, tuberculosis, radiation, syphilis)
Neoplasm
Congenital webs
Extrinsic compression (thyromegaly, cervical spine hyperostosis, adenopathy)
Radiation or caustic damage

Upper esophageal sphincter disorders
Primary cricopharyngeal dysfunction
Cricopharyngeal bar
Zenker diverticulum

Esophageal dysphagia
Motor disorders
Achalasia
Scleroderma
Diffuse esophageal spasm
Other spastic motor disorders
Other rheumatic conditions
Chagas disease

Intrinsic mechanical lesions
Benign stricture (peptic, lye, radiation)
Schatzki ring
Carcinoma
Eosinophilic esophagitis
Esophageal webs
Esophageal diverticula
Benign tumors
Foreign bodies

Extrinsic mechanical lesions
Vascular compression
Mediastinal abnormalities
Cervical osteoarthritis

Table 1.1 (*cont'd*)

Odynophagia
Mechanical
Trauma
Inflammatory
Pill-associated ulceration
Infectious
CMV, HSV, HIV

CMV, cytomegalovirus; HIV, human immunodeficiency virus; HSV, herpes simplex virus.

In patients with odynophagia, risk factors for opportunistic infection should be assessed and a careful medication history is warranted if pill esophagitis is a consideration.

Physical examination

The head and neck must be examined for sensory and motor function of the cranial nerves, masses, adenopathy, or spinal deformity. The patient should be observed swallowing water to visualize the co-ordinated symmetrical action of the neck and facial musculature. Evidence of systemic disease, including sclerodactyly, telangiectasias, and calcinosis in scleroderma, neuropathies or muscle weakness from generalized neuromuscular disease, and hepatomegaly or adenopathy due to esophageal malignancy should be sought. The presence of thrush suggests candidal infection as a cause of odynophagia.

Additional testing

If dysphagia is believed to be oropharyngeal, barium swallow radiography or endoscopy of the pharynx and esophagus may show occlusive lumenal lesions. Transnasal or peroral endoscopy also may reveal vocal cord paralysis, indicating neural dysfunction. Videofluoroscopy of mastication and swallowing of three different preparations (thin liquid, thick liquid, solid) is helpful in examining the co-ordination of the swallowing process in patients with suspected neuromuscular disease. In some instances, specialized manometry can reveal abnormal upper esophageal sphincter (UES) relaxations.

Endoscopy has become the preferred mode for assessing suspected esophageal dysphagia; however, contrast esophageal radiographic testing remains more sensitive for subtle structural lesions. Endoscopy is also optimal for identifying the etiology of odynophagia.

Differential diagnosis

Esophageal dysphagia
Obstructive esophageal lesions

Esophageal dysphagia is most commonly caused by structural lesions that physically impede bolus transit. Patients with esophageal strictures secondary to acid peptic damage may present with progressive dysphagia after a long history of heartburn. These strictures usually are located in the distal esophagus. More proximal strictures develop above the transition point to columnar mucosa in patients with Barrett esophagus. A Schatzki ring, a thin, circumferential mucosal structure at the gastroesophageal junction, causes episodic and nonprogressive dysphagia that often occurs during rushed ingestion of poorly chewed meat. Eosinophilic esophagitis should be considered in younger patients who present with intermittent solid food dysphagia or food impaction. Patients with squamous cell carcinoma also report progressive dysphagia, similar to peptic disease, but affected patients often are older and have had long-standing exposure to tobacco or alcohol and no prior pyrosis. Esophageal adenocarcinoma develops in areas of Barrett metaplasia resulting from prolonged gastroesophageal reflux. Other mechanical lesions (e.g. abnormal great vessel anatomy, mediastinal lymphadenopathy, and cervical vertebral spurs) can cause dysphagia.

Motor disorders of the esophagus

Primary and secondary disorders of esophageal motor activity represent the other main etiology of esophageal dysphagia. Primary achalasia is an idiopathic disorder characterized by esophageal body aperistalsis and failure of lower esophageal sphincter (LES) relaxation on swallowing with or without associated LES hypertension. Conditions that mimic primary achalasia include secondary achalasia, a disorder with identical radiographic and manometric characteristics caused by malignancy at the gastroesophageal junction or by paraneoplastic effects of a distant tumor, and Chagas disease, which results from infection with *Trypanosoma cruzi*. Other spastic esophageal dysmotilities, such as diffuse esophageal spasm, have also been associated with dysphagia. Systemic diseases (e.g. scleroderma and other rheumatic diseases) also cause dysphagia because of reduced rather than spastic esophageal motor function.

Odynophagia

Oropharyngeal odynophagia most commonly results from malignancy, foreign body ingestion, or mucosal ulceration. Esophageal odynophagia usually is a consequence of caustic ingestion, infection (e.g. *Candida albicans*, herpes simplex virus, cytomegalovirus), radiation damage, pill esophagitis, or ulcer disease induced by acid reflux (see Table 1.1).

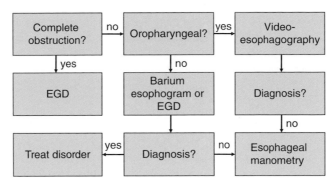

Figure 1.1 Evaluation of dysphagia or odynophagia. EGD, esophagogastroduodenosocpy.

Diagnostic investigation

Patients who present with complete obstruction should undergo upper endoscopy (Figure 1.1). Contrast radiography is not only associated with an aspiration risk but lesions found on radiography may be obscured by the contrast media. Airway protection is mandatory so there should be a low threshold for endotracheal intubation.

In the absence of complete obstruction, the history further dictates the next step in investigation. For dysphagia of presumed esophageal origin, barium swallow radiography or endoscopy may reveal occlusive lesions such as carcinomas, strictures, rings, or webs. Barium swallow testing also can show the characteristic bird's beak deformity of achalasia. The addition of a solid bolus (e.g. a marshmallow or barium pill) can increase the detection of subtle abnormalities during contrast radiography. Upper endoscopy affords the additional capability to perform a biopsy of any suspicious areas, including evaluation for eosinophilic esophagitis. If structural testing is nondiagnostic, manometry of the esophageal body and LES may detect the characteristic findings of achalasia, systemic diseases such as scleroderma, and other primary and secondary esophageal motor disorders.

Oropharyngeal dysphagia is best evaluated by video-esophagography. Endoscopy is rarely diagnostic so further evaluation of oropharyngeal symptoms should be directed towards manometric testing.

Since mucosal lesions are common, endoscopy is the procedure of choice for odynophagia. In addition, plain radiography of the neck may detect pharyngeal foreign bodies.

Management

Dysphagia
Selected causes of oropharyngeal dysphagia, including Parkinson disease, hypothyroidism, polymyositis, and myasthenia gravis, may have specific

Less invasive   More invasive

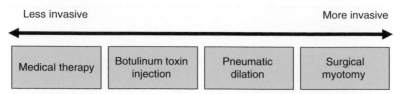

Figure 1.2 Treatment of achalasia.

therapies. Surgical myotomy may benefit patients with Zenker diverticulum or cricopharyngeal achalasia. A few limited studies suggest that myotomy also may be useful in treating selected cases of neuromuscular disease. For untreatable neuromuscular conditions, consultation with a speech pathologist may afford development of a rehabilitation program to improve swallowing. Techniques include altering food consistency, motor retraining, controlled breathing, coughing, and head positioning. When adequate nutrition cannot be maintained, alternative enteral feedings through a gastrostomy may be indicated.

Management of esophageal dysphagia depends on its cause. Benign strictures, webs, and rings are dilated by bougienage. Rigid dilators or through-the-scope (TTS) balloon dilators have equivalent efficacy in treating strictures. Eosinophilic esophagitis may improve with elimination diets or topical steroids. Early malignancies may be surgically resected, whereas palliation via endoscopic stenting or laser therapy, or radiation therapy may be used for unresectable lesions. Achalasia can be treated with botulinum toxin injection into the LES, large-caliber balloon endoscopic dilation, or surgical myotomy (Figure 1.2). Other primary esophageal dysmotilities may respond to nitrates, calcium channel antagonists, and, in rare instances, botulinum toxin or surgical myotomy.

Odynophagia

Therapy for odynophagia secondary to opportunistic infection relies on anti-infective treatments, whereas pill esophagitis and caustic ingestion may be managed with medications to reduce acid reflux and to coat the irritated esophagus.

Complications

The most serious complication of oropharyngeal dysphagia is tracheal aspiration, with development of cough, asthma, or pneumonia. Esophageal dysphagia may also result in aspiration, especially in the case of complete obstruction, and for more chronic symptoms in a failure to thrive because of reduced oral intake.

Complications from odynophagia are related to the underlying etiology. Bleeding or perforation from esophageal ulceration may occur.

Case studies

Case 1

A 32-year-old man with a history of gastroesophageal reflux disease presents to the emergency department with 3 h of difficulty swallowing. The symptoms were prompted by eating a steak and have progressed to the point where he can no longer swallow his own secretions. He states a prior history of similar symptoms 2 months earlier, which resolved after 1 h. He did not pursue medical evaluation at that time.

Physical examination reveals a healthy-appearing man who is sitting upright with a bucket into which he spits his saliva. No other abnormalities are noted. Laboratory tests are normal.

The patient is intubated and an upper endoscopy is performed at which time a large piece of steak is removed from the distal esophagus using a snare and net. A Schatzki ring is noted at 40 cm from the incisors, which is dilated using a 20 mm TTS balloon.

The patient is discharged and follow-up 1 month later reveals no recurrence of symptoms, although the patient is careful to cut his food into small pieces and chew his food thoroughly before swallowing.

> ### Discussion and potential pitfalls
>
> "Steakhouse syndrome" caused by food impaction is a common problem encountered by gastroenterologists. The key feature of this presentation is the intermittent symptoms triggered by injestion of large solid food items and the absence of symptoms in intervening periods. The inability to swallow one's own secretions is a red flag indicating complete esophageal obstruction – in these cases it is important to avoid contrast radiography, which not only interferes with the endoscopic visualization but is also potentially hazardous due to the risk of pulmonary aspiration. Endoscopic removal of the food bolus should be conducted in a manner that ensures airway protection by the use of an esophageal endoscopic overtube, or mechanical ventilation via endotracheal intubation.

Case 2

A 22-year-old woman is referred to your office for symptoms of dysphagia that have been present for 2 years. She is a recent immigrant to the US and has not previously sought healthcare for this problem. She describes intermittent difficulty with both liquids and solids; although she is able to swallow, the food and liquid feel as though they are "getting stuck in her chest." She also relates symptoms of halitosis and occasional regurgitation of undigested food.

Physical examination reveals a thin woman whose abdominal examination is normal. Upper endoscopy reveals a capacious esophagus with "sigmoid" appearance tapering to a narrowed esophagogastric junction but no mass or stricture. Esophageal manometry illustrates simultaneous (nonprogressive) contractions of the esophageal body with nonrelaxation of the lower esophageal sphincter, consistent with achalasia.

> **Discussion and potential pitfalls**
>
> The manometric findings of idiopathic achalasia are not specific and can be seen in Chagas disease and pseudoachalasia. The ganglion cell degeneration found in achalasia is presumed to be immune mediated, as opposed to pseudoachalasia where infiltration of the esophageal wall by tumor causes obstruction with proximal dilation. A smaller proportion of neoplasia-associated pseudoachalasia may be a result of a paraneoplastic process without direct tumor stenosis of the esophagogastric junction.

Case 3

A 26-year-old man known to be HIV positive presents with odynophagia. He has no prior AIDS-defining diagnosis and has not been taking highly active antiretroviral therapy (HAART). Painful swallowing with both liquids and solids has been noted for 2 weeks and is associated with a 10 lb weight loss. Physical examination is notable for the absence of oral candidiasis and no abdominal tenderness or masses. Laboratory tests include a CD4 count of 28.

The patient is prescribed oral antifungal medication but has no relief of symptoms after 7 days. Upper endoscopy is performed, which is notable for several well-demarcated ulcers in the mid to distal esophagus. Biopsies of the ulcer margin reveal large infected cells with intranuclear inclusions, consistent with cytomegalovirus infection. Ganciclovir and HAART are initiated and the patient improves within 5 days.

> **Discussion and potential pitfalls**
>
> Immunocompromised patients are at risk of opportunistic infections. Odynophagia in this group of patients is commonly due to fungal infections (*Candida albicans*), cytomegalovirus, and herpesvirus. Empiric therapy with an oral antifungal agent is a reasonable first step. If symptoms do not improve, investigation with upper endoscopy is indicated to evaluate for the presence of the viral infections. Idiopathic ulcerations associated with HIV are also a cause of odynophagia and are diagnosed by the exclusion of evidence of viral infection on biopsies of the ulcer.

> **Key practice points**
>
> *Dysphagia*
> * Complete obstruction requires emergency endoscopy – do not perform radiographic contrast studies.
> * Distinguish oropharyngeal from esophageal source through patient description of symptoms.
> * Oropharyngeal symptoms are best evaluated by fluoroscopic imaging, while esophageal symptoms can be evaluated by either barium swallow or endoscopy, followed by manometry to evaluate motility disorders.
>
> *Odynophagia*
> * If fungal etiology likely, empirical antimicrobial treatment is reasonable.
> * Endoscopy is the optimal test to evaluate odynophagia.

CHAPTER 2

Approach to the Patient with Chest Pain

Clinical presentation

History

Chest pain most often is attributed to cardiac etiologies. However, 20–30% of patients who undergo cardiac catheterization for chest pain exhibit patent coronary arteries. These patients with noncardiac chest pain experience symptoms as a consequence of diseases of the cardiopulmonary system, musculoskeletal structures, gastrointestinal tract, and central nervous system (Table 2.1). Less common causes include biliary tract disease, pleural and mediastinal inflammation, dissecting aortic aneurysm, and varicella zoster virus infection of the chest wall.

Chest pain from esophageal causes commonly is described as squeezing or burning, is substernal in location, and may last from minutes to hours. Noncardiac chest pain from esophageal sources may radiate in a pattern indistinguishable from angina and may not be related to swallowing. Symptoms can be exacerbated by ingesting cold or hot liquids or by stress and can awaken the patient from sleep. In contrast to cardiac chest pain, exertion only rarely triggers esophageal chest pain. Relief may be provided by antacid ingestion or nitroglycerin administration. Pain that lasts for hours, that is related to meals, that does not radiate laterally, and that is relieved by acid suppressants suggests an esophageal origin.

Physical examination

Physical examination occasionally helps to delineate the cause of chest pain. Reproduction of symptoms by chest wall palpation suggests a musculoskeletal source. Auscultation of pleural friction rubs or decreased breath sounds implies pleuropulmonary disease. Cutaneous eruptions in a dermatomal pattern indicate probable varicella zoster virus reactivation. A characteristic midsystolic click and murmur may suggest mitral valve prolapse. Abdominal tenderness raises concern for peptic or biliary tract disease.

Yamada's Handbook of Gastroenterology, Third Edition. Edited by Tadataka Yamada and John M. Inadomi.
© 2013 John Wiley & Sons, Ltd. Published 2013 by John Wiley & Sons, Ltd.

Table 2.1 Causes of chest pain

Cardiopulmonary disease
Coronary artery disease
Coronary artery spasm
Microvascular angina
Mitral valve prolapse
Aortic valve disease
Pericarditis
Dissecting thoracic aortic aneurysm
Mediastinitis
Pneumonia
Pulmonary embolus

Musculoskeletal causes
Costochondritis
Fibromyalgia
Arthritis
Nerve entrapment or compression

Esophageal disease
Gastroesophageal reflux
Achalasia
Diffuse esophageal spasm
Other spastic motor disorders
Infectious or pill-induced esophagitis
Food impaction

Neuropsychiatric causes
Panic disorder
Anxiety disorder
Depression
Somatization

Miscellaneous
Varicella zoster virus reactivation

Additional testing

The evaluation of a patient with chest pain is outlined in Figure 2.1. Initial diagnostic tests involve exclusion of cardiac disease. Most patients should undergo electrocardiography, exercise stress testing, echocardiography, or coronary arteriography, depending on their age and risk factors, because the presence of coronary artery disease cannot be established reliably from the history. An ergonovine test may be used to elicit coronary spasm in some patients. Once cardiac disease is excluded, noncardiac sources for chest pain may be evaluated. Musculoskeletal causes usually are detected on physical examination, whereas psychogenic causes may require referral to a mental health specialist for assessment.

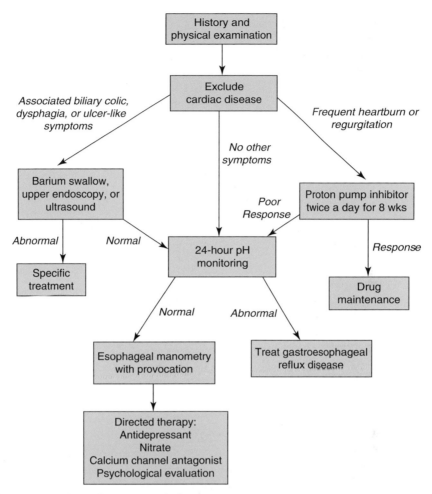

Figure 2.1 Work-up of a patient with chest pain.

Barium swallow radiography or upper endoscopy is used to exclude esophageal mucosal sources of chest pain. Radiographic techniques may observe subtle strictures or dysmotilities, whereas endoscopy is superior for detecting esophagitis and affords the capability to perform a biopsy of suspicious mucosa. When structural studies are normal, gastroesophageal reflux disease should be excluded because of its prevalence as a cause of chest pain. The best test for correlating symptoms with acid reflux is ambulatory pH monitoring of the esophagus using a probe positioned 5 cm above the lower esophageal sphincter. With this procedure, episodes may relate temporally to periods in which esophageal pH decreases. An esophageal pH less than 4 for longer than 5% of total exposure time suggests a diagnosis of gastroesophageal reflux disease with a sensitivity of 85% and a specificity of 95%. The addition of impedance testing allows for the detection of non-acid reflux events. An empirical trial of high-dose proton pump inhibitor therapy is an alternative to this test and can be expected to relieve symptoms in 80% of patients with noncardiac chest pain and underlying acid reflux.

Esophageal manometry may define an underlying esophageal dysmotility syndrome. By itself, manometry detects potentially pathogenic motor abnormalities in only a minority of patients with noncardiac chest pain. The diagnostic accuracy of manometry may be enhanced by pharmacological challenge with the α-adrenergic stimulant erogonovine, the cholinergic agonist bethanechol, or the cholinesterase inhibitor edrophonium. However, these agents provoke significant side-effects, especially in those individuals with underlying cardiac disease. Furthermore, their clinical utility is unproved. Thus, provocative testing is falling out of favor at many institutions. In some patients, balloon distension of the esophagus reproduces the presenting complaint, which suggests a visceral afferent disturbance as a cause of symptoms. Some centers use this test in their diagnostic evaluations.

Differential diagnosis

Cardiac disease

Cardiac etiologies must be considered in a patient with unexplained chest pain, even in the absence of coronary atherosclerosis. Coronary artery spasm in response to ergonovine is reported in some individuals with chest pain. Exertional chest pain may be a consequence of abnormalities of the smaller endocardial vasculature without evidence of fixed lesions or spasm of the epicardial vessels, a condition termed *microvascular angina* or *syndrome X*. Diagnosis of this disorder requires measuring cardiac lactate production and coronary sinus blood flow during fasting and after rapid atrial pacing followed by intravenous ergonovine challenge. Microvascular angina should be considered in patients with ischemic ST segment changes on electrocardiography or if left ventricular ejection fractions decrease in response to exercise on echocardiography or radionuclide ventriculography. The relationship of chest pain to mitral valve prolapse is controversial. Furthermore, esophageal motor abnormalities may coexist with both microvascular angina and mitral valve prolapse that make the cause of chest pain uncertain in affected individuals.

Musculoskeletal causes

Musculoskeletal conditions account for 10–30% of cases of noncardiac chest pain. Chest pain from musculoskeletal sources (e.g. costochondritis [Tietze syndrome], fibromyalgia, inflammatory arthritis, osteoarthritis, thoracic spinal disease) is characterized by localized chest wall tenderness and definable trigger points and may be reported at rest, with movement, or during sleep.

Neuropsychiatric causes

Panic disorder presents with at least three attacks in as many weeks of intense fear or discomfort accompanied by at least four of the following symptoms: chest pain, restlessness, choking, palpitations, sweating, dizziness, nausea or abdominal distress, paresthesia, flushing, trembling, and a sense of impending doom. Of all cases of noncardiac chest pain, 34–59% result from panic disorder. In addition to increased anxiety, these patients also exhibit increased incidence of depression and somatization.

Esophageal disease

Esophageal disorders, the most common causes of noncardiac chest pain, account for 20–60% of cases. Although heartburn is more prevalent, chest pain is a common atypical symptom of gastroesophageal reflux disease. In some cases, acid reflux may be induced by exercise. A small percentage of these patients exhibit altered esophageal motor patterns on acid perfusion. In most patients, however, there is a poor correlation between chest pain and acid reflux episodes. Primary spastic esophageal motor disorders are found in less than 50% of patients with noncardiac chest pain. One such condition, diffuse esophageal spasm, accounts for 5% of cases and is characterized by the presence of high-amplitude, nonperistaltic esophageal contractions on manometry. Esophageal hypersensitivity to balloon distension may correlate better with symptoms in patients with noncardiac chest pain than motor disturbances, which suggests that a primary disturbance of esophageal afferent neural function is pathogenic. Miscellaneous gastroesophageal sources of chest pain include infectious or pill-induced esophagitis, food impaction, and proximal gastric ulcers.

Management

Treatment of esophageal chest pain may be unsatisfactory because of diagnostic uncertainties, the intermittent nature of symptoms, the side-effect profiles of available pharmaceutical agents, and the awareness that many of these conditions improve spontaneously without treatment. After a careful diagnostic examination, many patients respond to physician reassurance that no dangerous condition exists.

For underlying gastroesophageal reflux disease, long-term treatment with a potent acid-suppressing medication such as a proton pump inhibitor (e.g. omeprazole) may be needed. Patients who respond poorly to medical therapy can be considered for antireflux surgery. For painful esophageal dysmotility, nitrates and calcium channel blockers may be considered, although response rates for these agents are low. Many of these patients respond instead to antidepressant agents (e.g. amitriptyline, imipramine, desipramine, trazodone) at doses lower than those used to treat endogenous depression. One study has shown improvement in chest pain with the selective serotonin reuptake inhibitor sertraline.

Uncontrolled studies suggest that injecting botulinum toxin into the esophageal body may decrease symptoms caused by diffuse esophageal spasm. Similarly, sildenafil has been suggested to improve symptoms of esophageal motor disorders. In rare cases of refractory esophageal motor dysfunction, esophageal dilation or surgical myotomy may relieve symptoms. For panic disorders, anxiolytics (e.g. benzodiazepines or buspirone) may be effective. However, these agents have abuse potential, may induce tolerance, and may exacerbate underlying depression. Cognitive behavioral therapy may produce significant improvements in chest pain, functional disability, and psychological distress in selected patient populations with psychogenic etiologies of chest pain.

Complications

Chest pain of esophageal origin rarely has long-term sequelae. The major risk in evaluating a patient with unexplained chest pain is the premature exclusion of coronary ischemia, which may have life-threatening consequences.

Case studies

Case 1

A 56-year-old woman with a history of hypertension and diabetes controlled by oral agents presents to her primary care physician reporting intermittent substernal squeezing chest pain, radiating up the neck, lasting approximately 30–90 min. Her symptoms generally occur at rest and are not clearly related to meals. She has taken over-the-counter antacids with intermittent improvement in her symptoms. Physical examination reveals an obese woman in no distress and with no significant abnormalities noted. Laboratory tests are normal other than a mildly elevated fasting blood glucose. An electrocardiogram (ECG) is normal.

The patient is referred for a stress echocardiogram which is read as normal. The patient is referred to a gastroenterologist who performs upper endoscopy. The esophagus, stomach and duodenum are normal. The patient is started on twice-daily omeprazole with improvement in her symptoms.

Discussion

Nonerosive reflux disease is a common cause of noncardiac chest pain and symptoms can mimic angina. While approximately 80% of patients will respond to high-dose proton pump inhibitor therapy, 24-h ambulatory pH monitoring off medications may be necessary to make the diagnosis of gastroesophageal reflux disease. It is important to exclude coronary ischemia in patients with chest pain.

Case 2

A 25-year-old man with a history of depression is referred to the gastroenterology clinic for evaluation of recurrent atypical chest pain, described as a nonradiating, squeezing pressure in the midsternum, occurring after meals and lasting for 2 h. Prior evaluation was unremarkable, including cardiac stress testing and esophagogastroduodenoscopy (EGD). A trial of high-dose proton pump inhibitors had no effect on his symptoms. The patient underwent esophageal manometry and 24-h pH testing (on high-dose omeprazole) which revealed high-amplitude, nonperistaltic esophageal contractions and normal esophageal acid exposure. The patient was tried on diltiazem up to 360 mg daily without benefit. He was then started on isosorbide dinitrate but had moderate side-effects and no significant relief. He was not interested in trying botox therapy. He was started on low-dose imipramine with modest improvement in his symptoms.

Discussion

This case highlights some of the challenges of treating noncardiac chest pain. Diffuse esophageal spasm accounts for approximately 5% of cases. Unfortunately, the evidence to support any particular therapeutic approach is limited. Some patients have an esophageal hyperalgesia syndrome and will respond to tricyclic antidepressants.

Key practice points

Chest pain

- Cardiac etiologies must be considered in a patient with unexplained chest pain, even in the absence of coronary atherosclerosis.
- Esophageal disorders are the most common causes of noncardiac chest pain.
- Although heartburn is more prevalent, chest pain is a common atypical symptom of gastroesophageal reflux disease.
- Chest pain from musculoskeletal sources is characterized by localized chest wall tenderness and definable trigger points and may be reported at rest, with movement, or during sleep.
- Barium esophagography and/or EGD can exclude an esophageal mucosal source of pain.
- The best test for correlating symptoms with gastroesophageal reflux is ambulatory pH monitoring, ideally with impedence testing, though an empirical trial of high-dose proton pump inhibitor therapy is a reasonable alternative.
- Esophageal manometry may define an underlying esophageal dysmotility.

CHAPTER 3

Approach to the Patient with Gastrointestinal Bleeding

Gastrointestinal (GI) bleeding is a common problem, ranging in severity from insidious occult blood loss to life-threatening hemorrhage. In approaching the patient with GI bleeding, it is important to assess the severity as well as the site of blood loss. Hematemesis (vomiting of bright red blood or coffee grounds-colored matter) indicates an upper GI source proximal to the ligament of Treitz. Melena (black, malodorous, tarry stools that indicate intestinal degradation of blood) usually results from acute upper GI bleeding, although bleeding from the small intestine and the right colon also produces melena. Hematochezia (bright red rectal bleeding) usually indicates a colonic source, although brisk bleeding from an upper GI site may also produce hematochezia or maroon-colored stools.

Acute Upper Gastrointestinal Bleeding

Clinical presentation

History

In a patient with hemodynamically significant upper GI bleeding, volume replacement with intravenous fluids and blood products is of paramount importance. While resuscitation is under way, a directed history usually can be obtained. Prior peptic disease or dyspeptic symptoms suggest ulcer bleeding. Recent ingestion of aspirin, nonsteroidal anti-inflammatory drugs (NSAIDs), alcohol, or caustic substances should be ascertained. Chronic ethanol consumption or known liver disease raises the possibility of varices or portal gastropathy. Prior aortic surgery, coagulopathies, neoplasm, or recent nosebleeds may suggest specific diagnoses.

Yamada's Handbook of Gastroenterology, Third Edition. Edited by Tadataka Yamada and John M. Inadomi.
© 2013 John Wiley & Sons, Ltd. Published 2013 by John Wiley & Sons, Ltd.

Physical examination

Various physical findings point to the cause of upper GI bleeding. Cutaneous stigmata of cirrhosis or malignancy may be present. Multiple cutaneous telangiectases suggest hereditary hemorrhagic telangiectasia. Lymphadenopathy, hepatosplenomegaly, and abdominal masses raise the possibility of malignancy. Hepatosplenomegaly, ascites, or dilated abdominal wall vessels suggest portal hypertension. Demonstration of maroon or melenic stools on rectal examination in the patient with upper GI bleeding indicates significant hemorrhage.

Additional testing

Laboratory studies

A hematocrit, platelet count, and coagulation studies should be part of the initial laboratory evaluation. The first hematocrit may not reflect the degree of blood loss because acute hemorrhage produces loss of both erythrocytes and volume, and thus the ratio of the two parameters is not altered. A low hematocrit with microcytosis suggests chronic blood loss, which can be confirmed with iron studies or ferritin measurement. With massive upper GI bleeding, azotemia reflects intestinal absorption of nitrogenous breakdown products of blood, although azotemia with creatinine elevation suggests renal insufficiency. Abnormal liver chemistry levels raise concern about possible cirrhosis with portal hypertension.

Potential pitfalls

Hematochezia is not always a sign of lower gastrointestinal hemorrhage; therefore, nasogastric lavage should be performed to evaluate for the presence of an upper gastrointestinal source. Note that a "clear" lavage indicates the absence of duodenal sampling, so only the presence of bile in the lavage fluid rules out active duodenal hemorrhage.

Upper endoscopy

Urgent upper endoscopy is indicated for hemorrhage that does not stop spontaneously or in patients with suspected cirrhosis or aortoenteric fistulae. Upper endoscopy is contraindicated when perforation is suspected and is relatively contraindicated in patients with compromised cardiopulmonary status or depressed consciousness. In such cases, endotracheal intubation with mechanical ventilation may enhance the safety of the technique. Upper GI barium radiography is not performed in the acute setting in a potentially unstable patient because it offers no therapeutic capability and may obscure endoscopic or angiographic visualization of the bleeding site.

Scintigraphy and angiography

When hemorrhage is so brisk that it obscures endoscopic visualization, scintigraphic and angiographic studies may be indicated. Scintigraphic ^{99m}Tc-sulfur colloid- or ^{99m}Tc-pertechnetate-labeled erythrocyte scans can localize bleeding to an area of the abdomen if the rate of blood loss exceeds 0.5 mL/min. They are used to determine if angiography is feasible and to direct the angiographic search and minimize any dye load. Angiography can localize the bleeding site if the rate of blood loss is greater than 0.5 mL/min and can offer therapeutic capability.

Other radiographic studies

If an aortoenteric fistula is suspected, a vigorous diagnostic approach, including abdominal computed tomographic or magnetic resonance imaging studies, should be pursued after endoscopy has excluded other bleeding sources.

Obscure GI bleeding

Obscure GI bleeding is defined as bleeding that is either persistent or recurrent and is of unknown origin after an appropriate endoscopic evaluation. Obscure GI bleeding may be overt (i.e. blood is visible, such as with melena or hematochezia) or occult (i.e. no gross blood is evident but there is either iron deficiency anemia or occult blood detectable in the stool). A suggested algorithm for the evaluation of obscure, overt GI bleeding is shown in Figure 3.1.

Differential diagnosis

The most common causes of upper GI hemorrhage are peptic ulcer disease, gastropathy (or gastric erosions), and sequelae of portal hypertension (i.e. esophageal and gastric varices, portal gastropathy). Other disorders comprise a small minority of cases (Table 3.1).

Peptic ulcer disease

Duodenal, gastric, and stomal ulcers cause 50% of upper GI bleeding. Bleeding occurs if an ulcer erodes into the wall of a vessel, which may loop into the floor of the ulcer crater, forming an aneurysmal dilation. Most cases of peptic ulcer disease result from gastric infection with *Helicobacter pylori* or from chronic use of aspirin or NSAIDs. Stigmata of recent bleeding from ulcer sources on endoscopy that are predictors of poor outcome include active arterial spurting, oozing of blood, a visible vessel (an elevated red, blue, or gray mound that resists washing), and adherent clot. Other prognostic indicators include amount of blood lost, patient age, concomitant disease, onset of bleeding while hospitalized, giant ulcers larger than 2 cm, and need for emergency surgery.

Gastropathy

Gastropathy may be produced by several mechanisms. Endoscopically, gastropathy may be visualized as mucosal hemorrhages, erythema, or erosions. An erosion, in contrast to an ulcer, represents a break in the mucosa of less than

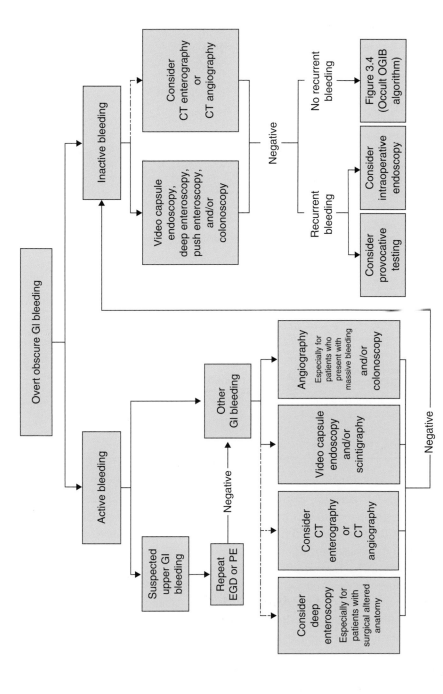

Figure 3.1 Suggested diagnostic approach to overt obscure GI bleeding. Dashed arrows indicate less preferred options. Positive test results should direct specific therapy. Because diagnostic tests can be complementary, more than one test may be needed, and the first-line test may be based upon institutional expertise and availability. CT, computed tomography; EGD, esophagogastroduodenoscopy; OGIB, obscure GI bleeding; PE, push enteroscopy. (Source: ASGE Standards of Practice Committee. The Role of Endoscopy in the Management of Obscure GI Bleeding, Gastrointest Endosc 2010; 72:475; with permission from the American Society for Gastrointestinal Endoscopy.)

Table 3.1 Causes of gross gastrointestinal hemorrhage

Upper gastrointestinal sources
Peptic ulcer disease (duodenal, gastric, stomal)
Gastritis (NSAID, stress, chemotherapyinduced)
Varices (esophageal, gastric, duodenal)
Portal gastropathy
Mallory–Weiss tear
Esophagitis and esophageal ulcers (acid reflux, infection, pill induced, sclerotherapy, radiation induced)
Neoplasms
Vascular ectasias and angiodysplasias
Gastric antral vascular ectasia
Aortoenteric fistula
Hematobilia
Hemosuccus pancreaticus
Dieulafoy lesion

Lower gastrointestinal sources
Diverticulosis
Angiodysplasia
Hemorrhoids
Anal fissures
Neoplasms
Inflammatory bowel disease
Ischemic colitis
Infectious colitis
Radiation-induced colitis
Meckel diverticulum
Intussusception
Aortoenteric fistula
Solitary rectal ulcers
NSAID-induced cecal ulcers

---

5 mm that does not traverse the muscularis mucosae. In addition to causing ulcers, NSAIDs produce erosions most often in the antrum that usually resolve after removing the offending agent. Ethanol is a gastric mucosal irritant when administered in high concentrations. Stress gastritis develops in patients in the intensive care unit who have underlying respiratory failure, hypotension, sepsis, renal failure, burns, peritonitis, jaundice, or neurological trauma. Although most patients in the intensive care unit have gastric mucosal abnormalities on endoscopy, only 2–10% develop gross hemorrhage. The hallmark of stress gastritis is the presence of multiple bleeding sites, which limit the therapeutic options.

Hemorrhage secondary to portal hypertension

Patients with portal hypertension are predisposed to hemorrhage from esophageal and gastric varices and portal hypertensive gastropathy. However, up to

50% of upper GI bleeds in patients with cirrhosis do not result from these causes. Variceal size is the best predictor of esophageal variceal hemorrhage because wall tension is determined by the diameter of a hollow vessel. Other predictors of esophageal variceal bleeding include the red color sign, which is the result of microtelangiectasia; red wale marks, which appear as whip marks; hemocystic spots, which appear as blood blisters; and diffuse redness. The white nipple sign, a platelet-fibrin plug, is diagnostic of previous hemorrhage but does not predict rebleeding.

Gastric varices are present in 20% of patients with portal hypertension and develop in another 8% after esophageal variceal obliteration. Isolated gastric varices suggest splenic vein thrombosis, which may be a consequence of pancreatic disease and is treated by splenectomy. Portal hypertensive gastropathy appears endoscopically as a mosaic, snakeskin-like mucosa as a result of engorged mucosal vessels that may bleed briskly or produce insidious iron deficiency anemia.

Miscellaneous causes of upper gastrointestinal bleeding

Mallory–Weiss tears are linear breaks in the mucosa of the gastroesophageal junction that are induced by retching, often in patients who have consumed alcohol. Most Mallory–Weiss tears resolve spontaneously with conservative management. Esophagitis and esophageal ulcers result from acid reflux, radiation therapy, infections with *Candida albicans* and herpes simplex virus, pill-induced damage, or iatrogenic sources (e.g. sclerotherapy). Hemorrhage from erosive duodenitis is similar to duodenal ulcer bleeding but usually is less severe because the lesions are shallower. Neoplasms most commonly bleed slowly, but occasionally exhibit massive hemorrhage. Vascular ectasias occur less commonly in the stomach and duodenum than in the colon and cause recurrent acute GI hemorrhage that may require frequent blood transfusions. Vascular ectasias often occur as a consequence of advanced age, but also are associated with chronic renal failure, aortic valve disease, and prior radiation therapy.

Hereditary hemorrhagic telangiectasia, or Osler–Weber–Rendu syndrome, is an autosomal dominant disorder with telangiectasia of the tongue, lips, conjunctiva, skin, and mucosa of the gut, bladder, and nasopharynx. Gastric arteriovenous ectasia (GAVE), or watermelon stomach, has the appearance of columns of vessels along the tops of the antral longitudinal rugae. Biopsies show dilated mucosal capillaries with focal thrombosis and fibromuscular hyperplasia of lamina propria vessels. Aortoenteric fistulae may produce fatal hemorrhage from the third portion of the duodenum in patients who have undergone prior synthetic aortic graft surgery. This patient may present with a minor "herald" hemorrhage before fatal exsanguination occurs.

Hematobilia and hemosuccus pancreaticus present with hemorrhage from the ampulla of Vater and are complications of liver trauma or biopsy, malignancy, hepatic artery aneurysm, hepatic abscess, gallstones, and pancreatic pseudocyst.

Bleeding in a Dieulafoy lesion results from pressure erosion of the overlying epithelium by an ectopic artery in the proximal stomach without surrounding ulceration or inflammation. Some patients present with upper GI bleeding from epistaxis, hemoptysis, oral lesions, or factitious blood ingestion.

Management

Resuscitation

The first step in managing a patient with upper GI bleeding is to assess the urgency of the clinical condition (Figure 3.2). Hematemesis, melena, or

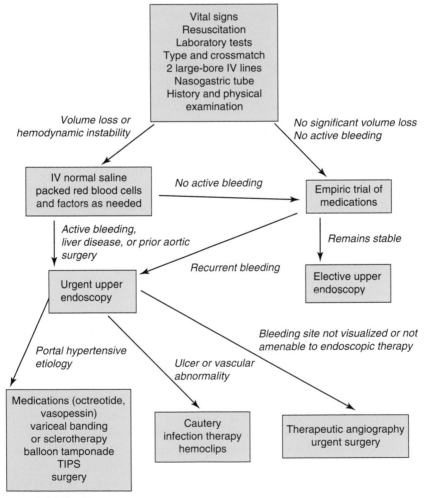

Figure 3.2 Work-up of a patient with acute upper gastrointestinal bleeding. IV, intravenous; TIPS, transjugular intrahepatic portosystemic shunt.

hematochezia suggest major hemorrhage, whereas pallor, hypotension, and tachycardia indicate substantial blood volume loss (>40% of total volume) and mandate immediate volume replacement. A patient with GI bleeding and postural or supine hypotension must be admitted to an intensive care unit. Two large-bore intravenous catheters should be inserted. A nasogastric tube should be placed. A bright red aspirate that does not clear with lavage of room temperature water is an indication for urgent endoscopy because it is associated with a 30% mortality, whereas coffee grounds-colored material that clears permits further assessment in a hemodynamically stable patient. A clear aspirate is found in some patients with duodenal bleeding. Thus, the clinician cannot be complacent if unstable hemodynamic parameters indicate ongoing blood loss. In addition to diagnostic laboratory testing, blood samples are sent for blood typing and cross-matching. Intravascular volume should be replenished with normal saline while awaiting the availability of blood products.

Transfusion of blood products

The need for blood transfusion is influenced by patient age, coexistent cardiovascular disease, and persistent hemorrhage. Generally, the hematocrit should be maintained above 30% in elderly patients and above 20% in younger patients with active hemorrhage. Packed erythrocytes are preferred for blood transfusion to avoid fluid load. If coagulation studies are abnormal, as in cirrhosis, fresh-frozen plasma or platelets also may be needed. Patients without coagulopathy may need fresh-frozen plasma and platelet transfusion if multiple transfusions have been given, because transfused blood is deficient in some clotting factors. Warmed blood should be transfused in patients with massive blood loss (>3 L) to prevent hypothermia. Some individuals with massive bleeding also require supplemental calcium to counter the calcium-binding effects of preserved blood.

Medications

Empiric medical treatment is often given before the evaluation is complete. For presumed peptic disease, intravenous proton pump inhibitor therapy may be given as studies have demonstrated reduced rates of rebleeding from ulcers and it may downstage the severity of the bleeding source. Proton pump inhibitors also play prominent roles in prophylaxis against development of erosions in patients on NSAIDs. Patients with *H. pylori* infection should be given combined therapy including antibiotics to eradicate the organism, even those who may have mucosal injury secondary to NSAIDs. Prophylaxis against stress gastropathy should be provided for patients at risk in intensive care units. For presumed varices or portal gastropathy, intravenous octreotide is begun when bleeding is diagnosed. Antibiotics (e.g. quinolones or ceftriaxone) should be administered to cirrhotics with acute GI bleeding, irrespective of the presence or absence of varices or the cause of bleeding, as they have been proven to reduce morbidity and mortality in this setting.

Therapeutic endoscopy

Before endoscopy, it may be beneficial to lavage the stomach through a large-bore orogastric tube with room temperature saline or water to enhance mucosal visualization. Alternatively, intravenous erythromycin can be administered to help clear the stomach of retained blood. Bleeding esophageal varices may be managed by endoscopic placement of rubber bands to constrict the bleeding site or by direct injection of a sclerosant solution such as sodium morrhuate. These therapies have initial success rates of 85–95% for controlling active hemorrhage. Band ligation may exhibit lower complication rates compared to sclerotherapy. Multiple courses of banding or sclerotherapy can be recommended to reduce rates of rebleeding. The role of endoscopy in managing gastric varices is less well established, although sclerotherapy, thrombin injection, cyanoacrylate injection, and snare ligation have been reported to be effective in small studies.

For nonvariceal hemorrhage, local injection, placement of hemoclips, or cautery may provide effective initial hemostasis and reduce the risk of rebleeding. Meta-analyses suggest reductions in mortality with endoscopic therapy. Solutions that stop bleeding from nonvariceal disease when injected include sclerosants (ethanolamine), vasoconstrictors (epinephrine), and normal saline. Thermal methods of cautery include bipolar electrocautery, heater probe application, argon plasma coagulation, and Nd:YAG laser therapy. Endoscopic visualization of a nonbleeding visible vessel or an adherent clot increases the risk of rebleeding in the patient with ulcer hemorrhage. Thus, for major hemorrhage secondary to ulcer disease, endoscopic therapy should be performed for active bleeding sites as well as visible vessels and adherent clots, which, when washed off, reveal visible vessels or active bleeding. Other sources amenable to cautery include refractory Mallory–Weiss tears, neoplasms, angiodysplasia, or Dieulafoy lesions. Patients with stress gastritis, gastropathy resulting from analgesics, and portal gastropathy usually present with multiple bleeding sites that cannot be controlled endoscopically. Fortunately, bleeding stops spontaneously in many of these individuals.

Mechanical compression

When endoscopic therapy of variceal hemorrhage fails, balloon tamponade with a Sengstaken–Blakemore or Linton–Nachlas tube achieves initial hemostasis in 70–90% of cases. However, rebleeding rates are high after removing the device. Most patients benefit from prophylactic endotracheal intubation before balloon tamponade.

Therapeutic angiography

Angiography is effective for many cases when endoscopic therapy fails or is not indicated. In peptic ulcer hemorrhage refractory to endoscopic control, angiographic embolization with microcoils, absorbable gelatin sponge, or autologous clot may be attempted. Intra-arterial vasopressin or embolization is useful for some patients with stress gastritis bleeding, as well as in those with bleeding from esophageal sources, refractory Mallory–Weiss tears, neoplasms, hematobilia, and hemosuccus pancreaticus. Angiographic placement of a portocaval shunt (transjugular intrahepatic portosystemic shunt, TIPS) can effectively control bleeding secondary to gastric varices, portal hypertensive gastropathy, and esophageal varices. With TIPS, an expandable metal stent is placed between the hepatic and portal veins to reduce portal pressure.

Surgery
When endoscopy or angiography fail, emergency surgery may be required.

Complications

The most serious complication of upper GI bleeding is exsanguination and death. Mortality from acute upper GI hemorrhage increases from 8–10% to 30–40% in patients with persistent or recurrent bleeding. Thus, a major focus of research has been on means to prevent initial or recurrent hemorrhage. For bleeding from ulcers, treatments directed to causes such as *H. pylori* are indicated. Prostaglandin analogs (e.g. misoprostol) and proton pump inhibitors have demonstrated efficacy in preventing NSAID-induced gastropathy and ulcers. Stress gastritis prophylaxis includes proton pump inhibitors, H_2 receptor antagonists, high-dose antacids, or sucralfate.

Because of the high mortality of hemorrhage secondary to portal hypertension, prevention of rebleeding is crucial. Obliteration of varices with multiple courses of endoscopic variceal band ligation or sclerotherapy reduces rebleeding rates. Meta-analyses suggest that propranolol therapy to reduce portal pressures reduces the probability of initial and recurrent hemorrhage from esophageal varices. Propranolol has also shown efficacy in preventing rebleeding from portal gastropathy.

Acute Lower Gastrointestinal Bleeding

Clinical presentation

History and physical examination
A thorough history and physical examination may point to the correct diagnosis. A history of hemorrhoids or inflammatory bowel disease is important to note. Abdominal pain or diarrhea suggests colitis or neoplasm. Malignancy also may be indicated by weight loss, anorexia, lymphadenopathy, or palpable masses.

Additional testing

Endoscopy

When lower GI bleeding is slow or has stopped, colonoscopy is the diagnostic procedure of choice because it is highly accurate in detecting potential bleeding sites and affords therapeutic capability. Colonoscopy can document the presence of diverticula; however, it frequently does not identify the actual bleeding site. With brisk bleeding, colonoscopy attempted after a rapid purge may provide diagnostic accuracy similar to or greater than angiography. In contrast, barium enema radiography may miss up to 20% of endoscopically identifiable lesions, especially angiodysplastic lesions, and can prevent therapies directed by colonoscopy or angiography. Thus, the technique is rarely useful in patients with unexplained lower GI bleeding. In patients with presumed GI bleeding distal to the ligament of Treitz who have undergone a colonoscopy with negative results, peroral enteroscopy or capsule endoscopy may detect small intestinal angiodysplastic lesions or other subtle lesions. As capsule endoscopy is purely a diagnostic modality, therapy may be provided by deep enteroscopy (e.g. balloon-assisted enteroscopy).

Scintigraphy and angiography

For cases with rapid hemorrhage where colonoscopy is nondiagnostic or cannot be performed, angiography can provide important information. With bleeding rates greater than 0.5 mL/min, lumenal blood extravasation from diverticula, angiodysplasia, neoplasia, Meckel diverticula, or aortoenteric fistulae may be observed. In rare cases, angiodysplasia or neoplasms in the small intestine and colon may be detected from the angiographic blush pattern in the absence of active bleeding. Prior to angiography, a scintigraphic bleeding scan may be needed to confirm ongoing bleeding and to direct the angiographer to the anatomical region where bleeding is occurring. When a bleeding site cannot be defined, some have advocated an aggressive angiographic approach with administration of heparin or streptokinase to increase the bleeding rate with the hope of enhancing the detection rate of the test. Helical computed tomography angiography also can detect angiodysplasia. Meckel diverticula can be diagnosed with Meckel scanning, which uses a radiolabeled technetium compound that accumulates in acid-producing mucosa in the diverticulum.

Other radiographic studies

Barium enema radiography may be useful for both diagnosing and treating intussusception. Detection of selected unusual bleeding sites in the small intestine may require enteroclysis, a barium study of the small intestine that involves perfusing barium, water, and methylcellulose through a tube fluoroscopically advanced to the ligament of Treitz to create a double-contrast image.

Differential diagnosis

Bleeding colonic diverticula, angiodysplasia, and ischemic colitis are the major causes of acute lower GI bleeding (see Table 3.1). Chronic or recurrent lower GI hemorrhage is most often due to hemorrhoids and colonic neoplasia. Unlike upper GI bleeding, most lower GI bleeding is slow and intermittent and does not require hospitalization.

Diverticulosis

Diverticular bleeding usually is painless and occurs in 3% of patients with diverticulosis. Red or maroon stools usually are passed, although melena may occur. Despite the preponderance of diverticula in the sigmoid colon, many bleeding diverticula are right-sided. Most cases spontaneously resolve and do not recur.

Angiodysplasia

Angiodysplasia is responsible for 10–40% of acute lower GI bleeding episodes. Angiodysplasia is also a common cause of chronic blood loss. Colonic angiodysplasias usually are multiple in number, small (<5 mm in diameter), and localized to the right colon and cecum. As with gastroduodenal vascular ectasia, colonic lesions are associated with advanced age, renal insufficiency, prior irradiation, and aortic valve disease, although the latter association has been questioned.

Ischemic colitis

Most cases of ischemic colitis present in the setting of reduced visceral blood flow and do not involve any underlying fixed narrowing of the mesenteric vasculature. Nevertheless, most patients with ischemic colitis are elderly with significant concurrent disease. Other causes include sepsis, hemorrhage from other causes, and dehydration.

Perianal disease

Hemorrhoids and anal fissures usually result in small volumes of bright red blood on toilet paper or on but not mixed in stool. In contrast, hemorrhage from rectal varices in patients with portal hypertension may be life-threatening. Because polyps and carcinoma may present similarly to hemorrhoids or fissures, these causes need to be excluded in appropriate patient populations.

Colonic neoplasia

Benign and malignant colonic neoplasms are common in elderly patients and usually are associated with small degrees of intermittent bleeding or occult blood loss. In contrast, small intestinal neoplasms are rare disorders that have increased incidence in inflammatory conditions (e.g. Crohn's disease or celiac sprue).

Miscellaneous causes of lower gastrointestinal bleeding

Colitis secondary to inflammatory bowel disease, infection (e.g. *Campylobacter jejuni*, *Salmonella* spp., *Shigella* spp., *Escherichia coli*), and radiation therapy rarely leads to bleeding that is more than small to moderate in volume. Meckel diverticulum, a congenital ileal diverticulum resulting from incomplete obliteration of the vitelline duct, may bleed profusely because acid-producing gastric-type mucosa within the lesion causes peptic ulceration. Patients usually present in childhood with painless red or melenic bleeding, which has been described as having a "redcurrant jelly" appearance. Intussusception presents with maroon stools and crampy pain and usually occurs at the site of a polyp or malignancy in adults. Portal hypertension may predispose to development of ileocolonic and anorectal varices, which may cause voluminous, brisk, blood loss. Portal colonopathy appears as multiple colonic vascular ectasias. Other rare causes of lower GI bleeding include aortoenteric fistulae, solitary rectal ulcers (caused by constipation-induced rectal prolapse), and cecal ulcers (most often caused by NSAIDs).

Management

Resuscitation

Resuscitation in acute lower GI bleeding follows protocols similar to those for upper GI hemorrhage, with prompt correction of volume deficits and stabilization of hemodynamic variables (Figure 3.3). Because extremely brisk upper GI hemorrhage also may present with red rectal bleeding, a nasogastric tube may need to be placed and upper endoscopy performed in any patient with a potential upper GI source. Laboratory studies provide the same information as with upper GI sources, although azotemia resulting from intralumenal blood degradation usually does not occur.

Medications

Certain lower GI sources are amenable to specific medication therapy. Hemorrhoids, anal fissures, and solitary rectal ulcers benefit from bulk-forming agents, sitz baths, and avoidance of straining. Steroid-containing ointments and suppositories are often used, but their efficacy is questioned. Inflammatory bowel disease usually responds to specific anti-inflammatory drug therapy. Intrarectal formalin may reduce bleeding secondary to radiation proctitis. Similar responses to hyperbaric oxygen have been anecdotally noted.

Therapeutic endoscopy

Diverticular bleeding can be treated with cautery or endoscopic clip placement. Colonoscopic bipolar cautery, monopolar cautery, heater probe application, argon plasma coagulation, and Nd:YAG laser have all been used successfully to

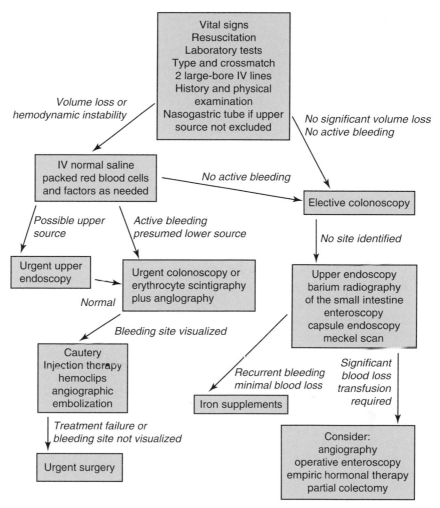

Figure 3.3 Work-up of a patient with acute lower GI bleeding. IV, intravenous.

treat angiodysplasia and the vascular changes that occur with chronic radiation proctocolitis. Colonoscopy also may be used to ablate or resect bleeding polyps or to reduce hemorrhage associated with colonic malignancy. Sigmoidoscopy can treat bleeding internal hemorrhoids with banding or thermal techniques.

Therapeutic angiography

When colonoscopy fails or cannot be performed, angiography may offer important therapeutic capability. Selective arterial embolization with polyvinyl alcohol particles or microcoils is replacing intra-arterial vasopressin to control lower GI bleeding. Angiographic embolization in the colon is considered a last resort because of a 13–18% risk of bowel infarction.

Surgery

For certain diagnoses (e.g. Meckel diverticulum or some malignancies), surgery is the appropriate primary therapy after stabilizing a patient. Emergency surgery carries high morbidity and mortality that increase as the clinical condition deteriorates. For cases of recurrent significant bleeding without a defined source of hemorrhage, right hemicolectomy or subtotal colectomy may be indicated in some patients with good overall prognoses.

Complications

As with upper GI sources, massive lower GI bleeding can have profound sequelae. Chronic or recurrent lower GI bleeding is associated with significant morbidity and subjects the patient to the risks of frequent transfusions.

Key practice points

- Hematochezia does not always arise from a lower GI source; therefore, evidence of upper GI bleeding should be sought (hematemesis or melenemesis, elevated blood urea nitrogen, blood in nasogastric lavage).

- While emergency upper endoscopy is indicated for acute upper GI hemorrhage, acute lower gastrointestinal hemorrhage may be appropriately managed initially with erythrocyte scintigraphy, angiography or emergency colonoscopy. The latter may not always be appropriate due to the necessity of a colonic lavage, the difficulty of visually locating the source of bleeding (diverticular and vascular ectasias in particular), and the limitations of endoscopic therapy.

- Occult GI hemorrhage (i.e. positive fecal occult blood test) without iron deficiency anemia warrants a colonoscopy only. An upper endoscopy is indicated only if iron deficiency is present.

Occult Gastrointestinal Hemorrhage

Clinical presentation

History

Patients with chronic occult blood loss most often are asymptomatic or report fatigue secondary to anemia. Palpitations, postural light-headedness, and exertional dyspnea suggest more significant anemia. Some patients exhibit pica, or compulsive ingestion of ice or soil, with iron deficiency. Dyspepsia, abdominal pain, heartburn, or regurgitation suggests possible peptic causes, whereas weight loss and anorexia raise concern for malignancy. Recurrent episodes of occult blood loss in elderly patients without other symptoms are consistent with vascular ectasias.

Physical examination

Profound iron deficiency may present with pallor, tachycardia, postural or supine hypotension, and a hyperdynamic heart caused by high cardiac output. Other rare findings include papilledema, hearing loss, cranial nerve palsies, retinal hemorrhages, as well as koilonychia (brittle, furrowed, and spooned nails), glossitis, and cheilosis. Lymphadenopathy, masses, hepatosplenomegaly, or jaundice suggest possible malignancy, whereas epigastric tenderness is found with peptic disease. Splenomegaly, jaundice, or spider angiomata raise the possibility of blood loss secondary to portal hypertensive gastropathy. Numerous cutaneous telangiectasias are suggestive of possible hereditary hemorrhagic telangiectasia.

Additional testing

Fecal blood testing

Fecal testing for occult blood can be performed with either guaiac preparations or immunochemical tests. The leuco dye guaiac is a colorless compound that turns blue on exposure to blood. However, peroxidase-containing foods such as radishes, turnips, cantaloupe, bean sprouts, cauliflower, broccoli, and grapes also cause the color change, as can medications (sucralfate, cimetidine), halogens, and toilet bowl sanitizers. Iron, however, causes a green, not blue, color change. Conversely, ascorbic acid, antacids, heat, and acid pH inhibit guaiac reactivity and obscure the diagnosis of fecal blood loss. Immunochemical tests are very sensitive to fresh blood. However, these techniques are less useful for upper GI sources because gut metabolism of globin compromises its immunological detection.

Tests for iron deficiency

Hypochromic, microcytic anemia, determined by visual or automated peripheral smear analysis, provides evidence of occult GI bleeding, although it may not develop until significant blood loss has occurred. Anisocytosis, or variability of cell size reflected by the red cell distribution width, also often increases with iron deficiency. In addition to these measured variables of complete blood count analysis, values of serum iron, ferritin and transferrin may be obtained. Serum ferritin levels correlate better with tissue iron stores and may decrease before anemia develops, although inflammatory conditions can falsely elevate ferritin levels because this marker is an acute-phase reactant. With iron deficiency, the iron level is low with a compensatory increase in transferrin concentration, resulting in a reduced percentage of transferrin saturation. Low values for serum iron and transferrin saturation also may be seen in anemia of chronic disease. In questionable cases, determination of bone marrow iron stores remains the gold standard for diagnosing iron deficiency anemia.

Endoscopy and radiography

For the patient with asymptomatic occult blood-positive stools with no anemia and normal ferritin, colonoscopy is the appropriate diagnostic procedure because

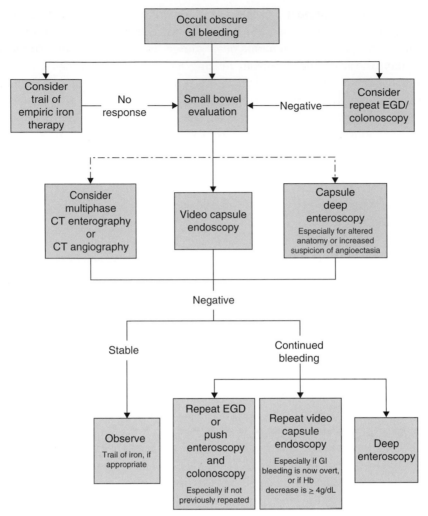

Figure 3.4 Suggested diagnostic approach to occult obscure GI bleeding. Dashed arrows indicate less preferred options. Positive test results should direct specific therapy. Because diagnostic tests can be complementary, more than one test may be needed, and the first-line test may be based upon institutional expertise and availability. CT, computed tomography; EGD, esophagogastroduodenoscopy; Hb, hemoglobin. (Source: ASGE Standards of Practice Committee, The Role of Endoscopy in the Management of Obscure GI Bleeding, Gastrointest Endosc 2010; 72:475; with permission from the American Society for Gastrointestinal Endoscopy.)

most studies show little risk of upper GI malignancies in this setting. In large, population-based screening studies, 2–10% of patients with guaiac-positive stools have colorectal cancer, although a much higher percentage have nonmalignant polyps. Sigmoidoscopy plus barium enema radiography is inferior to colonoscopy because it has significantly lower sensitivity in detecting colonic neoplasia. With occult, obscure GI bleeding, the approach shown in Figure 3.4 is recommended.

In cases of unexplained iron deficiency anemia but no positive fecal blood testing, small intestinal biopsies may be performed to exclude celiac disease. In patients with specific GI symptoms, the sequence of diagnostic testing should be directed to the anatomical site from which symptoms appear to arise. If no lesion is found using this protocol, further evaluation is indicated only if oral iron fails to correct the patient's anemia.

Differential diagnosis

Occult gastrointestinal (GI) hemorrhage is bleeding that is not apparent on visual stool inspection. Its prevalence is as high as 1 in 20 adults. Up to 150 mL of blood may be lost in the proximal gut without reliably producing melena. Most occult GI bleeding is chronic and, if significant, can produce marked iron deficiency anemia. An extensive list of disorders, including inflammatory disorders, infectious causes, vascular diseases, neoplasms, and other conditions, may produce occult bleeding with or without iron deficiency anemia (Table 3.2).

Inflammatory causes

Acid peptic diseases, including erosions or ulcers of the esophagus, stomach, and duodenum, are the most common causes of occult GI bleeding and are associated with iron deficiency in 30–70% of cases. Longitudinal erosions within the large hiatal hernia sac, known as Cameron erosions, may cause up to 10% of cases of iron deficiency anemia. Other inflammatory causes of occult bleeding include inflammatory bowel disease, celiac sprue, Meckel diverticulum, eosinophilic gastroenteritis, radiation enteritis, colorectal ulcers, and Whipple disease.

Infectious causes

In the United States, infectious causes of occult GI bleeding are uncommon, but organisms such as hookworms, *Mycobacterium tuberculosis*, amebas, and *Ascaris* species cause chronic blood loss in several hundred million people worldwide.

Vascular causes

Vascular ectasias cause up to 6% of all cases of iron deficiency anemia. In patients with portal hypertension, portal hypertensive gastropathy commonly causes occult blood loss and iron deficiency.

Tumors and neoplasms

Gastrointestinal tumors are the second most prevalent cause of occult bleeding in the United States after acid peptic disease. Colorectal carcinoma and adenomatous polyps are the most common neoplasms, followed by gastric, esophageal, and ampullary malignancies. Other tumors, such as lymphomas, metastases, leiomyomas and leiomyosarcomas, and juvenile polyps, also produce occult blood loss.

Table 3.2 Causes of occult gastrointestinal blood loss

Tumors and neoplasms
Primary adenocarcinoma
Metastases
Large polyps
Lymphoma
Leiomyoma
Leiomyosarcoma
Lipoma

Infectious causes
Hookworm
Strongyloidiasis
Ascariasis
Tuberculous enterocolitis
Amebiasis

Miscellaneous causes
Medications (NSAIDs)
Long-distance running
Gastrostomy tubes and other appliances

Vascular causes
Vascular ectasia
Portal hypertensive gastropathy
Hemangiomas
Blue rubber bleb nevus syndrome
Gastric antral vascular ectasia (GAVE)

Inflammatory disorders
Acid peptic disease
Hiatal hernia (Cameron erosions)
Inflammatory bowel disease
Celiac sprue
Whipple disease
Eosinophilic gastroenteritis
Meckel diverticulum
Solitary rectal ulcer
Cecal ulcer

Other causes of occult gastrointestinal bleeding

Medications are important causes of occult bleeding. Ulcerations and erosions of the stomach, small intestine, and colon can result from NSAIDs. Other drugs that cause occult bleeding include potassium preparations, certain antibiotics, and antimetabolites. Anticoagulants (e.g. warfarin) cause an increased incidence of occult bleeding, although anticoagulants more commonly increase the rate of blood loss from pre-existing lesions. Esophageal webs, as in the

Plummer–Vinson or Paterson–Kelly syndrome, are associated with iron deficiency. Iron deficiency anemia also develops in long-distance runners, possibly secondary to mechanical jarring or to subclinical mesenteric ischemia. Non-GI causes such as hemoptysis, oral bleeding, epistaxis, and factitious blood ingestion can mimic occult GI blood loss.

Management

Treatment of occult GI bleeding is dictated by the diagnostic evaluation. Some conditions of chronic blood loss require long-term iron supplementation. Oral ferrous sulfate at a dose of 325 mg three times daily is preferred in most patients because it is inexpensive, effective, and well tolerated. Other oral preparations include ferrous fumarate, ferrous gluconate, and preparations with added ascorbic acid to enhance absorption. Repletion of iron stores may take 3–6 months, although reticulocytosis peaks within 10 days and the hemoglobin level normalizes within 2 months. Parenteral iron, in complexed form, is indicated for patients who cannot absorb or do not tolerate oral iron. In some instances, iron may be administered intravenously. Parenteral preparations may result in rare anaphylaxis, and 10% of patients develop serum sickness-like reactions.

Complications

Chronic occult GI blood loss usually is well tolerated in young individuals; however, older patients or those with underlying cardiorespiratory disease may deteriorate because of the reduced oxygen-carrying capacity of their blood.

Case studies

Case 1

A 63-year-old man with a long history of hepatitis C virus infection and alcohol dependence presents to the emergency department with several hours of light-headedness and dark stool. He reports a 1-week history of back pain for which he has been taking ibuprofen several times a day. On physical examination, his pulse is 115 beats per min with a blood pressure of 98/50 mmHg. Skin exam reveals a few spider angiomata on the chest. There is melena on rectal exam. Laboratory studies are notable for a hemoglobin of 12 g/dL, platelets of 85,000, BUN 18 mg/dL, creatinine 0.8 mg/dL, INR 1.5, albumin 2.8 g/dL, bilirubin 1.7 mg/dL. Ethanol level is undetectable. A type and cross-match for blood is sent. Nasogastric (NG) aspirate reveals clear fluid without blood or bile.

Two 18 gauge intravenous catheters are placed and normal saline is given as a 1 L bolus with improvement of the patient's heart rate to 98 beats per min. Proton pump inhibitor and octreotide infusions are initiated. Ceftriaxone is administered intravenously and the patient is admitted to the intensive care unit (ICU). Additional saline boluses are given with normalization of his vital signs. A repeat hemoglobin is 8.5 g/dL. Urgent endoscopy reveals a 2 cm duodenal bulb ulcer with a visible vessel. Old blood is seen in the duodenum. Bipolar cautery therapy is applied with excellent results. No varices are seen. The octreotide drip is discontinued, but proton pump inhibitor therapy and antibiotics are continued. The patient is transferred out of the ICU on day 3. A stool antigen for *Helicobacter pylori*, sent on the second day of hospitalization, is positive. The patient is prescribed omeprazole, amoxicillin and clarithromycin for 14 days. Ibuprofen is discontinued. The omeprazole is continued for a total of 8 weeks. The patient is referred for outpatient evaluation in the hepatology clinic and for assistance with alcohol cessation. Repeat stool antigen testing for *H. pylori* is negative at 3 months.

Discussion and potential pitfalls

This case highlights many important points in the management of acute upper GI bleeding. First, although this patient has physical and laboratory evidence of cirrhosis, most GI bleeding in this setting is not due to varices. Nevertheless, it is reasonable to initiate empirical octreotide therapy. Second, proton pump inhibitor therapy is reasonable in the setting of melena (despite the negative NG lavage), though melena may also result from bleeding as far down the GI tract as the right colon. If endoscopy does not find an acid-related upper GI source of bleeding, then this therapy should be discontinued. Third, antibiotics are indicated because they have been shown to reduce morbidity and mortality in randomized, placebo-controlled trials of cirrhotics with GI bleeding. Fourth, despite the lack of anemia or blood on gastric aspirate, the hemodynamic alterations suggest significant blood loss, indicating a need for ICU monitoring and urgent endoscopy. Nasogastric tube lavage commonly does not reveal blood in the setting of duodenal bleeding and the hemoglobin does not reflect acute blood loss. Finally, testing for *H. pylori* is indicated for patients with peptic ulcer disease. In the setting of complicated peptic ulcer disease (i.e. with bleeding, perforation, or obstruction), documentation of eradication is recommended.

Case 2

A 76-year-old woman presents to the emergency department reporting sudden onset of hematochezia with presyncope 2 h early. She takes furosemide for hypertension, but is otherwise healthy. On physical examination, her pulse is 107 beats per min with a blood pressure of 102/56 mmHg. There are dark red clots on rectal exam. Laboratory studies are notable for a hemoglobin of 11.8 g/dL, platelets of 315,000, BUN 7 mg/dL, creatinine 1.0 mg/dL, INR 1.0, albumin 4.1 g/dL, bilirubin 0.8 mg/dL. A type and cross-match for blood is sent. Nasogastric tube aspirate reveals clear fluid.

Two 18 gauge intravenous catheters are placed and normal saline is given as a bolus with normalization of her vital signs after 2 L. The patient is admitted to the ICU. A repeat hemoglobin is 9.6 g/dL. She is given a polyethylene glycol (PEG)-electrolyte colonic lavage solution via the nasogastric tube in preparation for colonoscopy. Urgent colonoscopy reveals sigmoid diverticulosis. One diverticulum contains a clot which, when aggressively washed, reveals a small ulcer with a visible vessel. An endoscopic clip is successfully applied to the ulcer. She has no further bleeding during her 3-day hospitalization.

Discussion and potential pitfalls

Diverticular hemorrhage is a common cause of acute lower GI bleeding. Despite a negative NG lavage, studies have shown that up to 15% of hemodynamically significant hematochezia cases are due to a source found on upper GI endoscopy. Therefore, it is appropriate to consider doing this exam prior to colonoscopy. Some practitioners will perform esophagogastroduodenoscopy (EGD) prior to initiating the bowel preparation. Others will perform EGD only if the colonoscopy is negative. There are observational data suggesting that endoscopic therapy improves outcomes (e.g. length of stay, transfusion requirement) of patients with acute lower GI bleeding.

Case 3

A 50-year-old woman with adult-onset diabetes and chronic renal insufficiency is found to have iron deficiency anemia (hemoglobin 8.3 g/dL, ferritin 28 ng/mL, total iron-binding capacity (TIBC) 426 μg/dL, iron 12 μg/dL, iron saturation 20%, creatinine 2.0 mg/dL). She has no history of gross bleeding, takes no NSAIDs and has an unremarkable physical exam. The patient undergoes colonoscopy to the terminal ileum, with an excellent preparation, and is normal. EGD with biopsies of the duodenum is also normal. Iron therapy is started with modest improvement of the hemoglobin to 9.7 g/dL. Capsule endoscopy is performed, revealing scattered vascular ectasias in the proximal to mid-small bowel. Balloon enteroscopy is performed with cautery of over a dozen vascular ectasias. Iron therapy is continued with improvement of anemia to 11.5 g/dL at 3-month follow-up.

Discussion and potential pitfalls

When the initial evaluation of iron deficiency anemia with colonoscopy and EGD with biopsies (to rule out celiac sprue) is negative, the patient is said to have occult, obscure GI bleeding. Some practitioners will elect to proceed directly to small bowel evaluation with capsule endoscopy, while others will elect for a trial of iron replacement. Given the history of chronic renal insufficiency, there is a higher pretest probability of vascular ectasia. Ultimately, capsule endoscopy is only a diagnostic test and deep enteroscopy is required to deliver endoscopic therapy. Some advocate use of estrogen-progesterone therapy or subcutaneous octreotide injections to help control bleeding from vascular ectasia though evidence to support these approaches is limited.

CHAPTER 4

Approach to the Patient with Unexplained Weight Loss

Clinical presentation

History

The first step in evaluation is documenting weight loss because objective records cannot corroborate the reported weight loss in 50% of patients. Once documented, the history can provide important clues to the etiology of weight loss. Medications (e.g. procainamide, theophylline, thyroxin, and nitrofurantoin) may be factors in older patients. Fever or chills may suggest infectious causes, whereas selected risk factors raise the possibility of AIDS. Nausea or pain is reported with gastrointestinal (GI) obstruction, whereas masses or jaundice suggests underlying malignancy. Bulky, foul-smelling, greasy stools indicate probable malabsorption. Other systemic diseases are suggested by specific symptom profiles.

The history should also include a search for psychiatric causes, including alcoholism and depression. Psychomotor retardation or lack of interest in daily activities is characteristic of depression. A denial of significant weight loss is common in anorexia nervosa, whereas secretive purging is classic in bulimia. Anorexia nervosa may also be associated with symptoms of altered gut function (e.g. early satiety, bloating, vomiting, constipation) and endocrine activity (e.g. amenorrhea, loss of libido, symptoms of hypothyroidism).

Physical examination

Physical findings of weight loss relate to its cause and the degree of malnutrition. Attention should be paid to overall appearance as well as to mood and affect. Cutaneous examination may suggest endocrine disease or AIDS (e.g. Kaposi sarcoma). Jaundice reflects hepatic disease. Malignancy is suggested by lymphadenopathy, occult fecal blood, or masses, whereas obstruction produces abdominal distension and high-pitched bowel sounds. Demonstrably impaired mental function may be an underlying factor in older patients. Gross GI bleeding may be seen as a result of emesis-induced esophageal damage.

Yamada's Handbook of Gastroenterology, Third Edition. Edited by Tadataka Yamada and John M. Inadomi.
© 2013 John Wiley & Sons, Ltd. Published 2013 by John Wiley & Sons, Ltd.

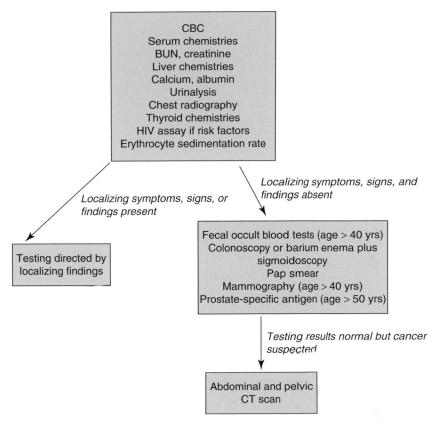

Figure 4.1 Work-up of a patient with unexplained weight loss. BUN, blood urea nitrogen; CBC, complete blood count; CT, computed tomography; HIV, human immunodeficiency virus.

Manifestations of severe malnutrition include hypothermia, bradycardia and other arrhythmias, hypotension, hypothermia, and dehydration, especially in patients with anorexia nervosa. Brittle hair or nails, decreased fat stores, acrocyanosis, downy hair, yellow cutaneous discoloration (from hypercarotenemia), and loss of secondary sexual characteristics may be seen, especially in young patients with anorexia nervosa. Self-induced vomiting or regurgitation produces halitosis, pharyngitis, gingival or dental erosions from reflux of gastric acid, and also may lead to parotid swelling and abrasion or scarring of the knuckles from inserting the fingers into the mouth.

Additional testing

Laboratory, radiological, and endoscopic evaluations are guided by the history and physical examination, including associated symptoms, patient age, symptom duration, prior medical conditions, degree of malnutrition, and emotional factors (Figure 4.1). Laboratory studies should include a complete blood count; sedimentation rate, electrolytes, blood urea nitrogen (BUN), creatinine, total protein, and albumin; urinalysis; and liver chemistries. Radiography of the chest and abdomen can detect malignancy or obstruction. Specific blood testing can screen for thyroid disease, and human immunodeficiency virus (HIV) assays, tuberculosis quantiferon or placement of a purified protein derivative can test for infectious causes (i.e. AIDS and tuberculosis, respectively). In the absence of specific findings, routine screening for malignancy is indicated, including Papanicolaou smear in women, colonoscopy in persons older than 50 years, mammography in women older than 40 years, and prostate-specific antigen in men older than 50 years.

Other tests for organic disease may be indicated in some patients. If malabsorption is suspected, screening tests such as qualitative fecal fat, serum carotene, and prothrombin time may be obtained. Specific tests for small intestinal or pancreatic causes of malabsorption are ordered if results of screening tests are positive or if suspicion of malabsorption is high. If structural disease is suspected, abdominal computed tomography or ultrasonography may detect underlying malignancies, whereas barium radiography and endoscopy may define sites of obstruction. In patients with suspected anorexia nervosa, structural evaluation of the GI tract is considered because Crohn's disease is in the differential diagnosis. Upper endoscopy or barium radiography should be performed with suspected rumination because esophageal disease can mimic this disorder.

When biological disease has been excluded, referral to a mental health specialist should be contemplated to exclude psychiatric causes of weight loss. Establishing a specific diagnosis using strict criteria (e.g. *Diagnostic and Statistical Manual of Mental Disorders IV*) benefits the patient by directing psychosocial treatment of the underlying condition.

Differential diagnosis

Unexplained weight loss may result from combinations of biological and behavioral factors. Hunger is a consequence of physiological processes, whereas appetite is more heavily influenced by environmental and psychological input, including the aroma and appearance of food and a person's mood. Weight loss may result from decreased caloric intake, increased metabolism, or urinary or fecal loss of calories. In general, a person's weight fluctuates by as much as 1.5% per day. A sustained weight loss greater than 5% warrants concern and possible investigation. In addition to anorexia, other symptom complexes contribute to weight loss, including nausea, vomiting, early satiety, postprandial abdominal pain, and altered consciousness. A variety of general medical, GI, and behavioral illnesses produce unexplained weight loss (Table 4.1). About half of all cases of unexplained weight loss are attributable to organic disease, whereas psychiatric conditions, especially in the elderly, comprise the majority of the remaining cases. Parkinson disease and Alzheimer disease are common neurological etiologies of weight loss.

Table 4.1 Causes of weight loss

General medical disorders
Endocrinopathies (thyrotoxicosis, diabetes mellitus, Addison disease)
Chronic infections (tuberculosis, fungal infections, endocarditis, AIDS)
Malignancy (carcinoma, lymphoma, leukemia)
Medications
Inadequate intake (immobility, impaired consciousness, dementia)

Behavioral disorders
Depression
Schizophrenia
Anorexia nervosa
Bulimia nervosa
Adult rumination syndrome

Gastrointestinal disease
Gastrointestinal obstruction (stricture, adhesions, neoplasm)
Motility disorders (achalasia, gastroparesis, intestinal pseudo-obstruction)
Pancreaticobiliary disease (biliary colic, chronic pancreatitis, pancreatic carcinoma)
Chronic hepatitis
Malabsorption in the small intestine
Bacterial overgrowth
Chronic mesenteric ischemia

General medical disorders

Because of its gravity, malignancy should be considered early in evaluating weight loss, although neoplasm is not prevalent in patients without specific signs or symptoms. Endocrinopathies such as thyrotoxicosis, diabetes, and Addison disease produce weight loss by varying mechanisms. Chronic infections (e.g. tuberculosis, fungal diseases, subacute bacterial endocarditis, and AIDS) can cause weight loss. In elderly patients, weight loss results from physiological changes, reduced taste or smell, neuropsychiatric syndromes, effects of medication, poor dentition, and lack of available food. Chronic obstructive lung disease and congestive heart failure produce weight loss by increasing caloric demands, by causing anorexia, or by increasing the work of eating.

Gastrointestinal disorders

Abdominal diseases cause weight loss in several ways. Lumenal obstruction usually is associated with exacerbation of symptoms on meal ingestion, either immediately (esophageal stricture or cancer, achalasia), 1–3 h postprandially (gastric or proximal intestinal blockage), or several hours later (distal ileitis, colon cancer). Motor disorders such as gastroparesis have similar effects. Likewise, pain from pancreaticobiliary sources may worsen after food ingestion, thus reducing intake. Malabsorption may result from disease of the small intestine or pancreas. Weight loss occurs in ulcer disease because of meal-evoked pain. Constipation may cause anorexia.

Behavioral disorders

Depression is the most common behavioral disorder that decreases food intake and also is characterized by mood changes, sleep disruption, anhedonia, and low self-esteem. Alcoholism produces weight loss by mechanisms independent of its common association with depression. Weight loss may also occur with thought disorders (e.g. schizophrenia) as a consequence of distorted perception about food or eating.

Eating disorders

Eating disorders such as anorexia nervosa and bulimia nervosa, both of which may affect up to 5–10% of young women, are distinguished by the patient's desire to maintain thinness and an altered body image. Adult rumination syndrome also produces weight loss and is often unrecognized.

Anorexia nervosa

Anorexia nervosa is characterized by distortion of body image and an inability to interpret hunger and satiety, with a preoccupation with eating and a sense of ineffectiveness. Patients are not truly anorectic but struggle against hunger to achieve an unrealistic degree of weight loss through dietary restriction and exercise, as well as self-induced vomiting or laxative abuse. The condition affects predominantly young women of all ethnic groups and socio-economic levels. There is significant concordance of anorexia nervosa in identical twins and a 6% prevalence in siblings of affected patients, suggesting genetic components as well. Other psychosocial factors, including low self-esteem, obsessive-compulsive and avoidant personality traits, and perfectionistic tendencies, participate in disease pathogenesis.

Bulimia nervosa

Bulimia nervosa is characterized by repetitive binges of overeating followed by acts to avert weight gain (e.g. self-induced emesis, laxative or diuretic abuse, excessive exercise) and occurs almost exclusively in women younger than 30 years, with a prevalence of 1–10%. Partial syndromes with occasional binge eating then purging behavior may be present in up to 19% of college-age women. There is a strong association of bulimia with affective disorders, low self-esteem, and family histories of mood disturbances, alcoholism, and drug addiction. Binge episodes typically last for 1–2 h, during which up to 4000 calories can be ingested.

Adult rumination syndrome

Rumination syndrome, or merycism, is an eating disorder in which the patient repetitively regurgitates food from the stomach, rechews it, and then reswallows it. Adult patients generally report weight loss, regurgitation, and vomiting and are concerned about medical rather than psychiatric causes. The episodes are initiated by belching or swallowing and creating a common esophageal and gastric channel by reducing lower esophageal sphincter pressure. Diaphragmatic and rectus abdominis muscle contraction produces regurgitation, expelling gastric contents into the mouth, where they are rechewed and ingested. The differential diagnosis includes esophageal strictures, gastroesophageal reflux disease, GI dysmotility syndromes, and lumenal obstruction. Characteristic manometric patterns may be seen in some patients with rumination syndrome.

Management

Specific therapies are available for many organic diseases that cause weight loss. If test results are negative, a period of observation is indicated because more than 65% of these individuals do well on follow-up. For individuals with minor degrees of weight loss, offering favorite foods or snacks may be adequate. With severe malnutrition (<70–75% of ideal body weight), hospitalization is necessary. Enteral refeeding may be attempted. If enteral feedings are poorly tolerated or refused, central or peripheral parenteral nutrition may be required. In severe malnutrition, rapid refeeding should be avoided because of potential gastroduodenal dilation and refeeding pancreatitis or diarrhea. For anorexia nervosa, feedings are re-established at 200–250 calories above the intake at time of presentation and are increased by 250–300 calories every 5 days to ensure a weekly weight gain of 1.5 kg as an inpatient and 0.75–1.0 kg as an outpatient. The goal for refeeding is to achieve 90–100% of ideal body weight.

Medical and psychological management of behavioral disease should be initiated immediately along with any refeeding program. Potassium supplements may be needed for patients with anorexia or bulimia nervosa. Antidepressant medications may produce striking weight gain in depressed patients. Prokinetic medications and laxatives may reduce GI symptoms in anorexia nervosa, thus aiding the overall treatment plan. Antidepressants may reduce binge episodes and impulsive behavior in some patients with bulimia but play little role in anorexia nervosa.

Psychological therapy for eating disorders addresses distorted beliefs about weight and eating, body image, fear of weight gain, self-criticism, and poor self-regulation. Therapies that have been efficacious for carefully selected patients with eating disorders include individual psychotherapy, interpersonal therapy, family therapy, and cognitive behavioral therapy. For patients with adult rumination syndrome, behavior modification and biofeedback appear to be the most effective approaches.

Complications

Profound weight loss has significant complications regardless of its cause. Cardiac complications include arrhythmias and sudden death, caused by either the primary disorder or metabolic consequences secondary to purging. Electrocardiographic changes include bradycardia, decreased QRS amplitude, QT prolongation, ST segment changes, and U waves secondary to hypokalemia. Liver chemistry abnormalities result from hepatic steatosis. Fecal impaction can result from many of the causes of weight loss as well as from decreased oral intake and dehydration. Clinical features of hypothyroidism may develop, although free thyroxin levels usually are normal. Bulimia patients may develop pseudo-Bartter syndrome with fluid retention and peripheral edema after abruptly discontinuing diet pills and laxatives.

The prognosis of a patient with unexplained weight loss depends on the cause. Many organic conditions, especially malignancies, are fatal. For patients with anorexia nervosa, the recovery rate ranges from 32% to 71% at 20 years although up to 5% die from complications of malnutrition. Nearly 75% of adolescents with anorexia nervosa continue to suffer from psychiatric diseases. Recovery rates for bulimia are 50–60%, although the condition is fatal in 1–5%.

Key practice points

- Sustained unexplained weight loss of 5% or more warrants investigation.
- The history will often elucidate the cause of weight loss.
- Investigation for malignancy (e.g. colonoscopy in a patient over 50, chest x-ray) is recommended.
- Mental health disorders are a common cause of weight loss and often require a multidisciplinary approach to management.

Case studies

Case 1

A 67-year-old man with a 20-year history of daily heartburn presents with a 20 lb weight loss and progressive solid food dysphagia over the past 3 months. EGD reveals a circumferential mass in the distal esophagus. Histopathology from the esophageal biopsies confirms poorly differentiated adenocarcinoma. Contrast computed tomography (CT) scan of the chest and abdomen reveals a thickened distal esophagus and liver metastases.

> ### Discussion and potential pitfalls
>
> Any evaluation of weight loss should first be directed toward any symptoms. In this case, the long history of heartburn and recent onset of solid food dysphagia suggest an esophageal malignancy. A benign peptic stricture would be less likely to result in such rapid weight loss.

Case 2

An 82-year-old woman with hypertension, hyperlipidemia and coronary artery disease presents with a 32 lb weight loss over the past 4 months. Her review of systems is unremarkable, as are her labs, including complete blood count (CBC), serum chemistries, liver transaminases, bilirubin, alkaline phosphatase, and thyroid function tests. Mammography and pelvic examination, including Papanicolaou smear, were normal. Colonoscopy, EGD and chest x-ray are normal. Given ongoing weight loss, CT of the abdomen and pelvis is performed, revealing a 4 cm mass in the head of the pancreas with mild dilation of the common bile duct and pancreatic duct and encasement of the superior mesenteric artery. Endoscopic ultrasound with fine needle aspiration is performed, revealing cells suspicious for malignancy. The patient's bilirubin rises to 6 mg/dL. Endoscopic retrograde cholangiopancreatography (ERCP) is performed with placement of a self-expanding metal stent into the common bile duct. The patient is referred to medical oncology for consideration of palliative chemotherapy.

> ### Discussion and potential pitfalls
>
> In the absence of historical features or symptoms to direct the diagnostic evaluation, most practitioners will begin by attempting to exclude malignancy. For women, this includes performing mammography and Papanicolaou smear. Given that colorectal cancer is the third most common cancer and the second leading cause of cancer death in the United States, colonoscopy is also recommended. When colonoscopy is negative, many practitioners will perform EGD at the same setting. Given the high incidence of lung cancer, chest x-ray should also be performed. Other tests for organic disease may be indicated in some patients, such as screening tests for malabsorption. If structural disease is suspected, abdominal CT or ultrasonography may detect underlying malignancies, as in this case. Though pancreatic cancer is the fourth leading cause of cancer death, there is no effective screening test. When pancreatic cancer causes symptoms, including weight loss, the prognosis is generally poor.

CHAPTER 5

Approach to the Patient with Nausea and Vomiting

Clinical presentation

History

Acute vomiting (for 1–2 days) most often results from infection, a medication or toxin, or accumulation of endogenous toxins, as in uremia or diabetic ketoacidosis. Chronic vomiting (longer than 1 week) usually results from a long-standing medical or psychiatric condition. Vomiting soon after eating suggests gastric outlet obstruction or inflammatory conditions (e.g. cholecystitis and pancreatitis), whereas delayed vomiting is characteristic of gastroparesis or more distal obstruction. Psychogenic vomiting may occur soon after eating, but most patients control their emesis until the gastric contents can be expelled into a toilet or other receptacle. Early morning nausea characterizes endocrine conditions, such as pregnancy. Meals may relieve nausea associated with peptic ulcer or esophagitis. Patients with cannabinoid hyperemesis almost universally report relief of symptoms with hot showers or baths.

The character of the vomitus can provide diagnostic clues. Vomiting of undigested food is seen with Zenker diverticulum and achalasia. Partial digestion is observed with gastric obstruction and gastroparesis. Bilious vomiting excludes proximal obstruction, whereas vomiting of blood suggests mucosal damage. Voluminous acidic emesis is observed with gastrinomas, whereas feculent emesis occurs in distal obstructions, bacterial overgrowth, and gastrocolic fistulae.

Associated symptoms should be investigated. Pain is reported with ulcer disease, obstruction, or inflammatory disorders. Diarrhea, fever, or myalgias suggest possible infection. Weight loss occurs in many patients with chronic nausea. However, patients with psychogenic vomiting usually maintain stable weight. Headaches, visual changes, altered mentation, and neck stiffness raise the possibility of central nervous system etiologies, whereas tinnitus or vertigo indicate labyrinthine causes. Light-headedness, palpitations, and dry mucous membranes suggest severe dehydration.

Yamada's Handbook of Gastroenterology, Third Edition. Edited by Tadataka Yamada and John M. Inadomi.
© 2013 John Wiley & Sons, Ltd. Published 2013 by John Wiley & Sons, Ltd.

Physical examination

A physical examination assists in diagnosing and managing nausea and vomiting. Fever suggests inflammation or infection. Tachycardia, orthostatic hypotension, loss of skin turgor, and dry mucous membranes indicate dehydration. Oral examination may reveal loss of dental enamel, a common finding in bulimia. Sclerodactyly and jaundice are characteristic skin findings in scleroderma and hepatobiliary disease, respectively. Adenopathy and masses suggest malignancy; hepatomegaly is also found in malignancy and in benign hepatic disease. An absence of bowel sounds signifies ileus, whereas high-pitched hyperactive bowel sounds with a distended abdomen are consistent with intestinal obstruction. A succussion splash on side-to-side movement is found in gastric obstruction and gastroparesis. Abdominal tenderness is noted with inflammation, infection, and lumenal distension, whereas gross or occult fecal blood prompts evaluation for ulcer, inflammation, or malignancy. On neurological examination, focal signs, papilledema, and impaired mentation suggest central nervous system disease. Asterixis is present in metabolic conditions, such as uremia and hepatic failure. Gut motility disorders may be associated with peripheral and autonomic neuropathy.

Additional testing

A thorough history and physical examination will provide sufficient information to diagnose and treat most patients with nausea and vomiting. If there is a clear temporal association of the onset of vomiting with myalgias, cramps, and diarrhea or with initiation of a new medication, no further work-up is needed. However, some patients require blood studies, structural evaluation, or assessment of gut function for appropriate treatment.

Laboratory studies

Several blood tests assist in evaluating the patient with nausea and vomiting (Figure 5.1). With long-standing symptoms or dehydration, serum electrolytes may show hypokalemia or an elevated blood urea nitrogen (BUN) relative to creatinine. Metabolic alkalosis may result from loss of hydrogen ions in the acidic vomitus and contraction of the extracellular space from dehydration. A complete blood count rules out anemia from inflammation or blood loss, leukocytosis from inflammation, or leukopenia from viral infection. Hypoalbuminemia results from chronic disease and gut protein loss. Amylase, lipase, and liver chemistry determinations are obtained for suspected pancreaticobiliary or hepatic disease. Metabolic causes can be assessed through pregnancy and thyroid tests, BUN, creatinine, glucose, calcium, and plasma cortisol. Specific serological markers can screen for presumed collagen vascular diseases, and antineuronal antibodies are positive with malignancy-associated motility disorders. Meningitis may be confirmed by lumbar puncture.

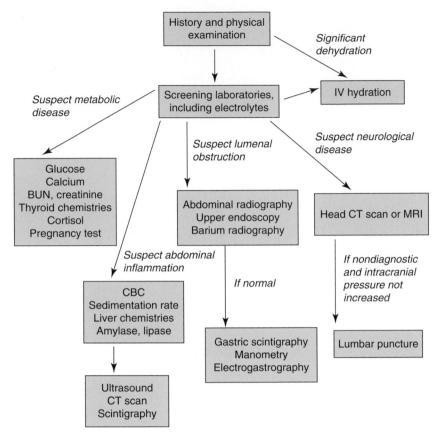

Figure 5.1 Work-up of a patient with nausea and vomiting. BUN, blood urea nitrogen; CBC, complete blood count; CT, computed tomography; MRI, magnetic resonance imaging.

Structural studies

Structural investigation may be needed to exclude organic illness as a cause of vomiting. Flat and upright abdominal radiographs are obtained as a screening examination. Small intestinal air–fluid levels with absent colonic air suggest obstruction, whereas diffuse distension is consistent with ileus. Contrast radiography of the small intestine may confirm partial obstruction. If symptoms are intermittent, enteroclysis may provide more detailed assessment of the small bowel. Upper endoscopy can assess possible gastric outlet obstruction and affords the ability to perform biopsy of suspicious lesions. Retained food in the absence of obstruction is seen in gastroparesis. For suspected pancreaticobiliary disease, ultrasound, computed tomography (CT), endoscopic ultrasound, hepatobiliary scintigraphy, or magnetic resonance cholangiopancreatography may be useful. Computed tomographic and magnetic resonance imaging (MRI) of the head may be indicated for suspected central nervous system sources. Angiography or MRI can detect mesenteric ischemia.

Functional studies

When lumenal obstruction is excluded, gastroparesis and intestinal pseudo-obstruction are considered causes of symptoms. Gastroparesis is diagnosed by demonstrating delayed emptying of an ingested meal. Scintigraphic measures of emptying of solid (^{99m}Tc-sulfur colloid in eggs) or liquid (^{111}In-DTPA in water) radionuclides are most commonly used, although office-based breath tests using ^{13}C-labeled foods show promise.

When scintigraphy incompletely characterizes the cause of nausea and vomiting, other functional tests may be offered in specialized gastrointestinal physiology laboratories. Manometry of the stomach and duodenum can evaluate motor patterns under fasting and fed conditions. These patterns are reasonably specific for neuropathic and myopathic causes of gastroparesis and pseudo-obstruction. Intestinal manometry complements findings from barium radiography of the small intestine, which can reveal slow transit and lumenal dilation in cases of severe dysmotility. Electrogastrography measures electrical pacemaker activity of the stomach through electrodes affixed to the abdomen. Some clinical conditions produce pacemaker rhythms that are too rapid (tachygastria) or slow (bradygastria) that are postulated to underlie development of nausea and vomiting. In rare cases of severe unexplained dysmotility, a surgical full-thickness intestinal biopsy is required to show degeneration of nerve or muscle layers.

Differential diagnosis

Nausea is the subjective sensation of an impending urge to vomit, and vomiting (emesis) is the forceful ejection of gastric contents from the mouth. Retching may precede vomiting but involves no discharge of upper gut contents. Other symptoms may be misinterpreted by the patient as nausea or vomiting. Regurgitation is the effortless return of gastric or esophageal contents in the absence of nausea or involuntary spasmodic muscular contractions. Rumination is characterized by regurgitation of food into the mouth, where it is rechewed and reswallowed. Anorexia refers to loss of appetite. Early satiety is the sensation of gastric fullness before a meal is completed. Nausea may be part of a general complaint of indigestion that includes abdominal discomfort, heartburn, anorexia, and bloating. The differential diagnosis of nausea and vomiting includes medications, gastrointestinal and intraperitoneal disease, neurological disorders, metabolic conditions, and infections (Table 5.1).

Medications

Drug reactions are among the most common causes of nausea and vomiting, especially within days after initiating therapy. Chemotherapeutic agents such as cisplatin and cyclophosphamide are potent emetic stimuli that act on central and peripheral neural pathways. Emesis from chemotherapy may be acute, delayed,

Table 5.1 Causes of nausea and vomiting

Medications
Nonsteroidal anti-inflammatory drugs
Cardiovascular drugs (e.g. digoxin, antiarrhythmics, antihypertensives)
Diuretics
Hormonal agents (e.g. oral antidiabetics, contraceptives)
Antibiotics (e.g. erythromycin)
Gastrointestinal drugs (e.g. sulfasalazine)

Central nervous system disorders
Tumors
Cerebrovascular accident
Intracranial hemorrhage
Infections
Congenital abnormalities
Psychiatric disease (e.g. anxiety, depression, anorexia nervosa, bulimia nervosa, psychogenic vomiting)
Motion sickness
Labyrinthine causes (e.g. tumors, labyrinthitis, Ménière disease)

Miscellaneous causes
Posterior myocardial infarction
Congestive heart failure
Excess ethanol ingestion
Jamaican vomiting sickness
Prolonged starvation
Cyclic vomiting syndrome
Chronic cannabis use (cannabinoid hyperemesis syndrome)

Gastrointestinal and peritoneal disorders
Gastric outlet obstruction
Obstruction of the small intestine
Superior mesenteric artery syndrome
Gastroparesis
Chronic intestinal pseudo-obstruction
Pancreatitis
Appendicitis
Cholecystitis
Acute hepatitis
Pancreatic carcinoma

Endocrinological and metabolic conditions
Nausea of pregnancy
Uremia
Diabetic ketoacidosis
Thyroid disease
Addison disease

Infectious disease
Viral gastroenteritis (e.g. Hawaii agent, rotavirus, reovirus, adenovirus, Snow Mountain agent, Norwalk agent)
Bacterial causes (e.g. *Staphylococcus* spp., *Salmonella* spp., *Bacillus cereus, Clostridium perfringens*)
Opportunistic infection (e.g. cytomegalovirus, herpes simplex virus)
Otitis media

or anticipatory. Analgesics such as aspirin or nonsteroidal anti-inflammatory drugs (NSAIDs) induce nausea by direct gastrointestinal mucosal irritation. Other classes of medications that produce nausea include cardiovascular drugs (e.g. digoxin, antiarrhythmics, antihypertensives), diuretics, hormonal agents (e.g. oral antidiabetics, contraceptives), antibiotics (e.g. erythromycin), and gastrointestinal medications (e.g. sulfasalazine).

Disorders of the gastrointestinal tract and peritoneum

Gut and peritoneal disorders represent prevalent causes of nausea and vomiting. Gastric outlet obstruction often produces intermittent symptoms, whereas small intestinal obstruction is usually acute and associated with abdominal pain. Disorders of gut motor activity (e.g. gastroparesis and chronic intestinal pseudo-obstruction) evoke nausea because of an inability to clear retained food and secretions. Gastroparesis occurs with systemic diseases (e.g. diabetes, scleroderma, lupus, amyloidosis, pancreatic adenocarcinoma, ischemia) or it may be idiopathic, occurring after a viral prodrome in some cases. Nausea is reported by half of patients with functional dyspepsia as well as some patients with gastroesophageal reflux, in individuals with both normal and delayed gastric emptying. Chronic intestinal pseudo-obstruction may be hereditary, result from systemic disease, or occur as a paraneoplastic response to malignancy (most commonly, small cell lung carcinoma). Superior mesenteric artery syndrome, developing after severe weight loss, recent surgery, or prolonged bed rest, occurs when the duodenum is compressed and obstructed by the superior mesenteric artery as it originates from the aorta.

Other rare mechanical causes of nausea and vomiting include gastric volvulus and antral webs. Inflammatory conditions (e.g. pancreatitis, appendicitis, and cholecystitis) irritate the peritoneal surface, whereas biliary colic produces nausea by activating the afferent neural pathways. Fulminant hepatitis causes nausea, presumably because of accumulation of emetic toxins and increases in intracranial pressure.

Central nervous system causes

Conditions with increased intracranial pressure, such as tumors, infarction, hemorrhage, infections, or congenital abnormalities, produce emesis with and without nausea. Emotional responses to unpleasant smells or tastes induce vomiting, as can anticipation of cancer chemotherapy. Psychiatric causes of nausea include anxiety, depression, anorexia nervosa, and bulimia nervosa. Young women with psychiatric illness or social difficulty may present with psychogenic vomiting. Labyrinthine etiologies of nausea include labyrinthitis, tumors, and Ménière disease. Motion sickness is induced by repetitive movements that result in activating vestibular nuclei.

Endocrinological and metabolic conditions

First-trimester pregnancy is the most common endocrinological cause of nausea. This condition, occurring in 50–70% of pregnancies, usually is transitory and is not associated with poor fetal or maternal outcome. However, 1–5% of cases progress to hyperemesis gravidarum, which may produce dangerous fluid losses and electrolyte disturbances. Other endocrinological and metabolic conditions associated with vomiting include uremia, diabetic ketoacidosis, thyroid and parathyroid disease, and Addison disease.

Infectious causes

Infectious illness produces nausea and vomiting, usually of acute onset. Viral gastroenteritis may be caused by rotaviruses, and the Hawaii, Snow Mountain, and Norwalk agents. Bacterial infection with *Staphylococcus* or *Salmonella* organisms, *Bacillus cereus*, and *Clostridium perfringens* also produces nausea and vomiting, in many cases via toxins that act on the brainstem. Nausea in immunosuppressed patients may result from gastrointestinal cytomegalovirus or herpes simplex infections. Infections not involving the gastrointestinal tract, such as hepatitis, otitis media, and meningitis, may also elicit nausea.

Miscellaneous causes of nausea and vomiting

Other common causes of symptoms include abdominal radiation therapy and postoperative nausea and vomiting. Nausea may be a manifestation of posterior wall myocardial infarction as well as of congestive heart failure. Acute graft-versus-host disease is the dominant cause of nausea and vomiting in bone marrow transplant recipients. Excess ethanol intake evokes nausea by acting on the central nervous system. Cyclic vomiting syndrome is a condition of unknown etiology characterized by episodes of emesis with intervening asymptomatic periods. While cannabis is often used to treat symptoms of nausea and vomiting, chronic use has been demonstrated to cause a syndrome of intermittent nausea, vomiting and abdominal pain similar in presentation to cyclic vomiting. Excess vitamin intake and prolonged starvation also cause nausea. Jamaican vomiting sickness results from ingesting unripe ackee fruit.

Management

The first decision in treating the patient with vomiting is to determine if intravenous resuscitation is needed. Poor skin turgor or orthostatic pulse or blood pressure changes indicate that more than 10% of body fluids have been lost, mandating intravenous infusion of saline. Potassium supplements may be started for hypokalemia when urine output is adequate. If prospects for oral replenishments are uncertain, hospitalization should be considered. The threshold for hospitalization is lower for diabetic patients, those with concurrent diarrhea or other chronic debilitating disease, and very young or old patients. Nasogastric suction may provide benefit in patients with obstruction or ileus. If the patient can be discharged, a liquid diet low in fat and indigestible residue is recommended because such a diet empties from the stomach more briskly. Medications that inhibit gastric motor function should be discontinued if possible. Diabetics should strive for optimal glycemic control because elevated blood glucose impairs gut motor function.

When feasible, medical treatment for nausea should be directed at the underlying illness. However, many patients benefit from medications that suppress emesis and correct aberrant gastrointestinal function. Antiemetic drugs acting on central nervous system muscarinic cholinergic, histamine, or dopamine receptors reduce symptoms in many cases. Antihistamines (e.g. meclizine, dimenhydrinate) are useful for labyrinthine disorders such as motion sickness or inner ear disease as well as uremic or postoperative vomiting. Sedation and dryness of the mouth may limit their use in some cases. Anticholinergic medications (e.g. scopolamine) also are effective in motion sickness when given orally or transdermally; however, these agents produce numerous side-effects, including dry mouth, headache, urinary retention, and constipation. Antidopaminergics (e.g. phenothiazines, butyrophenones) are commonly prescribed antiemetics that act directly on the brainstem regions that mediate emesis in response to a diverse range of peripheral stimuli and are thus useful for many causes of nausea and vomiting. Antidopaminergics produce many side-effects in the central nervous system, including sedation, agitation, mood changes, dystonias, parkinsonian symptoms, irreversible tardive dyskinesia, and hyperprolactinemic symptoms (galactorrhea, sexual dysfunction, amenorrhea). Other drug classes that have been suggested as generalized antiemetics include serotonin ($5\text{-}HT_3$) receptor antagonists (e.g. ondansetron, granisetron) and tricyclic antidepressants (e.g. nortriptyline, amitriptyline).

Gut motility disorders may respond to drugs known as prokinetic agents, which stimulate gastric emptying and intestinal transit. The most widely prescribed prokinetic medication is metoclopramide, which acts via serotonin ($5\text{-}HT_4$) receptor facilitation of gastric cholinergic function as well as by antidopaminergic effects in the stomach and brainstem. This drug enhances gastric emptying and reduces symptoms in gastroparesis but is poorly tolerated by 20% of patients because of significant antidopaminergic side-effects, including extrapyramidal reactions, dystonias, and galactorrhea. Domperidone is a peripheral dopamine antagonist with prokinetic properties that does not cross the blood–brain barrier and thus has fewer side-effects. This drug is prescribed throughout much of the world but is not approved for prescription in the United States by the Food and Drug Administration. The macrolide antibiotic erythromycin stimulates gastric emptying by action on receptors for the hormone motilin, which is the endogenous mediator of fasting gastrointestinal motility. However, erythromycin often is poorly tolerated because it can exacerbate nausea or induce abdominal pain. Pyloric injection of botulinum toxin reduces pylorospasm and improves symptoms in some patients with gastroparesis. The somatostatin analog octreotide is useful in some cases of intestinal pseudo-obstruction as a result of selective effects to stimulate contractile activity of the small intestine.

Extensive investigation has focused on drugs to prevent vomiting after cancer chemotherapy. $5\text{-}HT_3$ antagonists, such as ondansetron and granisetron, provide significant benefit with the most emetogenic treatments. Other drugs useful in this setting include high-dose metoclopramide, corticosteroids, and cannabinoids (e.g. tetrahydrocannabinol, nabilone), although as noted above chronic cannabis use may cause intermittent nausea and vomiting. Benzodiazepines (e.g. lorazepam) are especially effective for anticipatory nausea and vomiting. Neurokinin (NK$_1$) receptor antagonists (e.g. aprepitant) are useful for both acute and delayed emesis caused by chemotherapy.

Nonmedication therapies can be considered for some conditions of chronic nausea and vomiting. Acupuncture and acupressure have been used to treat nausea of pregnancy, motion sickness, and postoperative nausea. Ginger and pyridoxine have been proposed for nausea of pregnancy. Jejunostomy feedings may improve overall health in patients with advanced gastroparesis, whereas intravenous hyperalimentation may be needed for severe forms of intestinal dysmotility. Gastric neurostimulation delivered by an implantable device may reduce nausea and vomiting in patients with gastroparesis who are unresponsive to medications. Surgical resections only rarely benefit patients with nausea and vomiting secondary to dysmotility.

Complications

Chronic nausea and vomiting can produce dehydration, weight loss, and electrolyte abnormalities (e.g. hypokalemia and metabolic alkalosis), which may have significant morbidity in some patients. Increased intrathoracic pressure during vomiting produces purpura on the face and neck, whereas retch-induced Mallory–Weiss tears across the esophagogastric junction may present as upper gastrointestinal hemorrhage. The Boerhaave syndrome is a more severe complication that results when vomiting ruptures the esophagus, leading to mediastinitis or peritonitis. In patients with impaired mentation, emesis may cause pulmonary aspiration, producing chemical pneumonitis.

Key practice points

- The differential diagnosis of nausea and vomiting is very broad, including medication reactions, gastrointestinal and intraperitoneal diseases, neurological disorders, metabolic conditions and infections.
- The timing of vomiting in relation to meals and the character of the vomitus can provide key diagnostic clues as to the etiology.
- Flat and upright abdominal radiographs provide screening information concerning the presence or absence of intestinal obstruction.
- Contrast radiography of the small intestine can assess for partial intestinal obstruction.
- Upper endoscopy can assess for gastric outlet obstruction and perform diagnostic biopsies of suspicious lesions.
- The key initial step in the management of the patient with vomiting is determining whether intravenous resuscitation is required.
- Medical therapy of nausea and vomiting should be directed at the underlying illness whenever feasible.

Case studies

Case 1

A 55-year-old man presents with a 2-month history of epigastric pain with progressive early satiety, vomiting of partially digested food and approximately 10 lb weight loss. Physical examination is remarkable for dry mucous membranes and a succussion splash. Serum laboratories reveal mild hypoalbuminemia. An abdominal x-ray shows a mildly large stomach with a normal small bowel gas pattern. EGD is performed and demonstrates retained food in the stomach as well as edema, inflammation and ulceration in the gastric antrum. A thin gastroscope is able to pass into the duodenum with mild difficulty. Biopsies are taken to evaluation for malignancy and to assess for the presence of *H. pylori*. The patient is placed on a liquid diet and acid suppression therapy.

Discussion and potential pitfalls

This patient has classic symptoms of gastric outlet obstruction. The differential diagnosis includes a variety of benign and malignant etiologies, such as peptic ulcer disease, pancreatitis, gastric cancer, and pancreatic cancer. Psychogenic nausea and vomiting would not typically have associated weight loss. A barium study could be considered as an initial evaluation, but in the presence of significant vomiting and weight loss, many physicians would elect to perform EGD as it allows for direct visualization as well as biopsies to exclude malignancy. If malignancy is present, a staging CT scan would be appropriate. Nasogastric decompression should be considered prior to endoscopy to avoid the risk of aspiration of retained gastric contents. If the patient is unable to tolerate a liquid diet, parenteral nutrition is appropriate. In some cases of benign gastric outlet obstruction, surgical interventions are required (e.g. gastrojejunostomy), though this is uncommon since the introduction of acid suppression medications.

Case 2

A 40-year-old woman with type 1 diabetes mellitus presents with a 1–2-year history of intermittent vomiting of partially digested food. She denies weight loss and her physical exam is unremarkable except for changes of diabetic retinopathy. EGD is performed and shows retained food in the gastric body. A gastric emptying study reveals delayed gastric emptying.

Discussion and potential pitfalls

Diabetic gastroparesis is a difficult condition to manage. The initial approach involves attempting to improve glycemic control because gut motor function is impaired by elevated blood glucose. Dietary modification to reduce indigestible residue and increase low-fat liquids may relieve symptoms for many patients. Also, frequent, small meals can alleviate symptoms, though this can complicate insulin regimens. Therefore, close co-ordination with the patient's endocrinologist is advisable. Prokinetic medications may offer some benefit, though side-effects limit their overall utility. Gastric neurostimulation via an implanted device is currently being investigated for severe cases of gastroparesis.

CHAPTER 6

Approach to the Patient with Abdominal Pain

Clinical presentation

History

The location, character, intensity, and timing of pain as well as factors that enhance or minimize the pain are obtained from the history. Symptoms pertinent to past or present illnesses also are evaluated.

Pain localization

Pain from esophagitis, esophageal dysmotility, or esophageal neoplasm usually is substernal and may radiate to the back, jaw, and left shoulder and arm. The usual pain of peptic ulcer disease is epigastric. Radiation of ulcer pain to the back suggests a posterior penetrating duodenal ulcer. Small intestinal disease most commonly produces periumbilical pain, although ileal lesions may elicit hypogastric symptoms. Colonic pain may be perceived in any region of the abdomen or back. Liver capsular distension produces right upper quadrant pain. Gallbladder and bile duct pain is experienced in the epigastrium and right upper quadrant. Pancreatic pain typically is felt in the epigastrium with radiation to the back. Left upper quadrant pain suggests pancreatic disease but may also result from greater curvature gastric ulcers, splenic lesions, perinephric disease, and colonic splenic flexure lesions. Renal pain from acute pyelonephritis or obstruction of the ureteropelvic junction usually is sensed in the costovertebral angle or flank, although upper abdominal pain is not unusual. Ureteral pain may be referred to the testicle or thigh. Uterine lesions produce midline lower abdominal pain, whereas adnexal pain localizes to the ipsilateral lower quadrant. Pelvic pain may radiate to the back.

Migration of pain with disease evolution suggests underlying inflammation. Cholecystitis may begin in the epigastrium and migrate to the right upper quadrant, whereas appendicitis may start in the midline and then move to the McBurney point in the right lower abdomen.

Yamada's Handbook of Gastroenterology, Third Edition. Edited by Tadataka Yamada and John M. Inadomi.

Pain quality

Esophagitis produces burning or warm pain, whereas peptic ulcer pain is dull or gnawing. Pain from small intestinal obstruction or inflammation is colicky or crampy and may be associated with abdominal distension and audible bowel sounds. Pain from appendicitis may be colicky, but usually is a constant dull ache. Despite use of the terms biliary colic and renal colic, obstruction of these organs more often produces a steady rather than colicky pain. Acute cholecystitis leads to squeezing pain, whereas acute pancreatitis results in penetrating or boring pain. Nephrolithiasis evokes a sharp or cutting pain.

Pain intensity

Extremely severe abdominal pain is produced by peptic ulcer perforation, acute pancreatitis, or passage of a renal stone, whereas severe acute pain is evoked by small intestinal obstruction, cholecystitis, and appendicitis. Causes of more moderate acute pain include peptic ulcer disease, gastroenteritis, and esophagitis. Intensity of chronic abdominal pain is more difficult to assess because psychological factors can modify pain perception. Then, indirect questions about interference with sleep or daily function may provide useful information about pain severity.

Pain chronology

Peptic ulcer pain may be intermittent and often occurs in the morning or before meals. Posterior penetration should be considered when peptic ulcer pain becomes constant.

   Acute cholecystitis commonly develops during sleep and may be preceded by months of intermittent biliary colic. Nocturnal pain rarely occurs in patients with irritable bowel syndrome or functional abdominal pain. Appendicitis typically presents as progressive pain for 10–15 h without remission. Pain reaching peak intensity within minutes is more characteristic of ulcer perforation, abdominal aortic aneurysm rupture, passage of renal stones, or ruptured ectopic pregnancy. In acute pancreatitis, intestinal obstruction, cholecystitis, or mesenteric arterial occlusion, peak pain intensity is reached in 10–60 min. A gradual onset of pain for hours is reported in appendicitis, some cases of cholecystitis, diverticulitis, and mesenteric venous occlusion. The pain of irritable bowel syndrome is chronic and may be most intense after meals. In women, pain at monthly intervals suggests endometriosis or ovulation-related symptoms. Pain after starting medication raises the possibility of acute intermittent porphyria (barbiturates) or pancreatitis (steroids, tetracycline, thiazides).

Alleviating and aggravating factors

Antacids or acid-suppressing medications may relieve the pain of esophagitis or peptic ulcer disease. Ingesting food can relieve discomfort from a duodenal ulcer but may aggravate pain because of gastric body ulcers. The pain of pancreatic disease almost always is intensified by meal ingestion, as is discomfort from intestinal obstruction or mesenteric ischemia. Duodenal obstruction provokes pain within minutes of eating, whereas ileal lesions cause pain 1–2h after a meal. Pain from mesenteric ischemia is intensified after meals due to the inability of the impaired blood supply to satisfy the metabolic demands of the gut. Lactase deficiency may produce discomfort that is specific to consumption of dairy products. Heartburn may be aggravated by reclining or straining. Pancreatic pain is worse in the supine position and is relieved by leaning forward. In contrast, back pain in irritable bowel syndrome may be relieved by hyperextension of the spine. Psoas muscle irritation, as with a psoas abscess in Crohn's disease, often causes the patient to lie supine with the right leg flexed at the hip and knee. The pain of nerve root compressions and other musculoskeletal conditions may worsen with some movements. Abdominal pain in irritable bowel syndrome may be ameliorated by massaging the abdominal wall or by passing feces or flatus. Alternatively, irritable bowel pain is aggravated by eating or stress. Passage of diarrheal stools may reduce cramping in colitis.

Associated symptoms

Abdominal pain usually precedes nausea in conditions that ultimately require surgery, whereas nausea may occur first in disorders not requiring surgery. Diarrhea typically indicates a nonsurgical condition such as gastroenteritis, although appendicitis is an exception to this rule. In elderly patients with acute left-sided pain and bloody stools, ischemic colitis should be considered. Chronic abdominal pain with rectal bleeding suggests colonic neoplasm or inflammatory bowel disease. Abdominal pain with the recent onset of constipation is consistent with colonic obstruction, whereas long-standing constipation is a feature of irritable bowel syndrome. Anorexia and weight loss raise concern for malignancy, whereas high fevers (>39.5°C) early in the course of a painful condition suggest cholangitis, urinary tract infection, infectious enteritis, or pneumonia. Late fevers suggest a localized infection such as diverticulitis, appendicitis, or cholecystitis. Jaundice suggests disease of the liver, biliary tree, or pancreas. Many but not all women report abnormal or absent menses with ectopic pregnancy.

Risk factors

Heavy alcohol intake for prolonged periods can lead to acute pancreatitis, whereas analgesic intake predisposes to ulcer disease. Cocaine abuse may cause mesenteric ischemia. A patient with gallstones may present with distal intestinal obstruction secondary to gallstone ileus. Cardiovascular disease predisposes to mesenteric ischemia, whereas prior abdominal surgery increases the likelihood of intestinal obstruction. Patients with cirrhosis and ascites develop spontaneous bacterial peritonitis. During pregnancy, abdominal pain results from appendicitis, pyelonephritis, cholelithiasis, pancreatitis, and adnexal disease. The presence of a gravid uterus may modify the symptom presentation or findings of physical examination. Immunocompromised individuals are susceptible to common causes of abdominal pain as well as neutropenic enterocolitis, opportunistic infections such as cytomegalovirus, and graft-versus-host disease in patients who have undergone bone marrow transplantation. The typical signs of peritonitis may be absent in these patients.

Physical examination

A comprehensive extra-abdominal physical examination is required to provide insight into the cause of abdominal pain. A writhing, diaphoretic, pale patient usually is more ill than one who is resting comfortably, although some individuals with peritonitis may lie motionless to avoid abdominal irritation. Fever or tachycardia may point to an acute infectious or inflammatory process. Hypotension raises concern for an abdominal catastrophe such as a ruptured aneurysm. Scleral icterus or jaundice suggests cholestasis or biliary obstruction. Adenopathy, masses, and hepatomegaly suggest malignancy. A chest examination may reveal pneumonia as the cause of pain, whereas an irregular heart rhythm might suggest new-onset atrial fibrillation as a source of mesenteric arterial embolism. Radiculopathy as a cause of pain is suspected with asymmetrical strength or sensation on neurological examination. Peripheral or autonomic neuropathies are found in some patients with gastrointestinal dysmotility. The presence of occult fecal blood on rectal examination raises the possibility of malignancy, ischemia, ulcer disease, and inflammation. Right-sided tenderness on rectal examination may also be found with appendicitis. Perianal fistulae, fissures, and abscesses suggest Crohn's disease. In women, a pelvic examination is used to evaluate possible adnexal or uterine causes of abdominal pain. Dermatographia is a sign consistent with mast cell activation syndrome.

Abdominal, rectal, genital, and pelvic examinations are mandatory in a patient with acute abdominal pain. Intestinal obstruction is considered if scars are observed on inspection and if auscultation reveals high-pitched bowel sounds. In contrast, a silent distended abdomen suggests ileus secondary to intra-abdominal inflammation or peritonitis. A right upper quadrant friction rub or bruit suggests a possible hepatic tumor, whereas bruits elsewhere may indicate mesenteric insufficiency. Abdominal palpation should begin in an area distant from the reported site of pain to prevent conscious guarding. Involuntary guarding suggests peritonitis. Rebound tenderness suggests peritoneal inflammation but also may be elicited in noninflammatory conditions such as irritable bowel syndrome and thus has been considered an unreliable sign. It is often useful to shake the patient's bed gently from side to side, which may be a more subtle means of detecting peritonitis. Severe pain with little tenderness or guarding is consistent with intestinal infarction or early acute pancreatitis. The Carnett test can distinguish intra-abdominal discomfort from abdominal wall pain. Increased tenderness upon raising the head and tensing the abdomen suggests a superficial abdominal wall source. Discrepancies between tenderness

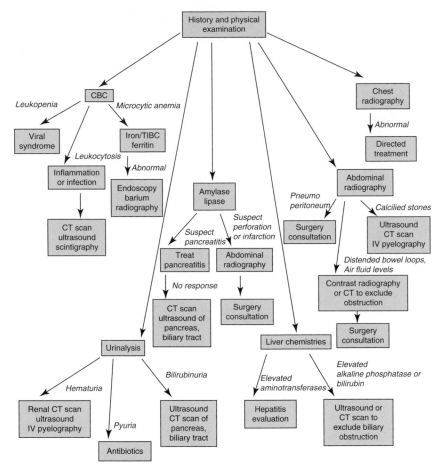

Figure 6.1 Work-up of a patient with abdominal pain. CBC, complete blood count; CT, computed tomography; IV, intravenous; TIBC, total iron-binding capacity.

elicited with pressure from the stethescope and that from the examining hand suggest possible functional abdominal pain.

Fecal occult blood raises concern for malignancy, ischemia, ulcer disease, or inflammatory conditions, whereas perianal fistulae, abscess, or inflammation suggests possible Crohn's disease. Rectal examination also may detect an intra-abdominal inflammatory process such as an appendiceal abscess that is not palpable over the anterior abdominal wall. Inguinal hernias as a cause of intestinal obstruction may be detected on genital examination, whereas pelvic examination of women is essential for diagnosing adnexal masses and pelvic inflammatory disease.

Additional testing

Determining the cause of abdominal pain commonly requires laboratory testing (Figure 6.1). However, diagnostic testing in the patient with chronic functional pain should be directed by alarm findings on exam and screening blood tests to avoid reinforcing the patient's conviction that there is something organically wrong. A complete blood count may show leukocytosis, indicating an inflammatory condition, or leukopenia, suggesting a viral syndrome. Microcytic anemia raises the possibility of gut blood loss. The sedimentation rate may be elevated in inflammatory conditions.

Electrolytes, blood urea nitrogen, and creatinine are measured to assess fluid status and renal function. Elevated serum amylase or lipase or both usually are observed early in acute pancreatitis. Perforated ulcers, diabetic ketoacidosis, or mesenteric infarction also may cause hyperamylasemia. Elevated levels of bilirubin or alkaline phosphatase suggest disease of the pancreas or biliary tract, whereas aminotransferase elevations indicate hepatocellular disease. Serum pregnancy testing is performed in women of reproductive potential who present with unexplained abdominal pain. Specific laboratory tests can assist in diagnosing acute porphyria or heavy metal intoxication. Tryptase levels are elevated in mast cell activation syndrome. Urinalysis may show erythrocytes or crystals, suggesting calculi; leukocytes or bacteria, suggesting infection; or bilirubin, suggesting pancreaticobiliary disease. Patients with ascites and abdominal pain should undergo paracentesis to exclude spontaneous bacterial peritonitis. Culdocentesis can aid in assessing intra abdominal hemorrhage.

Supine and upright (or decubitus) abdominal plain radiography is essential in all patients with acute abdominal pain and can detect pneumoperitoneum from lumenal perforation, calcified gallstones or renal stones, air–fluid levels with intestinal obstruction, generalized or localized distension with ileus, pneumobilia with biliary disease, and a ground-glass appearance with ascites. Barium radiographs may complement the findings of plain films when mechanical obstruction is suspected. Chest radiographs can eliminate pulmonary sources of acute abdominal pain.

Other imaging studies complement findings of the examination, laboratory testing, and plain films. Ultrasound is useful for suspected cholelithiasis, biliary dilation, ovarian cysts, abscess formation, and ectopic pregnancy, whereas computed tomography (CT) is more sensitive for pancreatic disease, retroperitoneal collections, intra-abdominal abscess, some vascular processes, trauma-induced hematomas, and changes in the mesentery or intestinal wall resulting from ischemia or inflammation (as with diverticulitis). Scintigraphy with ^{99m}Tc-iminodiacetic acid derivatives detects cystic duct obstruction from cholecystitis. Angiography or mesenteric resonance angiography may be indicated for suspected vascular occlusion. Ultrasound is sensitive for diagnosing the impending rupture of an abdominal aortic aneurysm, but further study with aortography may delay definitive therapy and should be performed in the operating room, if indicated, because of the risk of exsanguination. Upper endoscopy is performed for chronic epigastric pain that suggests uncomplicated peptic ulcer, but is contraindicated with suspected perforation.

Sigmoidoscopy or colonoscopy is helpful with lower abdominal pain secondary to suspected ischemia, infection, volvulus, drug-induced colitis, or inflammatory bowel disease. Endoscopic retrograde cholangiopancreatography (ERCP) may be required for suspected cholangitis, whereas ERCP and endoscopic ultrasound (EUS) are sensitive for detecting choledocholithiasis. ERCP, EUS, and magnetic resonance cholangiopancreatography may provide complementary information in diagnosing chronic pancreatitis. Laparoscopy may be performed on an emergency basis in extremely ill patients or electively for chronic abdominal pain where the diagnosis is elusive after extensive diagnostic testing.

Differential diagnosis

The differential diagnosis of abdominal pain includes pathological processes within and outside the abdomen (Table 6.1). Generally, pain from diseases of the hollow organs (e.g. gut, urinary tract, pancreaticobiliary tree) results from obstruction, ulceration, inflammation, perforation, or ischemia. Pain from disorders of solid organs (e.g. liver, kidneys, spleen) is caused by distension from infection, obstruction to drainage, or vascular congestion. In women, the adnexa and uterus are potential sources of pain. Lung or cardiac abnormalities may secondarily cause referred pain in the upper abdomen. Metabolic conditions (e.g. lead poisoning, diabetic ketoacidosis) cause diffuse or localized abdominal pain. Acute intermittent porphyria, a disorder of heme biosynthesis that results in accumulation of toxic intermediates, causes colicky abdominal pain, ileus, and psychiatric disturbances. Familial Mediterranean fever produces painful inflammation of joints, skin, and serosal surfaces in the abdomen and the chest. Mast cell activation syndrome represents an emerging process of immune dysfunction whereby degranulation of mast cells results in inflammation that causes abdominal pain, dermatographia, and other systemic symptoms. Degenerative disk disease, tabes dorsalis, and varicella zoster virus reactivation elicit superficial abdominal wall pain.

The acuity of the clinical presentation restricts the possible differential diagnoses. With acute abdominal pain, the clinician should quickly establish an accurate diagnosis and implement specific measures to reduce pain and treat the underlying cause if possible. Recurrent pain that lasts hours to days with intervening asymptomatic periods represents a diagnostic challenge in some cases. Many such patients are ultimately diagnosed as having a functional abdominal pain syndrome which is defined as at least 6 months of nearly continuous pain with poor relationship to physiological events such as eating or defecation, some loss of daily function, no evidence of malingering, and insufficient criteria to satisfy other functional or organic diagnoses. Patients with functional abdominal pain syndrome often exhibit evidence of psychosocial dysfunction, including anxiety, depression, somatization, or hypochondriasis. Functional abdominal pain often occurs in individuals with prior childhood

Table 6.1 Causes of abdominal pain

Intra-abdominal
Parietal inflammation
Perforated viscus
Spontaneous bacterial peritonitis
Appendicitis
Diverticulitis
Pancreatitis
Cholecystitis/cholangitis
Pelvic inflammatory disease
Familial Mediterranean fever

Visceral mucosal disorders
Peptic ulcer disease
Inflammatory bowel disease
Infectious colitis
Esophagitis

Visceral obstruction
Intestinal obstruction (adhesions, hernia, volvulus, intussusception, malignancy)
Biliary obstruction (stone, tumor, stricture)
Renal colic (stone, tumor)

Capsular distension
Hepatitis
Budd–Chiari syndrome
Pyelonephritis
Tubo-ovarian abscess
Ovarian cyst
Endometritis
Ectopic pregnancy

Vascular disorders
Intestinal ischemia
Abdominal aortic aneurysm
Splenic infarction
Tumor necrosis

Visceral motor and functional disorders
Irritable bowel syndrome
Functional dyspepsia
Esophageal dysmotility
Viral gastroenteritis

Extra-abdominal
Neurological
Radiculopathy
Varicellazoster virus reactivation

(*continued*)

Table 6.1 (*cont'd*)

Musculoskeletal
Trauma
Fibromyalgia

Cardiothoracic
Pneumonia
Myocardial infarction
Pneumothorax
Empyema
Pulmonary infarction

Toxic/metabolic
Uremia
Diabetic ketoacidosis
Porphyria
Lead poisoning
Reptile venom, insect bite
Addison disease

abdominal pain or with a history of physical or sexual abuse. Aberrant illness behaviors may be prominent in these patients. Chronic, continuous abdominal pain often has an obvious cause such as disseminated malignancy, chronic pancreatitis, or less serious illnesses with concurrent depression.

Management

Under ideal conditions, therapy is directed at eliminating the cause of abdominal pain. If this is not possible, efforts are aimed at decreasing pain perception and removing factors that exacerbate pain. Patients with pain from fever, vomiting, orthostatic hypotension, tachycardia, rebound, leukocytosis, new hyperbilirubinemia, or impaired mentation may need hospitalization. The threshold for hospital admission is lowered for the very young or old and for immunocompromised individuals.

Specific therapy exists for many conditions such as acid suppressants for gastroesophageal reflux or surgery for appendicitis or cholecystitis, but the diagnosis must be accurate. Some conditions that cause chronic pain may not be curable. Nonsteroidal anti-inflammatory drugs (NSAIDs) are often prescribed for chronic pain. However, because many chronic conditions have little tissue damage or inflammation, it is not surprising that NSAIDs are often ineffective. Opioid agents are useful for managing pain that is secondary to unresectable malignancy, but prescribing them for chronic nonmalignant states is controversial. Regardless of the indication, narcotics are best administered within an integrated treatment program. The use of opioids at regular intervals, rather than on an as-needed basis, is often more effective for treating severe pain. Pain cocktails that incorporate opioids, acetaminophen, and antiemetics allow flexible dosing that prevents mental clouding, respiratory depression, nausea, and constipation. Tricyclic antidepressants have analgesic effects that are independent of their mood-elevating effects. Agents with serotonergic and noradrenergic activity (e.g. amitriptyline, doxepin) exhibit the greatest effects, often at doses lower than required to treat depression. Conversely, although anxiolytics may reduce anxiety, they have little long-term efficacy in managing chronic abdominal pain and may actually worsen symptoms because of depleted brain serotonin levels.

Nonmedical treatments also are useful in treating chronic pain. Patients with pain secondary to unresectable neoplasm may benefit from referral to a multidisciplinary pain clinic. Celiac plexus blockade is effective therapy for selected patients with pancreatic adenocarcinoma but is less likely to control pain from chronic pancreatitis. Local neural blockade of trigger points may provide benefit in some cases of abdominal wall pain. Rhizotomy and cordotomy involve severing the neural pathways that sense pain and are indicated only for conditions in which life expectancy does not exceed 6 months because of significant complications, including bowel and bladder dysfunction, dysesthesias, and exacerbation of the pain. Transcutaneous electrical nerve stimulation and dorsal column stimulation reduce pain in some chronic conditions, presumably because pain inhibitory nerve fibers are stimulated and endogenous opioid production is activated. Acupuncture may work by similar mechanisms. Unfortunately, these techniques have not shown significant efficacy in treating chronic pain that is secondary to intra-abdominal causes.

Like most chronic illnesses, irritable bowel syndrome and functional abdominal pain have no cure. Thus, efforts should be directed to enhancing the quality of the patient's life. The physician must establish a good working relationship with the patient and acknowledge the reality of the pain and the suffering that it causes. Scheduling of frequent brief visits and directed appropriate diagnostic evaluation are important. The emphasis then shifts from diagnosis to treatment with a realization by the patient that a cure is not possible and an understanding that a major part of the treatment process will be to minimize the impact of the pain on daily life. Psychological or psychiatric consultation is appropriate when the clinician suspects a concurrent, major affective or personality disorder. Tricyclic agents represent the main form of medication therapy. Meta-analyses of tricyclic agents used to treat functional causes of abdominal pain have shown significant therapeutic benefits compared with a placebo. Most other drug classes provide little or no benefit in this condition. Opioid agents should be avoided in these patients because of drug dependency. Relaxation training, biofeedback, and hypnosis have shown benefit in small trials. Behavioral therapy reduces chronic pain behavior by rewarding the patient's expression of well behavior. Cognitive therapies promote healthy behavior by increasing the patient's awareness of situations that increase pain, with the goal of increasing the patient's control over these situations. Subsets of patients may benefit from formal psychotherapy.

Complications

The potential for complications depends on the cause of the pain. Failure to diagnose peritonitis, a ruptured ectopic pregnancy, or an aortic aneurysm can have fatal consequences. Other inflammatory conditions (e.g. pancreatitis, inflammatory bowel disease, or pelvic inflammatory disease) may require prolonged courses of treatment, producing debilitating symptoms and loss of productivity at home and work. Renal stones may lead to infection and renal insufficiency. The prognosis is excellent for many patients with chronic noninflammatory abdominal pain, including those with irritable bowel syndrome, endometriosis, and nerve root compression syndromes.

Case studies

Case 1

A 53-year-old man presents to the emergency department with complaints of worsening epigastric pain. The pain initially began 4 days before and started out as an intermittent dull ache in the epigastric region. The pain would be worse before meals and would improve slightly after a meal. However, over the last 5 h the pain has been constant and the patient is very uncomfortable. He denies any nausea or vomiting. He has been taking NSAIDs for the last week because of a knee injury. He has no other medical problems. On physical exam he appears uncomfortable. He has significant tenderness to palpation throughout the entire abdomen and also has rebound and guarding. Labs are significant for a leukocytosis and and elevated amylase. An abdominal series radiography with supine and upright views demonstrates evidence of free air within the abdomen. The patient is diagnosed with a perforated viscus and taken to surgery where he is found to have a perforated duodenal ulcer.

Discussion and potential pitfalls

Gastrointestinal perforation requires urgent surgical intervention; therefore, the diagnosis needs to be made rapidly. If a perforation is in the differential an abdominal series radiography with supine and upright or decubitus views should be obtained immediately. However, in gastroduodenal perforations free air may not be appreciated in one-third of cases on abdominal series radiography. If an abdominal series radiography is negative but perforation is still suspected, a CT scan should be performed. Failure to rapidly identify a gastrointestinal perforation leads to increased mortality.

Case 2

A 26-year-old man presents to the emergency department with a 3-day history of dull periumbilical pain. Over the past 24h the pain has become progressively worse and has migrated to the right lower quadrant. He also reports nausea, vomiting, and diarrhea over the past 24h. On physical exam he has a fever to 38.0°C, heart rate of 110, and is normotensive. Labs are only notable for a leukocytosis with a left shift. On physical exam the patient has McBurney point tenderness. A CT scan with IV and oral contrast demonstrates appendiceal wall thickening with periappendiceal fat stranding. The patient is diagnosed with acute appendicitis and is managed with surgical intervention with a laparoscopic appendectomy during which an inflamed appendix without evidence of perforation is identified and removed.

Discussion and potential pitfalls

Acute appendicitis is a common cause of acute abdominal pain seen in the emergency department. Classic symptoms include right lower quadrant abdominal pain, anorexia, nausea, and vomiting. However, patients may also present with nonspecific symptoms such as increased flatulence, diarrhea, and indigestion. If the diagnosis is suspected but unclear, a CT scan with IV and oral contrast should be performed. The diagnosis should be made early and managed with surgical intervention.

Key practice points

- An accurate history needs to be obtained, focusing on details of the abdominal pain, including location, quality, intensity, chronology, alleviating and aggravating factors, and associated symptoms.
- A thorough physical exam should be performed.
- Appropriate laboratory tests should be orderd based on the differential diagnosis.
- Rapid diagnosis of the etiology of the abdominal pain is essential, especially in cases of intestinal perforation, intestinal obstruction, appendicitis, and ruptured aortic aneurysm.

CHAPTER 7

Approach to the Patient with Gas and Bloating

Lumenal gas produces several clinical syndromes. Eructation, or belching, is the retrograde expulsion of esophageal and gastric gas from the mouth. Involuntary belching after eating is a normal phenomenon caused by the release of swallowed air during decompression of the distended stomach. It is exacerbated by foods that reduce lower esophageal sphincter tone. Most upper gastrointestinal air accumulates because of aerophagia, which is worsened by stimuli that evoke hypersalivation. Flatulence is the volitional or involuntary release of gas from the anus. On average, healthy young men pass flatus 14 times per day; some individuals report up to 25 daily gas expulsions. Bloating is the perception of retained excess gas within the gut lumen. Women more often report bloating than men. Although some conditions lead to increased gas production, many individuals with bloating exhibit normal gut gas volumes.

Clinical presentation

History

Patients with complaints of excess gas also commonly report associated symptoms including pain, bloating, halitosis, anorexia, early satiety, nausea, belching, loud borborygmi, constipation, and flatulence. Relief of symptoms with defecation or passage of flatus is consistent with a functional disorder, as is the absence of symptoms that awaken the patient from deep sleep. Conversely, the presence of associated vomiting, fever, weight loss, nocturnal diarrhea, steatorrhea, and rectal bleeding indicates probable organic disease. Medical conditions that predispose to bacterial overgrowth and use of medications that delay gut transit should be determined from the history. Selected carbohydrate malabsorptive conditions are hereditary, whereas others (e.g. lactase deficiency) are more prevalent in some ethnic groups. Anxiety disorders and other psychiatric conditions predispose to aerophagia and functional bowel disorders.

Yamada's Handbook of Gastroenterology, Third Edition. Edited by Tadataka Yamada and John M. Inadomi.
© 2013 John Wiley & Sons, Ltd. Published 2013 by John Wiley & Sons, Ltd.

A precise dietary history may correlate specific foods with symptoms. Ingestion of legumes, fruits, unrefined starches, and lactose-containing foodstuffs should be addressed, as should consumption of diet foods and candies and soft drinks containing fructose. Gum chewing, smoking, and chewing tobacco predispose to aerophagia.

Physical examination
Physical findings are usually normal in patients with complaints of excess gas. On assessment of general appearance, the patient with functional disease may exhibit anxiety, hyperventilation, and air swallowing. Other findings suggest organic disease, including sclerodactyly with scleroderma, peripheral or autonomic neuropathy with dysmotility syndromes, and cachexia, jaundice, and palpable masses with malignant intestinal obstruction. Visible scars on abdominal inspection may be evidence of prior fundoplication with subsequent induction of gas-bloat syndrome or other laparotomy with development of obstructing intra-abdominal adhesions. Abdominal auscultation can assess for absent bowel sounds with ileus or myopathic dysmotility, high-pitched bowel sounds with intestinal obstruction, or a succussion splash with gastric obstruction or gastroparesis. Abdominal percussion and palpation may reveal tympany and distension in mechanical obstruction or intestinal dysmotility. Ascites should be excluded on abdominal examination because patients occasionally misinterpret the fluid accumulation as excess gas. Occult fecal blood indicates mucosal damage, which may result from ulceration, inflammation or neoplasm.

Additional testing
Laboratory studies
Normal values for a complete blood count, electrolytes, glucose, albumin, total protein, and sedimentation rate exclude most inflammatory and neoplastic conditions. In selected patients, calcium and phosphate levels, renal function, liver chemistry values, and thyroid function tests may be needed. Patients with diarrhea should undergo stool examination for ova and parasites to rule out giardiasis. Tissue transglutaminase antibodies can screen for celiac disease.

Structural studies
Supine and upright plain abdominal radiographs may reveal generalized lumenal distension with ileus, diffuse haziness in ascites, and air–fluid levels in mechanical obstruction. Barium radiography and endoscopy are considered for patients with suspected obstruction, pseudo-obstruction, or an intralumenal inflammatory or neoplastic process. Small bowel biopsies are performed to confirm a diagnosis of celiac disease. Other tests such as ultrasound and computed tomography (CT) can be used to assess for other intra-abdominal disorders that might predispose the patient to complaints of excess gas.

Functional studies

Gastric emptying scintigraphy or manometry of the esophagus, stomach, and small intestine can be performed when an underlying motility disorder is considered. Hydrogen breath testing to detect monosaccharide or disaccharide malabsorption confirms associations between symptoms and specific foods. Conceptually, this technique relies on the ability of lumenal bacteria to produce hydrogen gas when metabolizing ingested substrates and the concurrent inability of human tissue to use similar metabolic pathways. Expired breath samples are obtained before and after ingesting an aqueous solution of the sugar that is presumed to be malabsorbed. An increase in breath hydrogen of greater than 20 parts per million within 120 min of lactose ingestion distinguishes biopsy-proven, lactase-deficient persons from lactase-sufficient persons with a sensitivity of 90%. Elevated fasting breath hydrogen prior to substrate ingestion and early rises within 30 min of sugar ingestion are consistent with small intestinal bacterial overgrowth. Glucose, the most commonly used sugar for breath hydrogen testing in suspected bacterial overgrowth, provides a diagnostic sensitivity of 70–90%. Patients can be tested for fructose or sorbitol malabsorption using hydrogen breath testing but the normal values of these tests are not well established.

Differential diagnosis

See Table 7.1.

Carbohydrate maldigestion

Malabsorption of small amounts of carbohydrates, demonstrated by increased breath hydrogen excretion, may produce eructation, bloating, abdominal pain, and flatulence. Lactase deficiency is the most common form of carbohydrate intolerance, affecting approximately 20% of the population in the United States. Fructose is naturally found in honey and fruits and is used as a sweetener in many commercial soft drinks. Sorbitol is also present in fruits and is used as a sweetener in dietetic candies and chewing gum. Malabsorption of as little as 37.5 g of fructose and 5 g of sorbitol may produce significant gaseous symptoms. Other poorly absorbed carbohydrates include xylitol and isomalt. To date, there is no convincing evidence to suggest that gaseous symptoms in irritable bowel syndrome (IBS) result from abnormal metabolism of these ingested simple carbohydrates. The autosomal recessive hereditary syndrome sucrase-isomaltase deficiency typically presents in infancy with malabsorption of sucrose.

   Of the complex carbohydrates, only rice and gluten-free wheat are completely absorbed in healthy individuals, whereas up to 20% of the carbohydrates from whole wheat, oat, potato, and cornflour are maldigested and can contribute to gas generation. Nondigestible oligosaccharides (e.g. stachyose, raffinose, and verbascose), abundant in beans and legumes, are avidly fermented by colonic

Table 7.1 Causes of gas and bloating

Eructation
Involuntary postprandial belching
Magenblase syndrome
Aerophagia (e.g. from gum chewing, smoking, oral irritation)
Gastroesophageal reflux
Biliary colic

Bacterial overgrowth
Intestinal or colonic obstruction
Diverticula of the small intestine
Hypochlorhydria
Chronic intestinal pseudo-obstruction
Cologastric fistula
Coprophagia

Functional bowel disorders
Irritable bowel syndrome
Nonulcer dyspepsia
Idiopathic constipation
Functional diarrhea

Carbohydrate malabsorption
Lactase deficiency
Fructose, sorbitol, and starch intolerance
Bean and legume ingestion

Gas-bloat syndrome
Postfundoplication

Miscellaneous causes
Hypothyroidism
Medications (e.g. anticholinergics, opiates, calcium channel antagonists, antidepressants)

bacteria to produce voluminous quantities of intestinal gas. Fiber intake correlates with flatus production in some individuals, although other studies suggest that fiber only increases the sensation of bloating without increasing gas production.

Small intestinal bacterial overgrowth

Small intestinal bacterial overgrowth may result from mechanical obstruction of the gut from postoperative adhesions, Crohn's disease, radiation enteritis, ulcer disease, or malignancy. Other organic abnormalities that predispose to bacterial overgrowth include small intestinal diverticula and gastric achlorhydria. Motor disorders of the gut are associated with overgrowth because of an impaired ability to clear organisms from the gut; 43% of cases of diabetic diarrhea are attributable to bacterial overgrowth. Disorders that increase bacterial delivery to the upper gut (e.g. cologastric fistulae and coprophagia) can overwhelm normal defenses against infection.

Dysmotility syndromes

Conditions that alter gut motor function produce prominent gas and bloating. Bloating is reported by patients with gastroparesis and by those with fat intolerance and rapid gastric emptying. A consequence of fundoplication for gastroesophageal reflux disease is an inability to belch or vomit secondary to an unyielding wrap of gastric tissue around the distal esophagus. In the initial months after fundoplication, up to 70% of patients experience bloating, upper abdominal cramping, and flatulence, a constellation of symptoms known as gas-bloat syndrome. Intestinal pseudo-obstruction leads to gaseous symptoms because of delayed small bowel transit of gas and development of bacterial overgrowth. Bloating also is reported by patients with chronic constipation.

Functional bowel disorders

Irritable bowel syndrome and functional dyspepsia may manifest with symptoms of gas and bloating. The pathogenesis is likely multifactorial and although some studies illustrate increased gas production and objective abdominal distension in irritable bowel syndrome, others do not. Abnormal gut motor and sensory function contribute to the symptoms of gas and bloating.

Miscellaneous causes

Aerophagia during gum chewing, smoking, or oral irritation produces significant gas symptoms, especially eructation. Patients who have undergone laryngectomy experience eructation from swallowing air for esophageal speech. Patients with intestinal obstructions may infrequently present only with symptoms of gas and bloating. Small bowel malabsorptive conditions including celiac disease may produce gaseous manifestations that may predominate or be part of a larger constellation of symptoms. Individuals with peptic ulcer, gastroesophageal reflux, or biliary colic may belch to relieve their other symptoms. Gaseous complaints may be reported as consequences of endocrinopathies such as hypothyroidism. Many medications (e.g. anticholinergics, opiates, calcium channel antagonists, and antidepressants) produce gas by retarding gut transit.

Diagnostic investigation

Evaluation of a patient with symptoms of gas and bloating should focus on the history, which should lead to directed use of laboratory, structural, and functional testing. Organic causes of symptoms may be indicated by objective findings of weight loss, fever, vomiting, nocturnal diarrhea, rectal bleeding or steatorrhea. Conversely, relief of symptoms with defecation or flatus is consistent with irritable bowel syndrome, as is the absence of symptoms that awaken the patient from sleep. Dietary intake should be assessed for legumes, fruits, unrefined starches, lactose, and many diet foods containing sorbitol or other nonabsorbable sugars. Chewing gum or tobacco and smoking predispose to aerophagia. Physical examination may reveal air swallowing or hyperventilation. Manifestations of systemic disease should be evaluated, such as dermatitis herpetifomis (celiac disease), sclerodactyly (scleroderma), neuropathy (dysmotility), cachexia/jaundice/masses (malignancy), surgical scars/distension/succussion splash (intestinal obstruction).

Laboratory tests should be limited. In addition to a complete blood count and chemistry, thyroid function tests, fasting cortisol, and serological testing for celiac (antitissue transglutaminase) may be considered. Rarely, antinuclear and scleroderma antibodies to screen for collagen vascular disease or antinuclear neuronal antibodies (anti-Hu) for paraneoplastic visceral neuropathy may be indicated. Stool analysis for *Giardia* may also be indicated in the correct clinical setting.

Imaging tests may reveal intestinal obstruction (plain abdominal radiography, ultrasonography, CT scan) but should not be routinely used. Endoscopy from above or below can be used if the clinical picture suggests celiac disease, inflammatory bowel disease or other structural intestinal disease.

Functional testing can be used to assess carbohydrate absorption, gut transit and motor function. Breath testing quantifies hydrogen production by luminal bacteria from metabolism of test substrates. Lactose, fructose, sucrose and sorbitol can be used to detect maldigestion or malabsorption of these sugars. Small intestinal bacterial overgrowth can also be detected by elevation of fasting hydrogen or early rises within 30 min of glucose consumption.

Gastric emptying tests use technetium 99 m sulfur colloid to measure emptying of solid meals. Radio-opaque markers may be detected using plain abdominal radiographs to document colonic transit. Finally, an ingested capsule (SmartPill, Buffalo, NY) that records pressure, temperature and pH can document gastric, small and large intestinal transit time.

Management

Medical
Underlying disorders responsible for symptoms of excess gas should be specifically managed whenever possible. Mechanical obstruction is usually managed surgically. Surgeries to vent the gut may help selected individuals with gas-bloat syndrome or intestinal pseudo-obstruction. Lactase deficiency is controlled by excluding lactose from the diet or by supplementing the diet with exogenous lactase. Acid-suppressive medications may reduce eructation associated with gastroesophageal reflux disease. Single or intermittent courses of oral antibiotics may control small intestinal bacterial overgrowth.

For complaints of excess gas for which no organic disorder is defined after appropriate diagnostic testing, attempts are made to decrease intestinal gas and to regulate bowel function. Aerophagia may be controlled by cessation of gum chewing and smoking and improving oral hygiene. The chronic belcher may be aided by self-observation in a mirror to demonstrate aerophagia. Dietary restriction of legumes, beans, fruits, soft drinks, dietetic candies and gums, and complex carbohydrates may benefit some individuals. Patients with constipation may experience reductions in gaseous symptoms when fiber products and gas-forming sugar laxatives such as lactulose, sorbitol, or prune juice are replaced by osmotic laxatives.

Medications may provide benefits for some individuals with gas and bloating. Simethicone alters the elasticity of mucus-covered intralumenal gas bubbles and promotes their coalescence. Activated charcoal sometimes reduces breath hydrogen and symptoms caused by ingesting indigestible carbohydrates. Bacterial α-galactosidase (Beano) has been marketed to reduce symptoms after ingesting legumes high in indigestible oligosaccharides. Probiotic compounds including *Bifidobacterium infantis* have been shown to reduce discomfort, bloating and distension in IBS patients. The nonabsorbable antibiotic rifaximin has also been shown in randomized clinical trials to reduce bloating and abdominal discomfort in IBS. Lubiprostone is a chloride channel activator approved for women with IBS and constipation that can reduce symptoms of gas.

Complications

Few complications occur in patients with gas and bloating caused by functional disease. However, complications from organic disease usually are manifestations of the underlying disease rather than of the gas itself. There have been rare case reports of explosions resulting from ignition by tobacco smoking of feculent gas expelled during eructation in patients with gastrointestinal obstruction and proximal bacterial overgrowth. Similarly, colonic explosions with perforation have been reported in patients undergoing colonoscopy with intracolonic cautery. In general, these vanishingly rare complications result from inadequate bowel cleansing or the use of mannitol or sorbitol purging solutions, both of which generate hydrogen gas.

Case studies

Case 1

A 32-year-old woman complains of excessive belching, in excess of 30 times per day. She denies abdominal pain, nausea, diarrhea, or weight loss. She has no medical problems including diabetes or thyroid disease and denies medication use. Physical examination is normal. Complete blood count, thyroid-stimulating hormone (TSH), and fasting cortisol are normal and antitissue transglutaminase is negative. The patient is queried further and her symptoms had increased when she tried to stop smoking by using nicotine gum, although she continues to smoke. She is counseled about aerophagia and over time is able to stop smoking and discontinue the gum, which results in substantial reduction in her symptoms.

Discussion

The most common cause of excessive eructation is aerophagia. Aerophagia is commonly exacerbated by smoking or gum chewing, but can be primary and is generally a learned behavior. Patients are often unaware of aerophagia so the use of a mirror to provide objective evidence of episodes of air swallowing can be useful. Self-awareness of this behavior can be therapeutic.

Case 2

A 48-year-old man with a 30-year history of type 1 diabetes complains of excessive gas and flatulence, with cramping abdominal pain and loose stools. He states that there had been a progressive increase in intestinal gas over the past 6 months despite no change in his diet, good glucose control, and regular exercise. His physical examination confirms reduced proprioception but the remainder of his examination is normal, including the abdomen. Laboratory tests reveal an elevated BUN and creatinine but a normal HbA1C and thyroid function. Stool is negative for *Giardia* antigen, ova and parasites examination. Glucose hydrogen breath testing reveals an abnormally elevated baseline level that increases significantly after carbohydrate ingestion. Ciprofloxacin 500 mg orally twice daily for 7 days is prescribed, which rapidly improves symptoms.

Discussion

Diabetes is associated with small intestinal bacterial overgrowth. Diabetic "enteropathy" is a neuropathy that interferes with normal intestinal motility; it rarely occurs in the absence of peripheral neuropathy so physical findings (reduced proprioception) are key to the diagnosis. The glucose hydrogen breath test is classically used to evaluate for the presence of bacterial overgrowth; however, it is insensitive and empirical therapy is often employed in lieu of diagnostic testing.

CHAPTER 8

Approach to the Patient with Ileus or Obstruction

Acute ileus is a potentially reversible state of inhibited motor activity in the gastrointestinal tract. Chronic pseudo-obstruction is a functional abnormality of longer duration that simulates mechanical obstruction but has no anatomical cause and may exhibit clinical manifestations similar to ileus. Toxic megacolon is a special form of ileus in which severe transmural inflammation produces colonic atony, systemic toxemia, and a high risk of spontaneous perforation. Obstruction implies complete or partial blockage of the gut at one or more levels.

Clinical presentation

History

Patients with ileus, obstruction and pseudo-obstruction may present with symptoms of abdominal pain, nausea, vomiting, abdominal distension or obstipation. Acute ileus or gastric or duodenal obstruction may be associated with little abdominal pain, whereas distal intestinal or colonic obstructions generally cause greater discomfort. The pain of mechanical obstruction is dull, ill defined, or squeezing. True colic (intermittent waves of pain) may be prominent. Upper and midabdominal pain are characteristic of obstruction proximal to the transverse colon, whereas left colonic obstruction is associated with lower abdominal discomfort.

Distension may be pronounced with ileus and with distal obstruction, but minimal with gastric obstruction. Audible bowel sounds are present and often increased with intestinal obstruction but are reduced or absent with acute ileus. Copious vomiting of clear liquid characterizes gastric obstruction, whereas marked bilious emesis occurs with duodenal blockage. Distal obstruction and ileus produce only mild nausea and vomiting. The pain of proximal, not distal, obstruction is often relieved by vomiting. If mechanical obstruction is incomplete or if ileus is mild, pain and distension may be intermittent and aggravated by fiber-rich, poorly digestible foods. Complete obstruction usually produces

Yamada's Handbook of Gastroenterology, Third Edition. Edited by Tadataka Yamada and John M. Inadomi.
© 2013 John Wiley & Sons, Ltd. Published 2013 by John Wiley & Sons, Ltd.

obstipation and the inability to expel flatus. Conversely, watery diarrhea is noted with partial obstruction and fecal impaction.

Careful family, medication, endocrine, immunological, and metabolic histories should be obtained from a patient with ileus, and the clinician should be alert to thyroid and parathyroid disorders, diabetes, scleroderma, heavy metal intoxication, and porphyria. Prior surgery raises the possibility of adhesions, and reports of abdominal wall bulging suggest hernias as a possible cause of obstruction. Histories of malignancy, radiation, inflammatory bowel disease, ulcer disease, gallstones, diverticular disease, pancreatitis, motility disorders, and foreign body ingestion suggest specific causes. Exacerbation of pain with menses is consistent with endometriosis.

Physical examination

A patient with obstruction usually appears to be in great distress, whereas a patient with ileus may be more comfortable despite pronounced abdominal distension. Inspection may reveal scars and visible distension. Auscultation usually reveals hypoactive or absent bowel sounds with ileus, whereas obstruction produces louder, high-pitched, hyperactive bowel sounds that may have a musical or tinkling quality. Shaking of the abdomen while listening through a stethoscope may reveal a succussion splash, which is associated with gastric obstruction or gastroparesis. Gentle palpation may detect subtle hernias that are not obvious on inspection. Hepatosplenomegaly, lymphadenopathy, and masses raise concern for malignancy, although tender masses may be present in inflammatory diseases (e.g. Crohn's disease). Tympany accompanies both ileus and obstruction, whereas shifting dullness and a fluid wave characterize ascites.

Rectal examination may detect occult fecal blood with inflammatory, neoplastic, infectious, or ischemic disease. Digital rectal and pelvic examinations may also detect subtle masses not found on abdominal palpation or may reveal obturator or sciatic hernias. Repeated abdominal examinations are essential to assess for development of complications such as perforation. If fever, hypotension, or signs of sepsis or peritonitis develop or if bowel sounds disappear, the viscus may be ischemic and operative intervention may be urgently indicated.

Key practice points

The physical examination can usually differentiate between ileus and obstruction. Ileus will present with absent or rare bowel sounds, whereas the physical examination in obstruction will reveal hyperactive, high-pitched (tinkling) bowel sounds.

Additional testing
Laboratory studies

Blood tests aid in establishing the cause of mechanical obstruction only in rare cases related to inflammation, infection, or neoplasm; in contrast, laboratory studies often indicate the cause of ileus. Abnormal electrolyte (including calcium, phosphate, and magnesium), blood urea nitrogen, or creatinine values support a clinical impression of dehydration. Leukocytosis may be present with inflammation or infection. Measurement of arterial blood gases may be necessary to evaluate the acid–base balance. With an ischemic or infarcted bowel, elevations in amylase, alkaline phosphatase, creatine phosphokinase, aspartate and alanine aminotransferase, and lactate dehydrogenase may be evident, although these enzymes also increase with hepatic and pancreaticobiliary disease.

Plain radiographic studies

Plain radiographs should be the initial structural studies performed on patients with suspected ileus or obstruction. Chest radiography can detect pneumonia, evaluate cardiorespiratory status, and detect free subdiaphragmatic air, whereas supine and upright abdominal plain films show intra-abdominal gas distribution. With complete occlusion of the small intestine, the lumen is widely distended and the valvulae conniventes are observed to span the lumenal air column; in addition, the colon empties within 12–24 h and no colonic air is radiographically visible. Upright or decubitus views commonly demonstrate air–fluid levels in a stepladder configuration.

With colonic obstruction, the colon proximal to the blockage dilates and the characteristic incomplete and scalloped indentations of the haustra are visible. With advanced strangulation, the bowel wall becomes edematous, exhibiting a thumbprint pattern on radiographs, and air in the intestinal wall, portal vein, and peritoneal cavity may be observed.

In ileus, lumenal dilation may be generalized or it may only manifest adjacent to an inflammatory site, producing a sentinel loop, as in appendicitis or pancreatitis. With concurrent peritonitis, the bowel wall may thicken. Colonic gas usually is more prominent in ileus than with small intestinal obstruction. Pure colonic dilation, most pronounced in the cecum, is the defining feature of acute colonic pseudo-obstruction. Stepladder air–fluid levels may be observed with either ileus or obstruction, but they are more well defined and longer with obstruction. A string-of-beads pattern of the air–fluid interfaces is most suggestive of high-grade obstruction of the small intestine. A diffusely hazy pattern with central localization of bowel loops is characteristic of ascites.

Additional structural studies

Computed tomographic scanning is used to define the site of obstruction and to exclude selected underlying disease processes (i.e. inflammation versus neoplasm). Conversely, ultrasound is generally not useful because of the obscuring effects of intralumenal gas. Upper endoscopy is useful with suspected esophageal, gastric, or duodenal lesions and offers the additional capability of therapeutic dilation of any stricture. Push enteroscopy provides similar diagnostic and therapeutic capabilities to the proximal jejunum. Angiography or magnetic resonance angiography may be useful for patients with suspected mesenteric ischemia and infarction.

Functional studies

Functional testing of gut motility may be considered for patients with prolonged ileus or suspected chronic intestinal pseudo-obstruction. Gastric emptying scintigraphy may document gastroparesis, whereas esophageal or gastroduodenal manometry may show the characteristic hypomotility pattern of visceral myopathy or the random, intense bursts of contractions in visceral neuropathy.

Differential diagnosis

Acute ileus, chronic pseudo-obstruction, and mechanical obstruction have numerous causes (Table 8.1).

Acute ileus

Several conditions have been associated with the development of acute ileus. Ileus is the normal physiological response to laparotomy. Gastric and small intestinal motility recover in the first postoperative day, whereas colonic contractions return in 3–5 days. Postoperative ileus beyond that time is considered pathological and warrants a search for surgical complications. Other intra-abdominal causes of acute ileus include abdominal trauma and inflammatory gut disorders. Noninflammatory conditions (radiation damage and mesenteric ischemia) and retroperitoneal disorders can also produce acute ileus. Extra-abdominal causes of ileus include reflex inhibition of gut motility by craniotomy, fractures, myocardial infarction, heart surgery, pneumonia, pulmonary embolus, and burns. Medications may inhibit motor activity, as may metabolic abnormalities.

Chronic intestinal pseudo-obstruction

Chronic intestinal pseudo-obstruction is a consequence of a variety of conditions. Chronic idiopathic pseudo-obstruction often presents after a viral prodrome, suggesting an infectious etiology. Hereditary conditions such as familial visceral myopathies and neuropathies produce pseudo-obstruction at early ages. In addition to gastroparesis, long-standing, poorly controlled diabetes mellitus may disrupt motor function in the small intestine. Rheumatological disorders and some endocrinopathies can lead to chronic pseudo-obstruction. Neuromuscular diseases chronically disrupt motor activity. In selected geographic locations, Chagas disease represents an infectious cause of pseudo-obstruction that occurs after exposure to *Trypanosoma cruzi*. Viral pseudo-obstruction in immunosuppressed patients has been reported as a consequence of infection

Table 8.1 Causes of ileus and obstruction

Acute ileus
Postoperative ileus
Abdominal trauma
Ulcer perforation
Bile or chemical peritonitis
Toxic megacolon
Pancreatitis
Cholecystitis
Appendicitis
Diverticulitis
Inflammatory bowel disease
Radiation therapy
Mesenteric ischemia
Retroperitoneal disorders (e.g. renal calculi, pyelonephritis, renal transplant, hemorrhage)
Extra-abdominal sources (e.g. craniotomy, fractures, myocardial infarction, cardiac surgery, pneumonia, pulmonary embolus, burns)
Metabolic disorders (e.g. electrolyte abnormalities, uremia, sepsis, diabetic ketoacidosis, sickle cell anemia, respiratory insufficiency, porphyria, heavy metal toxicity)
Medications (e.g. anticholinergics, opiates, calcium channel antagonists, chemotherapy, antidepressants)

Chronic intestinal pseudo-obstruction
Hereditary diseases (e.g. familial visceral neuropathy, familial visceral myopathy)
Diabetes mellitus
Rheumatological disorders (e.g. scleroderma, systemic lupus erythematosus, amyloidosis)
Endocrinopathies (e.g. hypothyroidism, hyperparathyroid disease or hypoparathyroid disease, Addison disease)
Neuromuscular diseases (e.g. muscular dystrophy, myotonic dystrophy)
Chagas disease
Infectious pseudo-obstruction
Pheochromocytoma
Paraneoplastic pseudo-obstruction

Mechanical obstruction
Adhesions
Congenital bands (e.g. Ladd bands)
Hernias (e.g. external, internal, diaphragmatic, pelvic)
Volvulus (e.g. colon, small intestine, stomach)
Obstructive lumenal tumors
Inflammatory bowel disease
Diverticulitis
Mesenteric ischemia
Radiation injury
Intussusception
Congenital conditions (e.g. hypertrophic pyloric stenosis, Hirschsprung disease, intestinal atresia/agenesis)
Fecal impaction
Gallstone ileus
Retained barium
Gastric bezoars

with cytomegalovirus and other agents. Pheochromocytoma produces chronic intestinal hypomotility, probably because of the motor inhibitory effects of circulating catecholamines. Chronic intestinal pseudo-obstruction can be a paraneoplastic manifestation of small cell lung carcinoma and, less commonly, other malignancies. Paraneoplastic pseudo-obstruction results from malignant invasion of the celiac axis or, alternatively, from plasma cell infiltration of the myenteric plexus, leading to the loss of enteric neural function.

Mechanical obstruction

The causes of mechanical intestinal obstruction may be divided into extrinsic lesions, intrinsic lesions, and intralumenal objects.

Extrinsic lesions

Extrinsic adhesions are the most common cause of small intestinal obstruction in adults, but they rarely occlude the colon. Congenital bands behave similarly and may occur in association with malrotation (Ladd bands). Hernias represent another extrinsic cause of obstruction that may be external (protruding through the abdominal wall), internal, diaphragmatic (usually paraesophageal), or pelvic.

Volvulus is an abnormal torsion of the bowel that produces a closed and obstructed loop of bowel, associated with an impairment of blood flow. Colonic volvulus involves the cecum in 10–20% and the sigmoid colon in 70–80% of cases and manifests as sudden abdominal pain followed by distension. Gastric volvulus occurs with diaphragmatic defects, congenital malformations, and large paraesophageal hernias.

Intrinsic lesions

Intrinsic lesions are less common causes of mechanical obstruction. Benign and malignant tumors can obstruct the lumen or provide a leading point for intus-susception. Primary small intestinal malignancies are rare and include lymphoma, adenocarcinoma, and carcinoids, whereas adenocarcinoma represents the most common obstructing colonic neoplasm. Metastatic tumors usually tether and fix the bowel rather than obstruct the lumen. Inflammatory processes and ischemia cause obstructing strictures, whereas blunt trauma may produce an intramural hematoma. In addition to neoplasm, a Meckel diverticulum may initiate intussusception. In children, there usually is no underlying mucosal or submucosal lesion that predisposes to intussusception.

Intralumenal objects

Intralumenal objects represent the least common causes of mechanical obstruction. Fecal impaction may produce colonic obstruction in patients who are dehydrated or immobile, who have underlying constipation, or who take medications that slow colonic transit. Rarely, large gallstones erode through the gallbladder into the gut lumen, where they migrate to obstruct the intestine, usually at the level of the distal ileum. Barium from radiographic procedures may obstruct the colon in patients with underlying colonic motility disorders. Gastric bezoars and ingested foreign bodies may occlude the gut lumen in select cases.

Diagnostic investigation

The diagnostic investigation of a patient with suspected ileus or obstruction is illustrated in Figure 8.1. The history and physical examination may direct the evaluation towards ileus or obstruction. Predisposing historical features modify the risk of either condition, and physical examination can indicate the presence of ileus (absent bowel sounds) or obstruction (hyperactive or high-pitched bowel sounds). Laboratory abnormalities may reveal the etiology of ileus, and radiographic tests usually differentiate obstruction from ileus.

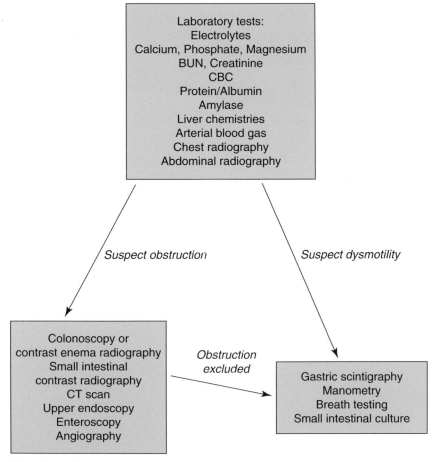

Figure 8.1 Work-up of a patient with ileus or obstruction. BUN, blood urea nitrogen; CBC, complete blood count; CT, computed tomography.

Obstruction generally requires assessment of the location by computed tomography (CT) scan, and accessible lesions can be identified and possibly sampled for tissue using appropriate endoscopic procedures. Ileus can be treated empirically with medication (see below) or more fully evaluated using gastric emptying tests and/or esophageal or gastroduodenal manometry.

Management

Medical
Fluid replacement
Correction of fluid, electrolyte, and acid–base imbalances is guided by the physical findings coupled with laboratory determination of hematocrit, electrolyte, blood urea nitrogen, creatinine, and blood gas levels. With severe hypovolemia, fluid resuscitation should be performed with concurrent monitoring of urine output, central venous pressure, and blood pressure. With gastric outlet obstruction, potassium chloride is often needed after establishing normal urine output because renal potassium losses are high in this condition.

Bowel decompression
Abdominal distension increases gastrointestinal secretion and causes nausea and vomiting, thereby increasing the risk of aspiration. Nasogastric suction is appropriate in ileus and obstruction. The patient should be given nothing by mouth, and intravenous fluids with or without parenteral nutrients should be administered to maintain adequate hydration and nutrition. Drugs that inhibit motor activity should be withheld. Placing a rectal tube or administering tap water enemas may reduce colonic distension in some patients.

In patients with documented ileus who do not have significant cardiovascular disease, the acetylcholinesterase inhibitor neostigmine may promote gas expulsion when administered in a controlled setting with cardiac monitoring. For patients with acute colonic pseudo-obstruction, some clinicians advocate therapeutic colonoscopic decompression, although few objective data support this practice. On the other hand, sigmoid volvulus is effectively treated by gentle endoscopic detorsion with aspiration of retained gas.

For patients with obstruction, endoscopic dilation of adhesions or radiation-induced strictures may be possible. Inoperable colorectal cancer may be palliatively treated by Nd:YAG laser recanalization of the colonic lumen or by placing expandable intralumenal stents.

Surgical
Complete intestinal obstruction is generally an indication for urgent surgery as soon as resuscitation is completed and nasogastric decompression is achieved

because strangulation cannot be excluded using clinical criteria in this setting. If strangulation is discovered, necrotic bowel should be resected.

With partial obstruction, immediate surgery and antibiotics are of no proven benefit. However, if fever, peritoneal signs, leukocytosis, or hyperamylasemia develop, laparotomy is indicated. Colonic obstruction nearly always requires surgery; nasogastric suction may have little effect in this setting. If the bowel cannot be cleansed, many surgeons perform a two-stage operation with initial resection of the obstructed segment and placement of a diverting colostomy followed by reanastomosis at a later date to reduce wound infection.

Complications

The most serious complication of obstruction or ileus is bowel infarction, with resulting peritonitis and possible death. Other complications include aspiration pneumonia, electrolyte abnormalities, and malnutrition. All may have serious consequences for unstable patients who have other concurrent disease. Many of the diseases that produce ileus and obstruction have serious sequelae, in addition to those that result from involvement of the bowel.

Case studies

Case 1

A 53-year-old man presents to the emergency department with abdominal pain for 5h. He has no prior history of abdominal pain, but awoke from sleep with gradual onset of diffuse upper abdominal pain in a colicky (intermittent) pattern. He mentions associated nausea and emesis of clear fluid. The pain does not radiate, and he has not had a bowel movement or passed gas since its onset. Physical examination reveals an uncomfortable man who is constantly shifting his position on the gurney. The abdomen is distended and high-pitched bowel sounds are present. An appendectomy scar is noted in the right lower quadrant. There is diffuse tenderness to palpation with voluntary guarding but no rebound. His rectal examination is notable for brown, heme-negative stool. His white blood count (WBC) is 16.3 and his Hb is 17.4 g/dL. Plain abdominal radiographs illustrate distended loops of small intestine with air–fluid levels and a transition point in the right lower quadrant. CT scan of the abdomen confirms distended small intestine with abrupt narrowing in the mid-ileum and a paucity of gas in the large intestine.

The surgical service performs a laparoscopic examination, which reveals adhesions in the right lower quadrant and small intestinal obstruction. The adhesions are taken down and the remainder of the bowel appears normal without signs of ischemia. Postoperatively the patient recovers quickly and is discharged in good condition.

Discussion

Obstruction of a hollow viscus such as the small intestine will create colicky pain, which increases and dissipates in a cyclical fashion. The physical examination should be sufficient to diagnose small bowel obstruction. Signs of prior surgery should be sought to determine the likelihood of adhesions causing obstruction. Unlike ileus or chronic pseudo-obstruction, the bowel sounds are hyperactive. Plain abdominal radiographs should be sufficient to illustrate dilated small intestinal loops that are generally fluid-filled with an air interface. CT scans will generally be able to identify the transition point, or site of obstruction.

Case 2

A 76-year-old woman recently underwent an open reduction with internal fixation for a hip fracture. A gastroenterologist is consulted to manage increasing abdominal distension with diffuse, continuous, pressure-like abdominal pain that is 3/10 in severity. The patient mentions associated nausea but no emesis. Her past medical history is notable only for diabetes mellitus (type 2). Physical examination reveals an obese woman who is in no acute distress. Vital signs are normal and her abdominal examination is notable for a distended abdomen, absence of bowel sounds, and no abdominal tenderness to palpation. WBC is 7.6 and Hb is 7.5 mg/dL. Plain abdominal radiographs reveal gas distension of the entire colon including the rectum, with the cecum 9 cm in diameter.

Discussion

This is a typical presentation of acute colonic pseudo-obstruction – a patient is admitted to hospital for a nongastrointestinal indication and during the hospital course is noted to have a distended abdomen and dilated large intestine. The abdominal examination differs from acute obstruction in that bowel sounds are absent and tenderness is generally absent to minimal. Significant tenderness is worrisome for perforation, which will usually occur in the cecum due to LaPlace's law, which stipulates that despite similar colonic wall thickness throughout the colon, the greatest wall tension will occur in the region with the greatest diameter (the cecum).

The patient is managed conservatively, with correction of serum electrolytes, discontinuation of narcotics, and frequent turning. A nasogastric tube is placed and set to intermittent suction, and the patient is not given anything by mouth. The next day her abdomen remains distended and tympanitic, with mild diffuse tenderness but no rebound or guarding. Her plain abdominal radiographs reveal a cecum that is 12 cm in diameter, without thumbprinting or perforation.

Based on her increased symptoms and enlarged cecal diameter, intervention is recommended. Intravenous neostigmine is administered under close cardiac monitoring. No bradycardia is noted and the patient responds appropriately with increased flatus and a reduction in abdominal distension. Although slow to recover, she is discharged 1 week later having had no further episodes of ileus.

Discussion

Neostygmine was shown in a randomized controlled trial to reduce colonic distension, symptoms and complications of acute colonic pseudo-obstruction. Since this is an acetylcholinesterase inhibitor, contraindications include cardiovascular disease (especially brady-dysrhythmias) and bronchospasm. Infusion of 2 mg neostigmine intravenously should be performed in a telemetry setting and atropine should be available for symptomatic bradycardia. (Source: Ponec RJ, Saunders MD, Kimmey MB. Neostigmine for the treatment of acute colonic pseudo-obstruction. N Engl J Med 1999;341(3):137–41.)

CHAPTER 9

Approach to the Patient with Constipation

Clinical presentation

History

Constipation, the most prevalent digestive complaint in the United States, is defined as a symptomatic decrease in stool frequency to fewer than three bowel movements per week. Some patients with normal stool frequency report constipation if they pass dry stools, strain during defecation, or experience a sense of incomplete fecal evacuation. A thorough history is required to elicit features suggestive of organic or functional etiologies of constipation. Constipation since childhood may suggest a congenital disorder of coloanal motor function. In adults, a recent change in bowel habits warrants exclusion of organic obstructive disease, whereas a several year history is more consistent with functional disease. Bleeding or anal pain suggests a structural cause of symptoms. Other symptoms (e.g. straining, abdominal pain, bloating, or incomplete evacuation) or associated extracolonic manifestations (e.g. heartburn, nausea, dyspepsia, early satiety, or genitourinary symptoms) are more common with functional disorders such as irritable bowel syndrome (IBS). Reports of skin or hair changes, temperature intolerance, or weight gain suggest possible hypothyroidism, whereas weight loss raises concern for malignancy. Underlying systemic illness (e.g. diabetes or a rheumatological condition) should be identified. A careful history of medication use, including laxative use, is essential. In children, inquiry should be made regarding nightmares, enuresis, school performance, and family tension.

Physical examination

Abdominal masses, hepatomegaly, or lymphadenopathy suggest possible obstructing malignancy. Peripheral or autonomic neuropathy may indicate a neuropathic motility disorder. The anorectal examination can detect tumors, strictures, fissures, hemorrhoids, and rectal prolapse. Occult or gross fecal blood warrants a search for neoplasm or inflammatory disease, although local anorectal

Yamada's Handbook of Gastroenterology, Third Edition. Edited by Tadataka Yamada and John M. Inadomi.

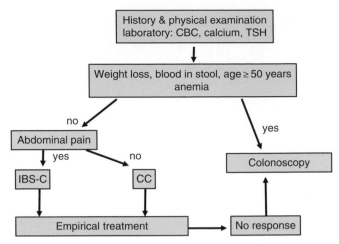

Figure 9.1 Constipation. CBC, complete blood count; CC, chronic constipation; IBS-C, irritable bowel syndrome-constipation predominant; TSH, thyroid-stimulating hormone.

disease commonly produces blood loss. Anorectal neuromuscular function is tested by assessing basal anal tone, adequacy of maximal anal squeeze, and perianal cutaneous sensation, including the anal wink. Long-standing constipation with straining and prolapse may produce anal or perineal nerve damage that leads to reduced anal pressure and fecal incontinence. Examination during attempted defecation maneuvers can suggest rectal prolapse and evidence of rectosphincteric dyssynergia. Pelvic examination in women may demonstrate a rectocele with straining.

Additional testing
Laboratory studies
If the history or examination suggests systemic or local anorectal disease, further evaluation may be needed (Figure 9.1). A microcytic anemia raises concern for colonic neoplasm or inflammatory disease. Other screening tests include measuring serum calcium to exclude hyperparathyroidism and thyroid-stimulating hormone levels to exclude hypothyroidism. Specific serological tests can detect rheumatological disease, Chagas disease, or paraneoplastic pseudo-obstruction, whereas other assays are used for catecholamines, porphyrins, and glucagon.

Structural studies
Endoscopic or radiographic evaluation is performed on any individual with suspected mechanical obstruction as a cause of constipation. In young patients, flexible sigmoidoscopy is sufficient. For patients older than 40–45 years or if alarm findings such as bleeding are present, it is important to evaluate the entire colon by colonoscopy because of the increased risk of colorectal neoplasm. Computed tomography (CT) scans or barium enema radiography can show proximal colonic dilation as well as persistent contraction of the denervated segment in Hirschsprung

disease. Deep rectal biopsy specimens obtained at least 3 cm above the anal verge are obtained to exclude Hirschsprung disease, when indicated.

Functional studies

In young patients without alarm symptoms, or patients in whom structural diseases have been excluded, empirical trials of medical therapy are offered. For a patient whose condition is refractory to standard treatment, additional evaluation may be indicated to assess the functional integrity of the colon and anorectum. Anorectal manometry with balloon expulsion should be performed in patients with chronic constipation who do not respond to empirical medical therapy. The transit of stool through different colonic regions can be quantified by obtaining serial abdominal radiographs after ingesting radio-opaque markers, or by newer technology involving a swallowed capsule that measures pH, temperature, and intralumenal pressure to determine intestinal transit time. These studies can distinguish between slow-transit constipation (colonic inertia), in which transit is delayed in all colonic regions, and functional outlet obstruction, where passage is selectively retarded at the level of the anorectum. In some cases, marker elimination is normal, even though the patient denies stool output. Such individuals often exhibit psychological disturbances that contribute to their symptoms.

Differential diagnosis

The causes of constipation are numerous, including secondary causes and idiopathic disorders, and relate to either impairment of colonic transit or to structural or functional obstruction to fecal evacuation (Table 9.1).

Mechanical colonic obstruction

Colonic obstruction may result from mechanical narrowing of the distal colon or anus or from functional outlet obstruction. The most important mechanical cause is colon carcinoma, which typically presents in individuals over age 50 or in selected high-risk groups. Although colon cancer often presents with gross or occult fecal bleeding, a subtle decrease in stool frequency or caliber for weeks to months may be the only initial complaint. Benign colonic strictures resulting from diverticulitis, ischemia, or inflammatory bowel disease produce similar symptoms. Anal strictures, foreign bodies, or spasm from painful fissures or hemorrhoids also may interrupt stool expulsion.

Neuropathic and myopathic disorders

Diseases of the extrinsic or enteric innervation of the colon and anus may produce constipation. Constipation may be caused by transection of the sacral nerves or cauda equina, lumbosacral spinal injury, meningomyelocele, or low spinal anesthesia. These may lead to colonic hypomotility and dilation, decreased rectal tone

Table 9.1 Causes of constipation

Colonic obstruction
Colorectal neoplasms
Benign strictures (e.g. diverticulitis, ischemia)
Inflammatory bowel disease
Endometriosis
Anal strictures or neoplasms
Rectal foreign bodies
Anal fissures and hemorrhoids

Neuropathic and myopathic disorders
Peripheral and autonomic neuropathy
Hirschsprung disease
Chagas disease
Neurofibromatosis
Ganglioneuromatosis
Hypoganglionosis
Intestinal pseudo-obstruction
Multiple sclerosis
Spinal cord lesions
Parkinson disease
Shy–Drager syndrome
Transection of sacral nerves or cauda equina
Lumbosacral spinal injury
Meningomyelocele
Low spinal anesthesia
Scleroderma
Amyloidosis
Polymyositis/dermatomyositis
Myotonic dystrophy

Metabolic and endocrine disorders
Diabetes mellitus
Pregnancy
Hypercalcemia
Hypothyroidism
Hypokalemia
Porphyria
Glucagonoma
Panhypopituitarism
Pheochromocytoma

Medications
Opiates
Anticholinergics
Tricyclic antidepressants
Antipsychotics
Anti-parkinsonian agents
Antihypertensives

Table 9.1 (*cont'd*)

Ganglionic blockers
Vinca alkaloids
Anticonvulsants
Calcium channel antagonists
Iron supplements
Aluminum antacids
Calcium supplements
Barium sulfate
Heavy metals (i.e. lead, arsenic, mercury)

Idiopathic constipation
Colonic inertia
Megarectum/megacolon
Rectosphincteric dyssynergia
Rectocele/rectal prolapse
Irritable bowel syndrome

and sensation, and impaired defecation. Colonic reflexes are preserved with high spinal lesions; thus, digital stimulation can trigger defecation. However, patients with spinal injury have reduced meal-induced colonic motor activity and impaired rectal sensation and compliance that can contribute to constipation. Constipation is prevalent with multiple sclerosis, cerebrovascular accidents, Parkinson disease, and dysautonomias, including Shy–Drager syndrome.

Hirschsprung disease is the best characterized enteric nervous system disease that presents with constipation. Most commonly, affected infants present with obstipation and proximal colonic dilation at birth. With Hirschsprung, the internal anal sphincter does not relax normally with rectal stimulation because of an absence of enteric ganglion cells which functionally blocks fecal expulsion. Some individuals with very short segment involvement present with constipation in adulthood or, in rare instances, incontinence. Other enteric nervous system diseases include zonal colonic aganglionosis (in which patchy areas of the colon are devoid of neurons either congenitally or secondary to ischemia), chronic intestinal pseudo-obstruction (myopathic and neuropathic), and Chagas disease (resulting from infection with *Trypanosoma cruzi*). Neurofibromatosis, long-standing laxative abuse, and diabetes mellitus may lead to enteric neuronal damage. Idiopathic megacolon is divided into primary and secondary disorders. Primary megacolon is thought to be associated with neuropathic dysfunction. Secondary megacolon and megarectum develop later in life, usually in response to chronic fecal retention. This disorder may be confused with Hirschsprung disease on anorectal manometry, if large enough volumes of rectal distension are not used to elicit anal relaxation on reflex testing.

Rheumatological disorders evoke a generalized slowing of colonic transit. Dermatomyositis and myotonic dystrophy produce myopathic dysfunction.

Amyloidosis and scleroderma may produce either myopathic or neuropathic disease. Constipation in systemic lupus erythematosus has multiple mechanisms, including local ischemia secondary to vasculitis.

Metabolic and endocrine disorders

The most common endocrine causes of constipation are diabetes, pregnancy, and hypothyroidism. Although symptoms usually are mild, life-threatening megacolon may develop in myxedema. Other endocrine causes of constipation include hypercalcemia, hypokalemia, porphyria, panhypopituitarism, pheochromocytoma, and glucagonoma.

Medications

Many medications produce mild or severe constipation that may limit their use. Drug classes that slow colonic transit include antispasmodics, tricyclic antidepressants, antipsychotics, anti-parkinsonian agents, opiates, certain antihypertensives, ganglionic blockers, vinca alkaloids, anticonvulsants, and calcium channel antagonists. Cation-containing agents include iron, aluminum antacids, calcium, barium, and heavy metals (i.e. arsenic, lead, mercury).

Idiopathic and functional causes

In most patients with constipation, no organic abnormality can be identified that causes their symptoms. The majority of young to middle-aged adults with chronic constipation are women. The most common cause of constipation in association with abdominal pain in this age group is irritable bowel syndrome, which is defined by specific symptom criteria. Thirty percent of patients who complain of infrequent defecation have normal colonic transit on quantitative testing; these individuals often exhibit evidence of psychosocial stress and have irritable bowel syndrome as a cause of symptoms. Many individuals with delayed colonic transit exhibit a generalized disorder of propulsion in the colon and are given a diagnosis of slow-transit constipation or colonic inertia. Some patients with colonic inertia also exhibit dysmotility of the esophagus, small intestine, or bladder that suggests the presence of a systemic disorder of smooth muscle function. Other persons with delayed colonic transit exhibit a functional impediment to defecation at the level of the anorectum. Causes of outlet obstruction include rectal prolapse, rectal intussusception, rectocele, megarectum, and dyssynergic defecation. Normal defecation involves the co-ordinated relaxation of the puborectalis muscle and anal sphincter. Dyssynergic defecation is characaterized by impaired relaxation or paradoxical contraction of the puborectalis muscle or anal sphincter.

Childhood constipation often manifests as fecal impaction with rectosigmoid dilation. The cause of childhood constipation is uncertain; impaired rectal sensation and altered anal tone are not reliably demonstrable. Many children exhibit evidence of rectosphincteric dyssynergia upon attempted defecation, which may be a learned behavior in response to prior painful defecation problems.

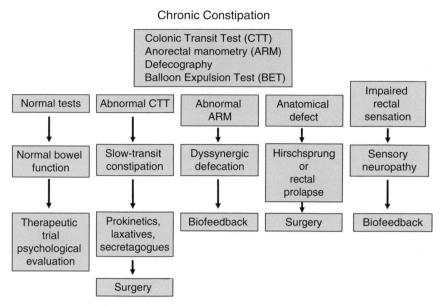

Figure 9.2 Work-up of a patient with constipation.

Constipation in the elderly also has several potential etiologies, including mechanical factors, hormonal disturbances, impaired motor function, and effects of medication. Straining with defecation is more commonly reported than infrequent stool passage in the elderly, possibly explaining the high rates of laxative use in this age group. In elderly institutionalized patients, fecal impaction is a common problem because of mental confusion, immobility, or inadequate toilet arrangements.

Diagnostic investigation (Figure 9.2)

Colonic transit tests include colonic marker studies or the SmartPill. Anorectal manometry assesses anorectal function in patients with straining and suspected functional outlet obstruction. Rectosphincteric dyssynergia is suggested by manometric demonstration of increased anal tone with attempted defecation. Manometry is complemented by electromyography of the anal sphincter in some centers. Rectal sensation is quantified during progressive rectal balloon inflation. Some patients with irritable bowel syndrome tolerate balloon distension poorly, whereas individuals with megarectum accommodate large balloon volumes without sensing a need to defecate. Measurement of anal tone during rectal balloon inflation detects a volume-dependent relaxation, a phenomenon known as the *rectoanal inhibitory reflex*: loss of this reflex suggests possible Hirschsprung disease. The diagnosis must be confirmed by deep rectal biopsy because falsely absent rectoanal inhibitory reflexes are present with megarectum if inadequate rectal volumes are delivered. Attempted defecation maneuvers, including expulsion of a rectal balloon, can help to assess for abnormalities of anal relaxation.

Defecography involves cinefluoroscopic recording of the attempted defecation of barium paste which is infused into the rectum. Structural abnormalities, including rectoceles and rectal prolapse or intussusception, can be diagnosed by this technique. Defecography also quantifies the anorectal angle at rest and with defecation. Rectosphincteric dyssynergia is characterized by a paradoxical decrease in this angle during defecation, which precludes evacuation of the rectal contrast material.

Management

Dietary and behavioral approaches

After structural and metabolic causes of constipation are excluded and offending medications are withdrawn, dietary and lifestyle changes can be offered. Many persons respond to increasing fiber intake to 20–30 g per day. Wheat bran is most effective in increasing stool weight and accelerating colonic transit, followed by fruits and vegetables, oats, corn, cellulose, soya, and pectin. In patients with irritable bowel syndrome, fiber should be gradually increased to minimize bloating. Establishing routine defecation after meals is recommended to take advantage of the gastrocolonic reflex, the increase in colonic motility that occurs in the initial postprandial hour. Daily exercise, such as walking or running, is encouraged.

Pharmacological therapy

Bulk-forming agents such as psyllium, methylcellulose, and polycarbophil may be given to patients who do not respond to dietary measures. These agents increase stool volume, improve fecal hydration, and increase colonic bacterial mass, leading to acceleration of colonic transit and reduced straining. If bulking agents are ineffective or produce unacceptable gas and bloating, hypertonic cationic and anionic (magnesium hydroxide), lubricant (mineral oil), or hyperosmotic sugar (sorbitol, lactulose) laxatives or stool softeners (docusate salts) may be useful. Cationic laxatives increase intralumenal water content by their osmotic effects. The use of magnesium products should be avoided in renal failure. Many such agents also can be given in the enema form to effect prompt defecation. Mineral oil penetrates and softens the stool but may reduce absorption of vitamins A, D, and K. Sorbitol and lactulose are nonabsorbable sugars that are degraded by colonic bacteria to increase stool osmolarity. Docusate salts are anionic surfactants that reduce fecal surface tension, allowing better mixing of aqueous and fatty substances and thereby softening the stool. Stimulant laxatives include castor oil, anthraquinones (e.g. cascara, senna, casanthranol, and danthron), and phenylmethanes (e.g. phenolphthalein and bisacodyl). Anthraquinones may produce melanosis coli, whereas danthron has reported hepatotoxic effects. Phenolphthalein has been associated with nongastrointestinal neoplasms in rodents and has been removed from the US market. The use of some stimulant laxatives purportedly produces long-term damage of colonic enteric nerves.

Other medications are useful in selected patients. Isotonic electrolyte solutions containing polyethylene glycol may promote a gentle laxative effect without uncomfortable side-effects in patients who develop cramping with hypertonic laxatives. For patients with more refractory constipation, the prostaglandin analog misoprostol and the antigout drug colchicine exhibit impressive stimulatory effects on colonic function. However, these agents may produce significant cramping in some individuals. Furthermore, misoprostol should be used with care in women of reproductive potential because of its abortifacient properties. Lubiprostone increases intestinal fluid secretion by activation of chloride channels, and is approved for women with constipation and constipation-dominant IBS. Its main adverse effects include nausea and headache. Finally, methylnatrexone is approved for opioid-associated constipation and alvimopan is approved for constipation after bowel surgery.

Nonpharmacological treatment

Nonmedication treatments are more appropriate for some causes of constipation. Biofeedback techniques using manometry or electromyography are indicated for selected conditions of anorectal dysfunction that do not respond to laxative therapy. With these methods, rectal sensation can be enhanced and paradoxical anal contractions with defecation can be corrected with learned behaviors.

Surgery is indicated for Hirschsprung disease. Anal myotomy may be beneficial with short segment involvement, whereas resection, bypass, or endorectal pull-through procedures are performed for more typical presentations of the disease. Subtotal colectomy with ileorectal anastomosis may be beneficial in carefully selected patients with severe colonic inertia that is unresponsive to medications. Surgical resection or reduction of large rectoceles is considered in patients when digital pressure on the pelvis or posterior vaginal wall results in improved fecal evacuation. Rectal prolapse may be surgically repaired with suspension or rectopexy, although these operations often have no effect on the underlying defecation problem. Surgery for rectosphincteric dyssynergia is contraindicated because of a high risk of postoperative incontinence.

Complications

Chronic constipation may lead to rectal prolapse, hemorrhoidal bleeding, or development of an anal fissure. Fecal impaction may produce colonic obstruction or stercoral ulcers, which can bleed or perforate. Large fecalomas may cause extrinsic ureteral compression, resulting in recurrent urinary infections. Fecal incontinence results from anal sphincter damage or perineal nerve dysfunction from straining or prolapse.

Case studies

Case 1

A 23-year-old woman presents with over 5 years of constipation. She describes having a bowel movement every week induced by stimulant laxatives, but these are associated with a sensation of incomplete evacuation. Without laxatives she will have a bowel movement perhaps once every other week. She describes abdominal bloating but no associated abdominal pain, and no weight loss or rectal bleeding. Physical examination reveals a well-developed woman with a normal examination of the abdomen and pelvis. Rectal examination has normal squeeze and anal wink is intact. Laboratory values include a normal complete blood count, calcium and thyroid-stimulating hormone (TSH).

Discussion

Chronic constipation in the absence of associated abdominal pain is classified as a separate entity from irritable bowel syndrome (Rome III criteria). In addition to not meeting criteria for IBS and the absence of loose stools, two or more of the following must be present to fulfill the diagnosis of chronic constipation: during at least 25% of defecations, have (a) straining, (b) lumpy or hard stools, (c) sensation of incomplete evacuation, (d) sensation of anorectal obstruction, (e) manual maneuvers to facilitate bowel movement, or (f) less than three defecations per week.

While some of the management is similar between IBS and chronic constipation, these are categorized differently due to potential differences in etiology and evaluation.

Case 2

A 53-year-old woman has a chief complaint of constipation for several years. She has a bowel movement once per week and often requires manual maneuvers to induce a movement. Her physical examination is normal and her laboratory tests including blood counts, albumin, and TSH are normal. She previously consulted another gastroenterologist who performed a colonoscopy, which was normal. You perform anorectal manometry, which is notable for increased anal contraction with attempted defecation. You follow this abnormality with defecography that illusrates paradoxical contraction of the puborectalis muscle and an inability to expel a 50 mL water-filled balloon. You provide her with a diagnosis of dyssynergic defecation.

Discussion

Dyssynergic defecation criteria include: (1) the diagnostic criteria for functional chronic constipation, (2) dyssynergia during repeated attempts to defecate defined as a paradoxical increase in anal sphincter pressure (anal contraction) or less than 20% relaxation of the resting anal sphincter pressure or inadequate propulsive forces based on manometry, imaging, or electromyography, (3) one or more of the following: (a) inability to expel an artificial stool (50 mL water-filled balloon) within 1 min, (b) prolonged colonic transit time, (c) inability to evacuate or >50% retention of barium during defecography.

CHAPTER 10

Approach to the Patient with Diarrhea

Patients may describe diarrhea as bowel movements that are increased in frequency, larger in size, loose in consistency, or associated with urgency or incontinence. The range of normal bowel patterns is broad, but 99% of the population in western societies defecates between three times a week and three times a day. The normal daily stool weight is 100–200 g, although individuals on high-fiber diets may pass 500 g per day. In the United States, a daily stool weight of more than 200 g is considered abnormal.

Clinical presentation

History
Diarrhea can be acute (<3 weeks in duration) or chronic (≥3 weeks). Acute diarrhea usually is due to an infectious agent, although drugs or osmotically active compounds may also be implicated. The patient should be questioned about recent travel, sexual practices, ingestion of well water or poorly cooked food and shellfish, and exposure to high-risk persons in day-care centers, hospitals, mental institutions, and nursing homes. The characteristics of the diarrhea provide clues to the causative organism. Watery diarrhea with nausea but little pain is most consistent with toxin-producing bacteria, whereas invasive bacteria may produce more pain and bloody diarrhea. Viruses induce watery diarrhea in association with pain, fever, and mild-to-moderate vomiting. Antibiotic-associated colitis must be suspected if the history is consistent. New medication or inadvertent use of over-the-counter drugs with laxative effects (e.g. antacids containing magnesium) should be identified.

The differential diagnosis of chronic diarrhea is more extensive. Frequent passage of voluminous stools that do not abate with food avoidance is consistent with a secretory process, whereas passage of low-volume, loose stools at a normal frequency may be secondary to a motor disturbance. Foul-smelling, bulky, greasy

Yamada's Handbook of Gastroenterology, Third Edition. Edited by Tadataka Yamada and John M. Inadomi.
© 2013 John Wiley & Sons, Ltd. Published 2013 by John Wiley & Sons, Ltd.

stools suggest fat malabsorption. Soft stools that float or disperse in the toilet water and resolve with fasting are reported by some patients with carbohydrate malabsorption, especially if they occur after ingesting specific foodstuffs such as dairy products or fruits. Fever, bleeding, pain, and weight loss raise concern for a mucosal injury. Severe pain also may be present with pancreatic disease. Fecal incontinence raises the question of a neuropathic disorder.

Identification of risk factors is important in diagnosing the cause of diarrhea. Diabetes and scleroderma are associated with intestinal dysmotility and bacterial overgrowth. Heat intolerance, palpitations, and weight loss suggest possible hyperthyroidism, whereas flushing and wheezing are reported by some patients with carcinoid syndrome. Chronic diarrhea may be a consequence of selected abdominal surgeries including vagotomy and cholecystectomy. Long-standing ethanol abuse impairs small intestinal function and promotes development of pancreatic exocrine insufficiency. A family history of diarrheal illness warrants evaluation for inflammatory bowel disease, celiac sprue, hereditary pancreatitis, or multiple endocrine neoplasia.

Physical examination

Orthostatic pulse or blood pressure changes, decreased skin turgor, and dry mucous membranes indicate severe diarrhea and the need for intravenous hydration and possible hospital admission. Emaciation, edema, peripheral neuropathy, cheilosis, and glossitis result from severe malabsorption. Relevant skin findings include dermatitis herpetiformis with celiac sprue, pyoderma gangrenosum with inflammatory bowel disease, and sclerodactyly with scleroderma. Arthritis may complicate inflammatory bowel disease or Whipple disease. Resting tachycardia suggests hyperthyroidism, whereas pulmonic stenosis and tricuspid regurgitation are found in carcinoid syndrome. Peripheral or autonomic neuropathy suggests diabetes or intestinal pseudo-obstruction. Neuropsychiatric findings are characteristic of Whipple disease. An abdominal mass suggests the presence of malignancy, Crohn's disease, or diverticulitis. Localized abdominal tenderness implicates an inflammatory condition. Rectal examination may reveal perianal disease with Crohn's disease, reduced sphincter tone that could lead to incontinence, and occult or gross fecal blood suggestive of mucosal injury.

Additional testing
Stool tests

Routine stool cultures are readily available for detecting *Salmonella*, *Shigella*, or *Campylobacter*. Special culture techniques are needed to diagnose enterohemorrhagic *E. coli*, *Yersinia* and *Plesiomonas*. If parasitic disease is suspected, stool should be examined for ova and parasites to find *Giardia*, *Cryptosporidium*, *E. histolytica*, or *Strongyloides*. Stool antigen tests also are available for *Giardia*. In individuals with recent antibiotic use, stools should be sent for *C. difficile* toxin determination.

Inflammatory etiologies are characterized by red and white blood cells in the stool. Noninflammatory diarrhea may be further evaluated by stool electrolytes, specifically sodium and potassium. Direct measurement of stool osmolality may be altered by bacterial degradation of carbohydrate so it is not routinely obtained; instead, normal plasma osmolality is assumed (290 mOsm/kg H_2O). A difference of >125 mOsm/kg between stool osmolality and twice the sum of stool sodium plus potassium concentrations suggests an osmotic cause, whereas a gap of <50 mOsm/kg is consistent with secretory diarrhea. Stool Osm gaps between 50–125 mOsm/kg are difficult to categorize with certainty. Osmotic diarrhea suggests ingestion of nonabsorbed solutes such as magnesium, phosphate or sulfate. Stool or urine samples can be analyzed for sulfate, magnesium, phosphate, bisacodyl, castor oil, or anthracene derivatives.

Key practice points

Stool electrolytes are used to differentiate osmotic from secretory diarrheas. Laxative use generally results in an osmotic diarrhea. However, sodium sulfate or sodium phosphate ingestion will not produce an osmotic gap. While direct examination of stool osmolality is difficult, it is helpful in some situations such as factitious diarrhea: stool osmolality >375–400 mOsm/kg H_2O suggests contamination of stool with concentrated urine, while values <200–250 mOsm/kg H_2O are seen when stool is contaminated with dilute urine or water.

Malabsorption is diagnosed by fecal fat detection, generally screened using qualitative tests and verified with quantified fat on a 72-h collection while the patient is ingesting >100g fat/day. Fecal fat exceeding 7 g/24 h is abnormal; however, severe diarrhea (>800 g stool/24 h) can wash fat from the bowel lumen and result in fat excretion as high as 14 g/24 h.

Lower endoscopy is indicated if there are signs of mucosal injury and even if the endoscopic appearance of the colon is normal, random biopsies should be performed to evaluate for collagenous and lymphocytic colitis. If a small intestinal etiology of malabsorption is suspected, upper endoscopy may be performed to evaluate for inflammation or malabsorption disorders such as celiac disease.

Breath testing also is used to detect bacterial overgrowth as well as lactase deficiency. Arteriography or mesenteric resonance imaging may be necessary to confirm the diagnosis of mesenteric ischemia. In selected instances, ^{14}C-triolein breath tests can provide evidence of fat malabsorption, whereas D-xylose testing can screen for small intestinal mucosal disease. Schilling tests help distinguish small bowel disease, bacterial overgrowth, and pancreatic disease as causes of malabsorption. Pancreatic etiologies, including chronic pancreatitis and pancreatic neoplasms, can be evaluated by abdominal radiography, endoscopic retrograde pancreatography, endoscopic ultrasound, or exocrine pancreatic function tests in selected referral centers.

Secretory diarrhea should be evaluated by serum gastrin, vasoactive intestinal peptide (VIP), serotonin, calcitonin, histamine, and prostaglandins and urine

5-hydroxyindoleacetic acid to detect endocrine neoplasia. Further evaluation with abdominal computed tomography (CT), endoscopic ultrasound, and somatostatin receptor scintigraphy is performed to localize the tumor(s) and direct therapy. Octapeptide (^{111}In-OTPA) cholecystokinin analog scanning has been used for medullary thyroid carcinoma. Rare patients will benefit from ^{111}In-labeled leukocyte tests for inflammatory disease or ^{51}Cr-albumin or α_1-antitrypsin tests that demonstrate protein-losing enteropathy.

Differential diagnosis

High-output diarrhea of more than 200 g daily arises from two pathophysiological mechanisms: increased anion secretion and decreased absorption of electrolytes. Increased anion secretion may result from enterotoxins, endogenous hormones or neuropeptides, inflammatory mediators, bile salts, laxatives, and medications. Decreased water and electrolyte absorption develop from enterotoxins, decreased mucosal absorptive surface area, acceleration of transit with inadequate time for absorption, impaired mucosal barrier function, and ingestion of poorly absorbed osmotically active solutes. Conditions that produce high-output diarrhea are divided into osmotic, secretory, and mucosal injury categories (Table 10.1) although some diseases produce diarrhea by more than one mechanism. Patients with normal stool output of less than 200 g daily may also complain of diarrhea. Normal-output diarrhea most often results from anorectal disease, hormonally induced hyperdefecation, or functional bowel disorders in which gut sensorimotor defects alter perception and transit of lumenal contents.

Osmotic diarrhea

Under normal conditions, most ingested food is absorbed before it reaches the colon. In many diarrheal disorders, undigested nutrients are not absorbed and act as osmotic agents to draw free water into the intestinal lumen. The most common cause of osmotic diarrhea is lactase deficiency. Other causes of osmotic diarrhea include nonabsorbable laxatives, magnesium-containing antacids, medications, and candies or soft drinks that contain the poorly absorbed sugars fructose and sorbitol. Congenital defects of carbohydrate absorption include sucrase-isomaltase deficiency, trehalase deficiency, and glucose-galactose malabsorption.

Some small intestinal diseases produce osmotic diarrhea from maldigestion or malabsorption. Celiac disease is caused by hypersensitivity to dietary gluten. Patients with this disease may be asymptomatic, exhibit iron deficiency anemia, or develop diarrhea and malabsorptive symptoms. Tropical sprue is an infectious disease of unknown origin that is observed on the Indian subcontinent, Asia, the West Indies, northern South America, central and southern Africa, and Central

Table 10.1 Causes of diarrhea

Osmotic diarrhea	
Nonabsorbed solutes	Magnesium, sulfate and phosphate laxatives
	Sorbitol, fructose, lactulose
Disaccharidase deficiency	Lactase deficiency
	Isomaltase-sucrase deficiency
	Trehalase deficiency
Small intestinal mucosal disease	Celiac disease
	Tropical sprue
	Viral gastroenteritis
	Whipple disease
	Amyloidosis
	Intestinal ischemia
	Lymphoma
	Giardiasis
	Intestinal radiation
	Mastocytosis
	Eosinophilic gastroenteritis
	Abetalipoproteinemia
	Lymphangiectasia
Pancreatic insufficiency	Chronic pancreatitis
	Pancreatic carcinoma
	Cystic fibrosis
Reduced intestinal surface area	Small intestinal resection
	Enteric fistulae
	Jejunoileal bypass
Bile salt malabsorption	Bacterial overgrowth
	Ileal resection
	Crohn's disease
Other medications	Olestra and orlistat
Secretory diarrhea	
Laxatives	Bisacodyl
	Ricinoleic acid
	Dioctyl sodium sulfosuccinate
	Senna and aloe
	Oxyphenisatin
Medications	Diuretics
	Thyroid supplements
	Theophylline
	Colchicine
	Quinidine
	Selective serotonin reuptake inhibitors
Bacterial toxins	*Vibrio cholerae*
	Enterotoxigenic *Escherichia coli*
	Staphylococcus aureus
	Bacillus cereus
	Clostridium perfringens

(continued)

Table 10.1 (*cont'd*)

Hormonally induced	Vasoactive intestinal polypeptide
	Serotonin
	Calcitonin
	Glucagon
	Gastrin
	Substance P
	Prostaglandins
Defective neural control	Diabetic diarrhea
Bile acid diarrhea	Ileal resection
	Crohn's disease
	Bacterial overgrowth
	Post cholecystectomy
Mucosal inflammation	Collagenous colitis
	Lymphocytic colitis
Defective transport	Congenital chloridorrhea
	Villous adenoma
Mucosal injury diarrhea	
Inflammatory bowel disease	Crohn's disease
	Ulcerative colitis
Acute infections	Viruses (rotavirus, Norwalk agent)
	Parasites (*Giardia, Cryptosporidium, Cyclospora*)
	E. coli (enteroinvasive, enterohemorrhagic)
	Shigella
	Salmonella
	Campylobacter
	Yersinia enterocolitica
	Entamoeba histolytica (amebiasis: acute or chronic)
Chronic infections	*Clostridium difficile*
	Nematode infestation
Ischemia	Atherosclerosis
	Vasculitis
Normal-volume diarrhea	
Functional bowel disorders	Irritable bowel syndrome
Endocrinopathies	Hyperthyroidism
Proctitis	Ulcerative proctitis
	Infectious proctitis
Fecal incontinence	Surgical and obstetrical trauma
	Hemorrhoids
	Anal fissures
	Perianal fistulae
	Anal neuropathy (diabetes)

America. It produces diarrhea and malabsorption due to villous atrophy in persons who have resided in these regions for as little as 1–3 months. Crohn's disease involving the small intestine may lead to malabsorption and diarrhea. Whipple disease, caused by infection with *Tropheryma whippelii,* is diagnosed by demonstration of characteristic periodic acid–Schiff (PAS)-positive macrophages on examination of small intestinal mucosal biopsies. Congenital or acquired (secondary to trauma, lymphoma, or carcinoma) intestinal lymphangiectasia causes protein-losing enteropathy with steatorrhea as a result of obstructed lymphatic channels. Bacterial overgrowth produces steatorrhea from bile salt deconjugation, brush border injury, and mucosal inflammation. Intestinal infection with *Giardia, Cryptosporidium, Isospora,* or *Mycobacterium avium* complex produces brush border and intramucosal damage. Systemic mastocytosis and eosinophilic gastroenteritis grossly distort the intestinal mucosa and promote nutrient malabsorption. Short bowel syndrome and fistulae reduce the villous surface area available for nutrient uptake. Other conditions (e.g. postvagotomy diarrhea and thyrotoxicosis) accelerate intestinal transit, leaving inadequate time for nutrient assimilation. Adrenal insufficiency causes generalized disturbances in mucosal absorption.

Pancreaticobiliary diseases also are common causes of osmotic diarrhea with maldigestion and malabsorption that manifest with steatorrhea. Cirrhosis and bile duct obstruction can produce maldigestion because of the impaired delivery of bile salt to the small intestine, which then leads to poor micelle formation with ingested fats.

Secretory diarrhea

The most common causes of acute secretory diarrhea are enterotoxins released by infectious organisms. Viruses (e.g. rotavirus, Norwalk agent) are also likely to act through toxins. In some AIDS patients, secretory diarrhea results from defined organisms (*Cryptosporidium, Mycobacterium avium* complex), but other cases are idiopathic. Laxatives represent the other common cause of secretory diarrhea.

Rare cases of secretory diarrhea result from overproduction of circulating agents that stimulate secretion. Carcinoid syndrome classically presents with watery diarrhea and flushing, which are consequences of secreting serotonin, histamine, catecholamines, kinins, and prostaglandins. Diarrhea is the major symptom in 10% of patients with gastrinoma and exhibits both secretory and osmotic characteristics. Overproduction of VIP by VIPoma tumors produces the syndrome of watery diarrhea, hypokalemia, and achlorhydria (WDHA), in which patients often pass more than 3 L of stool daily. Medullary carcinoma of the thyroid, which may be sporadic or part of the multiple endocrine neoplasia (MEN type IIA) syndrome, causes secretory diarrhea because of the release of calcitonin. Glucagonoma causes mild diarrhea as well as characteristic rashes (migratory necrolytic erythema), glossitis, cheilitis, neuropsychiatric manifestations, and thromboembolism. Systemic mastocytosis produces a mixed secretory and osmotic diarrhea associated with flushing. Villous adenomas larger than 3 cm in diameter produce secretory diarrhea, possibly secondary to prostaglandin production.

Other disorders also cause secretory diarrhea. Collagenous and lymphocytic colitis induce active colonic secretion of water and electrolytes. Bile salt diarrhea results from stimulation of colonic secretion. Multiple factors contribute to the pathogenesis of diabetic diarrhea; however, the response of this condition to the somatostatin analog octreotide suggests a prominent secretory component. Furthermore, improvement in diabetic diarrhea with the α-adrenoceptor agonist clonidine suggests a pathogenic imbalance between absorptive adrenergic and secretory cholinergic mucosal function. Diabetic diarrhea presents in patients with long-standing diabetes and characteristically is profuse, watery, nocturnal, and associated with severe urgency. Chronic alcoholics may develop severe watery diarrhea, which may be partly secretory. Ten percent to 25% of long-distance runners develop diarrhea, which is postulated to result from release of gastrin, motilin, VIP, or prostaglandins.

Mucosal injury diarrhea

Conditions that injure the small intestinal or colonic mucosa lead to passive secretion of fluids from damaged epithelia and alterations in electrolyte and water absorption. Small intestinal infections that produce mucosal injury diarrhea include yersiniosis, tuberculosis, and histoplasmosis. Chronic mucosal injury diarrhea may result from inflammatory bowel diseases such as Crohn's disease and ulcerative colitis, ischemic colitis, and radiation enterocolitis. Other diseases that manifest as inflammatory diarrhea include eosinophilic gastroenteritis, milk and soy protein allergy, Behçet syndrome, Cronkhite–Canada syndrome, graft-versus-host disease, and Churg–Strauss syndrome.

Normal-output diarrhea

It is not uncommon for patients with chronic diarrhea to present with stools of normal daily volume. Many of these individuals pass frequent, small, well-formed stools that are associated with urgency and a sense of incomplete evacuation. The most common cause of chronic diarrhea in the United States is irritable bowel syndrome. Endocrinopathies such as hyperthyroidism alter colonic motor activity, leading to passage of multiple low-volume stools. Proctitis also is a common cause of low-volume, frequent stools. Fecal impaction in institutionalized or hospitalized patients may cause diarrhea from flow of fluid around the obstructing bolus (pseudo-diarrhea).

Discussion and potential pitfalls

Irritable bowel syndrome (IBS) is the most common etiology of chronic diarrhea in the United States. In a young person without alarm symptoms or signs such as overt or occult gastrointestinal bleeding, weight loss or anemia, the presence of diarrhea and abdominal pain relieved with defecation is most likely diarrhea-predominant IBS. Basic laboratory tests to evaluate for anemia and malabsorption, and stool examination for chronic infection are generally sufficient to make a positive diagnosis of IBS. In the correct demographic, serology and/or genetic testing for celiac disease may also be obtained.

Diagnostic investigation

Acute diarrhea

The major focus of evaluation of acute diarrhea is exclusion of infectious etiologies. Stool cultures routinely examine for *Salmonella, Shigella,* and *Campylobacter*. It may be necessary to specify cultures to include enterohemorrhagic *E. coli, Yersinia* and *Plesiomonas*. Ova and parasites to detect *Giardia, Cryptosporidium, E. histolytica,* or *Strongyloides* may be considered. Stool antigen tests are available for *Giardia*. In individuals with recent antibiotic use, stools should be sent for *C. difficile* toxin determination. Twenty percent to 40% of cases of acute infectious diarrheas remain undiagnosed despite laboratory evaluation.

Chronic diarrhea

Most patients with chronic diarrhea require additional tests to complement the history and physical examination findings (Figure 10.1). Chronic infections should be excluded by stool examination for ova and parasites, *C. difficile* toxin, and selected bacterial cultures. If infection is present, directed therapy should be initiated. The next step is to differentiate inflammatory from noninflammatory etiologies of chronic diarrhea. An elevated erythrocyte sedimentation rate (ESR) or C-reactive protein (CRP) raises concern for inflammatory disease. The presence of leukocytes and erythrocytes in the stool confirms inflammatory diarrhea. Flexible sigmoidoscopy or colonoscopy should be performed to

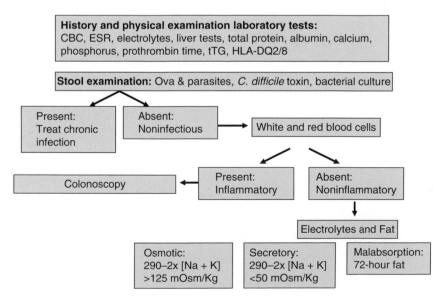

Figure 10.1 Chronic diarrhea. CBC, complete blood count; ESR, erythrocyte sedimentation rate; tTG, tissue transglutaminase.

evaluate for the presence of mucosal injury, which occurs in inflammatory bowel disease or invasive infections.

In the absence of inflammatory indicators, stool should be examined to rule out the presence of malabsorption. Steatorrhea is a separate entity from diarrhea but symptoms can overlap; therefore, stool should be examined for fat, initially qualitatively and if positive, verified quantitatively. Serum albumin and globulin may be reduced by malabsorption, malnutrition, or protein-losing enteropathy. Protein and hemoglobin levels tend to be lower with small intestinal versus pancreatic etiologies of malabsorption. Tissue transglutaminase antibodies are positive in many cases of celiac disease, and the diagnosis is excluded by the absence of HLA-DQ2/8 defects.

Discrimination of noninflammatory, nonmalabsorptive diarrhea into osmotic or secretory causes is performed by stool electrolytes. Osm gaps >125 mOsm/kg are consistent with osmotic diarrhea and gaps <50 mOsm/kg are normal, indicating secretory processes; gaps between these values are inconsistently classified and investigation into both categories may be warranted.

Finally, exclusion of structural/organic causes of chronic diarrhea is consistent with functional conditions, including irritable bowel syndrome. Note, however, that in the correct setting an IBS diagnosis can be made positively without the need for invasive testing.

Management

Acute diarrhea

Therapy for diarrhea depends on its severity and its cause. Fluid resuscitation is crucial in cases of severe diarrhea. Oral rehydration solutions maximize intestinal absorption and should be started early in the course of illness. Intravenous crystalloid solutions are indicated for hypotensive patients or those who cannot drink. Serum electrolytes should be closely monitored. Zinc and magnesium losses may be significant with chronic diarrhea, so specific replacement therapy may be needed. Acute infectious diarrhea without bleeding, severe dehydration, or host factors that impair the ability to clear the infection can be treated symptomatically with antidiarrheal agents and rehydration. The antidiarrheal effects of bismuth subsalicylate in traveler's diarrhea may stem from both antimicrobial and antisecretory properties. For complicated or prolonged infection unresponsive to supportive care, liquid stools should be sent for culture and positive results appropriately treated.

Antibiotic therapy of acute infectious diarrhea depends on the causative organism. Antibiotics are indicated for shigellosis, cholera, some cases of traveler's diarrhea, antibiotic-associated colitis, parasites, and sexually transmitted infections. Treatment with an antibiotic is usually recommended for noncholera vibrios, prolonged *Yersinia* infection, early *Campylobacter, Aeromonas,* and *Plesiomonas* infections, and day-care outbreaks of enteropathogenic *E. coli*. Antibiotic treatment of O157:H7 enterohemorrhagic *E. coli* infection is not recommended because it may predispose to development of hemolytic uremic syndrome. Antibiotics also are indicated for chronic diarrhea secondary to bacterial overgrowth, tropical sprue, and Whipple disease. Viral diarrhea and cryptosporidiosis usually are not treated specifically.

Chronic diarrhea

Lactose restriction is indicated for lactase deficiency, whereas a gluten-free diet is the appropriate treatment for celiac disease. Inflammatory bowel diseases are treated with specific anti-inflammatory medications, whereas pancreatic enzyme replacement is indicated for chronic pancreatitis. For secretory diarrhea secondary to endocrine neoplasia, AIDS, or diabetes, the somatostatin analog octreotide has antisecretory and motor-retarding properties that provide effective antidiarrheal action. Octreotide may also prevent other manifestations of hormone oversecretion such as flushing and tachycardia with carcinoid syndrome. Parenteral calcitonin has shown utility in controlling diarrhea from VIPoma and carcinoid tumors. The α-adrenoceptor agonist clonidine treats diabetic diarrhea and diarrhea associated with opiate withdrawal. Indomethacin is occasionally effective for diarrhea secondary to endocrine tumors and food allergy.

For diseases that do not have a specific treatment, therapy relies on medications that stimulate absorption, inhibit secretion, or retard transit to afford time for improved fluid absorption. The opiate derivatives loperamide, diphenoxylate, codeine, and paregoric are the most common nonspecific treatments for diarrhea and act to retard gut transit by evoking a segmenting motor pattern to promote increased fluid absorption. Cholestyramine binds bile acids and some toxins and may be useful in some cases. Diarrhea secondary to irritable bowel syndrome may be controlled with antispasmodic drugs such as hyoscyamine, a tricyclic antidepressant, or a serotonin receptor antagonist in cases refractory to opiate agents.

Complications

Most cases of diarrhea in the United States result only in loss of productive work and personal time. However, in other regions of the world and in high-risk patients in the United States (e.g. persons with AIDS), diarrhea is a major cause of morbidity and mortality, especially in children. Diarrhea causes up to 8 million deaths of children yearly because of severe volume depletion or electrolyte disturbances. This group requires aggressive fluid and electrolyte replacement, intravenously with crystalloid formulations or orally with glucose-electrolyte combinations (e.g. the World Health Organization solution) or commercial formulas (e.g. Pedialyte and Infalyte).

Case studies

Case 1

A 23-year-old man presents with 3 weeks of bloody diarrhea. He mentions 8–10 bowel movements daily that are watery and associated with tenesmus. Associated symptoms include bilateral lower quadrant abdominal pain, fatigue and low-grade fevers. He has lost 5 kg over the past 3 weeks and has diminished appetite. He has no recent travel and no prior history of prolonged diarrhea. On physical examination, he is pale and appears tired. His blood pressure is 95/60 with a pulse of 96 bpm and a temperature of 38°C. His examination is notable for dry mucous membranes and bilateral lower quadrant abdominal tenderness, left greater than right, without rebound or guarding. His rectal examination is notable for blood and stool with normal sphincter tone. Laboratory tests include a white blood count of 15.3, Hb 9.1 mg/dL, platelet count 475,000. Liver tests, INR and amylase are normal. Stool tests reveal white and red blood cells, negative *C. difficile* toxin, and negative bacterial cultures and examination for ova and parasites. Abdominal CT scan reveals thickening of the colonic wall from cecum to rectum, with a cecal diameter of 12 cm.

> **Discussion**
>
> This patient has evidence of mucosal injury diarrhea. After elimination of infectious etiologies, the most likely diagnosis is inflammatory bowel disease. The CT findings of pancolonic inflammation favor a diagnosis of ulcerative colitis. The preferred method for evaluating the presence of inflammatory bowel disease is lower endoscopy. With a patient as ill as depicted in this scenario, an unprepped flexible sigmoidoscopy is likely adequate for establishing the diagnosis. Colonoscopy may be hazardous even without evidence of toxic megacolon, and formal assessment of the extent of the patient's disease should be deferred until his condition improves.

Case 2

A 23-year-old woman presents with abdominal pain and diarrhea for over 1 year. She complains of multiple episodes of watery to loose bowel movements that occur 1–2 times per week. There is no blood in her stool, but she describes lower abdominal pain prior to the diarrhea, which is relieved with defecation. She has not lost weight and is eating normally. Between episodes she feels well, and the symptoms never awaken her from sleep. Physical examination reveals a well-developed woman with normal vital signs. Her abdominal examination is notable for minor bilateral lower quadrant tenderness without rebound or guarding and there are no masses or enlarged organs. Laboratory tests include a normal complete blood count, electrolytes, liver tests and amylase, with an albumin of 4.2 mg/dL. Stool tests are negative for white or red cells, *C. difficile* toxin, and ova and parasites × 3 evaluations.

Discussion

This patient has no evidence of mucosal injury or inflammation. The most likely diagnoses include irritable bowel syndrome and carbohydrate malabsorption. An acceptable management strategy would include an elimination diet trial, starting with lactose-containing foods. If this is unsuccessful, symptomatic treatment of diarrhea-predominant irritable bowel syndrome with antidiarrheals would be indicated. Persistent symptoms could be evaluated with lower endoscopy with biopsies to evaluate for inflammatory bowel disease, and/or HLA-DQ2/DQ8 to identify susceptibility for celiac disease, neither of which is likely based on the normal laboratory tests.

Key practice points

- Chronic diarrhea is generally defined as loose, watery or voluminous stools for 3 weeks or more.
- Stool should be examined for chronic infection and for evidence of mucosal injury or inflammation. If red or white cells are present, endoscopic evaluation is indicated to evaluate for inflammatory bowel disease, infections, ischemia and other ulcerating diseases.
- In the absence of mucosal injury, stool electrolytes are helpful to differentiate between osmotic and secretory causes of diarrhea.
- Fecal fat is used to identify patients with malabsorption.
- Motility and functional disorders such as irritable bowel syndrome will present without inflammation, malabsorption or osmotic markers.

CHAPTER 11

Approach to the Patient with an Abdominal Mass

Mass lesions in the abdomen may arise from localized infection or from inflammation, trauma, vascular disease, or neoplasm. These can be difficult to distinguish from the history and physical examination alone, given that the clinical presentation often is nonspecific. Careful radiological or endoscopic characterization of the lesion is important because the etiology determines the clinical management and prognosis.

Clinical presentation

History

The history provides important clues to the etiology of an abdominal mass. Pain related to meals or defecation suggests a lumenal origin, whereas gross or occult fecal bleeding or alterations in bowel function suggest either a primary source within or invasion of a lumenal site. Nausea and vomiting with abdominal distension raise concern for an obstructive process within the proximal gut. Dysuria or hematuria may indicate involvement of the urinary tract either by primary disease or by local irritation, as with Crohn's disease. Jaundice suggests benign or malignant obstruction at the level of the pancreas or bile ducts. Impingement of a large mass on surrounding vasculature may present with lower extremity edema or intestinal ischemia. Ascites may indicate peritoneal metastases from an intra-abdominal malignancy or a worsening of liver function in a cirrhotic patient with hepatocellular carcinoma. High fever points toward an intra-abdominal abscess, whereas unexpected loss of more than 5% of body weight raises suspicion of malignancy. Medications may predispose to selected liver masses (e.g. hepatic adenoma with oral contraceptive use). Paraneoplastic syndromes may suggest specific malignancies: pseudoachalasia may relate to hepatocellular carcinoma, dermatomyositis may develop with lumenal cancer, seborrheic keratoses (Leser–Trélat sign) or acanthosis nigricans are seen with gastric cancer, and deep venous thromboses (Trousseau

Yamada's Handbook of Gastroenterology, Third Edition. Edited by Tadataka Yamada and John M. Inadomi.
© 2013 John Wiley & Sons, Ltd. Published 2013 by John Wiley & Sons, Ltd.

syndrome) are found with intra-abdominal adenocarcinoma. A family history of neoplasia or inflammatory bowel disease may suggest these as etiologies.

Physical examination

A general physical examination as well as directed assessment of the mass complements the history. Scleral icterus or jaundice suggests liver infiltration versus biliary obstruction from a bile duct or pancreatic tumor. Temperature higher than 38°C is consistent with an infectious or inflammatory process such as an intra-abdominal abscess. Lower fevers may accompany some neoplasms. If the mass is tender, as with Crohn's disease, this suggests that the mass is inflammatory. Lymphadenopathy raises concern for metastatic malignancy. Palpable supraclavicular (Virchow) or periumbilical (Sister Mary Joseph) nodes are found with gastric cancer. Rectal examination detects approximately half of all rectal neoplasms. Occult fecal blood is highly predictive of malignancy in a patient with a known abdominal mass.

Additional testing

Laboratory studies

Laboratory tests are important in evaluating selected abdominal masses. A complete blood count can test for anemia due to blood loss or chronic disease or for leukocytosis with inflammation or localized infection such as an abscess. Liver chemistry levels are abnormal with some hepatobiliary neoplasms. Determination of chronic liver chemistry abnormalities with the new onset of a liver mass suggests possible hepatocellular carcinoma arising in pre-existing cirrhosis. Amylase and lipase values may be elevated in some pancreatic cancers. Endocrine neoplasms may secrete hormones that can be detected by specific blood tests or measurement of urinary metabolites. Serum tumor markers may provide adjunctive information in the diagnostic work-up. CA-19-9 and CA-242 are reasonably sensitive for detecting pancreatic adenocarcinoma but are not specific. Carcinoembryonic antigen is elevated with colon cancer as well as with benign liver and pancreatic diseases. α-Fetoprotein is secreted by larger hepatocellular carcinomas. Ovarian tumors are suggested by elevations of CA-125.

If ascites is present, cytological examination may reveal malignant cells. Serologies for infections such as echinococcosis may be obtained for suspicious cystic liver masses. A high level of triglycerides in the ascitic fluid indicates chylous ascites possibly due to lymphoma. Hematuria is worrisome for urological malignancy versus bladder or ureteral involvement by intra-abdominal tumors. Aspiration of pus with Gram stain and culture can provide both a diagnosis and treatment of selected intra-abdominal abscesses.

Structural studies

Endoscopy of the gastrointestinal tract is useful in evaluating suspected lumenal masses because of the ability to visualize suspicious lesions directly and to obtain biopsies. Routine upper endoscopy evaluates to the descending duodenum. Enteroscopy can be used to evaluate more distal small intestinal masses. Push enteroscopy can reach lesions in the upper jejunum. When there is no evidence of obstruction, capsule endoscopy may detect unsuspected small bowel tumors in patients with unexplained blood loss. Sigmoidoscopy examines the colon distal to the splenic flexure in optimally prepared patients, whereas colonoscopy visualizes the entire organ as well as the distal ileum. Endoscopic retrograde cholangiopancreatography defines filling defects within the pancreas or biliary tree and can obtain diagnostic brushings in approximately 50% of pancreatico-biliary neoplasms. Endoscopic ultrasound provides additional detail in characterizing tumors of the gut lumen and pancreaticobiliary tree and can determine if local disease extension precludes surgical resection.

Radiological and radionuclide imaging techniques are useful for evaluating suspected masses in the solid organs of the abdomen, pelvis, and retroperitoneum and in regions of the gut lumen that are poorly investigated by endoscopic techniques. Ultrasound is an effective screening examination for imaging the biliary tree and liver. Computed tomography (CT) provides a more detailed and comprehensive evaluation of suspected neoplasia in many organs. Specialized dedicated protocols have been developed to focus on selected regions such as the pancreas. Both techniques are of value in diagnosing intra-abdominal abscess as well. Both modalities can be used to direct needle aspiration or biopsy of suspected lesions. Magnetic resonance imaging is especially useful in the study of selected liver masses and can help delineate the presence of hemangiomas, focal nodular hyperplasia, adenomas, and other abnormalities. Magnetic resonance cholangiopancreatography can assess for abnormalities within the bile and pancreatic ducts. Selected nuclear medicine tests are indicated in evaluating certain abdominal masses. Octreoscanning has assumed a crucial role in investigating suspected endocrine neoplasia. ^{111}In-labeled leukocyte scans may define the extent and locations of intra-abdominal abscesses. ^{18}F-fluorodeoxyglucose positron emission tomography is emerging as a promising modality for characterizing selected intra-abdominal malignancies.

Histopathological evaluation

In many instances, tissue must be obtained to distinguish accurately between a malignant and a noncancerous etiology of a radiographically or endoscopically detected mass. For solitary liver lesions, a directed biopsy can be obtained under laparoscopic guidance. If radiographic testing suggests hepatic adenoma, surgical resection is advised rather than biopsy due to the risk of hemorrhage. When multiple liver lesions suggest metastases, computed tomography or ultrasound can be used to direct percutaneous biopsy. Percutaneous biopsy is not recommended for suspected renal cell cancer because of the risk of seeding the needle tract with malignant cells. For suspected resectable pancreatic cancer, tissue is best obtained using endoscopic retrograde cholangiopancreatography or endoscopic ultrasound.

Mucosal masses in the stomach, colon, and rectum often are easily accessible to endoscopy for biopsy. Tissue from submucosal masses may be obtained by fine needle aspiration under endoscopic ultrasound guidance.

Differential diagnosis

The differential diagnosis of abdominal masses is broad (Table 11.1). The likelihood of finding unresectable neoplasm also is highly variable, depending on the anatomical site of its origin. Many intra-abdominal masses present with pain, whereas others present with bleeding, systemic symptoms such as weight loss or fever, or obstruction. Others are detected while still asymptomatic as part of a routine healthcare surveillance program.

Liver masses
Both solid and cystic masses may develop in the liver. Causes of single solid hepatic masses include hemangiomas, adenomas, focal nodular hyperplasia, focal fatty infiltration, leiomyomas, teratomas, hepatocellular carcinoma, lymphomas, sarcomas, and solitary metastases from distant cancer. The presence of multiple solid lesions should prompt a search for extrahepatic malignancy, most commonly from the breast, colon, or lung. Cystic masses include benign cysts, bacterial liver abscesses (which may be multiple), amebic abscess, and echinococcal cysts.

Pancreaticobiliary masses
Most solid masses in the pancreas are malignant. Pancreatic adenocarcinoma usually arises from pancreatic ductal epithelium. Other solid pancreatic masses include lymphoma, solid and papillary epithelial neoplasms, and neuroendocrine tumors (insulinomas, gastrinomas, glucagonomas, somatostatinomas, VIPomas). Pancreatic masses with cystic components include pancreatic pseudocysts complicating pancreatitis, mucinous or serous cystadenoma, cystadenocarcinoma, and intraductal papillary mucinous tumors.

Masses of the biliary tree also may be cystic or solid. Cystic lesions include choledochal cysts and Caroli disease, which is characterized by segmental dilation of the intrahepatic bile ducts. Cholangiocarcinoma is the most common malignant tumor of the bile ducts. Other biliary tumors include gallbladder carcinoma, bile duct adenomas, cystadenomas, and granular cell tumors.

Gastrointestinal masses
Masses involving the lumenal gastrointestinal tract are prevalent. Adenocarcinoma accounts for 95% of gastric cancers. Lymphoma is the second most common cell type. Small intestinal masses more commonly are benign and include adenomas, hamartoma, fibromas, and angiomas. Adenocarcinoma,

Table 11.1 Causes of abdominal masses

Hepatic masses
Hemangioma
Adenoma
Focal nodular hyperplasia
Focal fatty infiltration
Hepatocellular carcinoma
Lymphoma
Sarcoma
Leiomyoma
Teratoma
Metastatic tumor
Abscess
Benign cysts
Echinococcal cyst

Pancreaticobiliary masses
Pancreatic adenocarcinoma
Lymphoma
Neuroendocrine tumors
Pseudocysts
Abscess
Mucinous and serous cystadenoma
Cystadenocarcinoma
Intraductal papillary mucinous tumors
Bile duct adenoma
Choledochocele
Cholangiocarcinoma
Gallbladder carcinoma
Granular cell tumor

Gastrointestinal masses
Adenocarcinoma
Adenoma
Lymphoma
Hyperplastic polyps
Hamartoma
Leiomyoma
Leiomyosarcoma
Leioblastoma
Kaposi sarcoma
Carcinoid
Colitis cystica profunda
Lipoma
Liposarcoma
Angioma
Neuroma
Schwannoma
Inflammatory mass (Crohn's disease, appendicitis)
Abscess

Table 11.1 (*cont'd*)

Miscellaneous masses
Renal cell carcinoma
Renal cyst
Transitional cell carcinoma of the renal pelvis
Renal lymphoma
Mesenteric cyst
Cystic teratoma
Mesothelioma
Hematoma
Abdominal aortic aneurysm
Ovarian carcinoma
Ovarian cyst
Uterine fibroma
Uterine carcinoma
Tubo-ovarian abscess
Ectopic pregnancy

leiomyosarcoma, and lymphoma are malignancies that arise from the small intestine. The most common colorectal masses are benign polyps, including non-adenomatous (hyperplastic, hamartoma) and adenomatous growths. Polyps may be sporadic, occur in those with risk factors such as a positive family history or long-standing colitis, or arise as part of a hereditary polyposis syndrome.

Adenocarcinomas constitute the majority of colorectal cancers, although lymphoma and Kaposi sarcoma also occur. Benign colonic masses may be due to perforation of an inflamed appendix, selected infections (e.g. amebiasis), or inflammation from Crohn's disease. The appearance of colorectal cancer can be mimicked by colitis cystica profunda, a benign disease characterized by submucosal mucus-filled cysts. Carcinoids arise most commonly in the appendix, followed by the ileum, rectum, and stomach. Gastrinomas may originate in the pancreas or in the proximal bowel wall. Tumors originating from smooth muscle (leiomyoma, leiomyosarcoma) or fat (lipoma, liposarcoma) may be seen throughout the digestive tract. Less common cell types include neurofibromas, schwannomas, and leioblastomas.

Miscellaneous masses

Miscellaneous lesions may present as abdominal masses. Renal masses may be infectious, neoplastic, or congenital. The most common malignancy is renal cell carcinoma. Other neoplasms include transitional cell carcinoma of the renal pelvis with parenchymal invasion, lymphoma, and renal oncocytoma. Renal cysts most commonly are benign but may harbor carcinoma, especially in patients with von Hippel–Lindau or tuberous sclerosis. Cystic masses in the mesentery include mesenteric cysts, cystic teratomas, and cystic mesotheliomas. A hematoma is considered in any patient with a history of blunt abdominal trauma. Abdominal aortic aneurysms may be detected as pulsatile abdominal masses. Gynecological masses involving the ovaries or uterus may be palpable on abdominal examination.

Management

Management of an intra-abdominal mass depends on the nature of the mass and whether it is malignant, has disseminated, and is no longer surgically resectable. In general, solitary neoplasms are best cured by operative removal. Additional benefit may be obtained with adjuvant chemotherapy with or without concomitant radiotherapy in some settings, as with certain colorectal carcinomas. Intra-abdominal carcinomas with local or distant spread that preclude resection may be subjected to systemic chemotherapy with variable, often disappointing results. Other multifocal neoplasms such as lymphomas may be more responsive to cytotoxic chemotherapy. Some endocrine tumors may respond to hormonal suppression using chronic therapy with the somatostatin analog octreotide. Abdominal abscesses should be drained percutaneously or surgically and therapy should be directed at the underlying cause (e.g. active Crohn's disease). Pancreatic pseudocysts can be drained percutaneously, endoscopically, or surgically. Finally, endoscopy can be used to remove large polyps (including some with superficial carcinoma) using a snare and retrieval technique.

Complications

The complications associated with an abdominal mass depend on its location and histological characteristics. Lumenal obstruction results from gut mucosal tumors, whereas biliary obstruction is a consequence of bile duct or pancreatic masses. Certain masses such as hepatic adenomas may rupture and produce life-threatening hemorrhage. Abscesses may not respond to antibiotic therapy and may have lethal outcomes if not appropriately drained. Similarly, many malignant tumors are fatal, especially if dissemination has already occurred when diagnosed.

Case studies

Case 1

A 58-year-old woman presents to her physician with complaints of a new fullness in her mid-abdomen and progressive fatigue. She denies any symptoms of abdominal pain, nausea, vomiting or altered bowel movements. She has not seen any blood in her stool. On physical exam, she has a nontender abdomen but there is a firm mobile mass palpable just to the left of the umbilicus. Labs are notable for a hematocrit of

30, mean corpuscular volume (MCV) of 70, low serum iron, elevated total iron-binding capacity (TIBC), and low ferritin. CT scan demonstrated a 5 cm mass adjacent to the small bowel. Surgery is performed to remove the mass. Histology demonstrates a tumor with spindle cell morphology that stains positively for CD117 (C-KIT). In addition, there are >5 mitoses per high-power field. The tumor is diagnosed as a gastrointestinal stromal tumor (GIST) with features that are high risk for malignancy due to the size, location (small bowel), and mitotic rate. The patient is referred to an oncologist for consideration of adjuvant therapy with imatinib.

Discussion and potential pitfalls

Gastrointestinal stromal tumors (GISTs) are mesenchymal neoplasms that can occur anywhere along the GI tract. A majority of GISTs occur in the stomach, with the next most common location being the small bowel. GISTs are often asymptomatic but can also present with vague abdominal pain, obstructive symptoms (nausea and vomiting), GI bleeding due to ulceration, and fatigue due to iron deficiency anemia from chronic blood loss. The risk of malignant potential depends on the tumor size, mitotic rate, and location. GISTs and leiomyomas can be difficult to differentiate based on histology alone so immunohistochemistry (IHC) for CD117 (C-KIT) is recommended. However, in ~5% of cases IHC for CD117 can be negative due to a platelet-derived growth factor receptor-α (PDGFR-α) mutation.

Case 2

A 45-year-old man is referred to a gastroenterologist for evaluation of abdominal pain and symptoms of chronic flushing and diarrhea. The patient states that the flushing episodes typically last for 1–5 min and involve the face, neck, and upper chest. He cannot identify any particular triggers to the flushing episodes. In addition, he experiences watery diarrhea 3–4 times daily. On physical exam, he appears healthy with normal vital signs. His abdomen is nontender and no masses are palpable. Laboratory studies demonstrate an elevated urinary 5-hydroxyindoleacetic acid (HIAA) 250 mg in a 24-h urine collection and an elevated serum chromogranin A. In addition, a 24-h stool collection is consistent with a secretory diarrhea. A CT scan is performed that demonstrates a 3 cm vascular mass in the terminal ileum and multiple mestatic lesions in the liver. The patient is diagnosed with metastatic carcinoid. He is treated with depot octreotide with monthly intramuscular injections and loperamide for management of his symptoms. The patient is also referred to oncology for consideration of chemotherapy.

Discussion and potential pitfalls

Carcinoid tumors are neuroendocrine tumors. Patients who present with carcinoid syndrome (chronic flushing and/or diarrhea) usually have metastatic disease to the liver. Carcinoid tumors may occur anywhere in the GI tract and can also originate from the lungs, and rarely the kidneys or ovaries. Occasionally localization of the tumor can be challenging using conventional imaging methods such as CT or MRI. In cases where localization of the tumor is difficult, somatostatin receptor scintigraphy can be performed since over 90% of carcinoids have somatostatin receptors, which can be imaged using radiolabeled octreotide.

Key practice points

- Mass lesions in the abdomen may arise from localized infection or from inflammation, trauma, vascular disease, or neoplasm.
- Cross-sectional imaging is essential in localizing the mass and can provide additional information regarding the etiology of the mass.
- Mass lesions in the pancreas are often malignant.
- A biopsy may be indicated if it will change surgical management of the lesion.

CHAPTER 12

Approach to the Patient with Jaundice

Jaundice, a yellow discoloration of the sclera, skin, and mucous membranes, results from the accumulation of bilirubin, a by-product of heme metabolism. Of the 250–300 mg of bilirubin produced daily, 70% results from the reticuloendothelial breakdown of senescent erythrocytes. Bilirubin is cleared by the liver in a three-step process. It is first transported into hepatocytes by specific membrane carriers. It is then conjugated to one or two molecules of glucuronide. Finally, the conjugated bilirubin moves to the canalicular membrane, where it is excreted into the bile canaliculus by another carrier protein. Once in the bile, most conjugated bilirubin is excreted in the feces, although a small amount is deconjugated by colonic bacteria and reabsorbed. Colonic bacteria also reduce bilirubin to urobilinogens that are reabsorbed and excreted in urine. Any disturbance of this pathway can lead to hyperbilirubinemia and jaundice.

Normal bilirubin levels are 0.4 ± 0.2 mg/dL, and more than 95% is unconjugated. Hyperbilirubinemia is defined as a total bilirubin level higher than 1.5 mg/dL, an unconjugated level higher than 1.0 mg/dL, and a conjugated level higher than 0.3 mg/dL. Generally, the serum bilirubin level must exceed 2.5–3.0 mg/dL for jaundice to be visible. Hyperbilirubinemia is separated into two classes: unconjugated (>80% of total bilirubin) and conjugated (>30% of total bilirubin) (Table 12.1). With prolonged jaundice, circulating bilirubin may bind covalently to albumin, which prevents its elimination until the albumin is degraded. Therefore, with certain cholestatic disorders, measurable hyperbilirubinemia persists after the disease is resolved. Conjugated bilirubin is cleared by renal glomeruli; in renal failure, bilirubin levels may increase.

Conjugated hyperbilirubinemia

Causes of conjugated hyperbilirubinemia are listed in Table 12.1.

Yamada's Handbook of Gastroenterology, Third Edition. Edited by Tadataka Yamada and John M. Inadomi.

Table 12.1 Causes of conjugated hyperbilirubinemia

Congenital conjugated hyperbilirubinemias
Rotor syndrome
Dubin–Johnson syndrome

Intrahepatic cholestasis
Familial and congenital
Progressive familial intrahepatic cholestasis types 1–3
Benign recurrent intrahepatic cholestasis
Cholestasis of pregnancy
Choledochal cysts, Caroli disease
Congenital biliary atresia

Hepatocellular conditions
Alcohol-related disorders
Viral hepatitis
Autoimmune hepatitis
Cirrhosis
Drug-related hepatitis
Wilson disease
Hereditary hemochromatosis

Infiltrative conditions
Granulomatous
Carcinoma
Hematological malignant disease
Amyloidosis

Cholangiopathies
Primary biliary cirrhosis
Idiopathic adult ductopenia
Autoimmune (overlap) cholangiopathies

Infections
Bacterial
Fungal
Parasitic
HIV related

Miscellaneous causes
Postoperative sepsis
Pregnancy
Total parenteral nutrition
Cholestasis after liver transplantation
Drug hepatotoxicity

Extrahepatic cholestasis
Inside bile ducts
Calculi
Parasites

Table 12.1 (*cont'd*)

Inside wall
Stricture
Cholangiocarcinoma
Sclerosing cholangitis
Choledochal cysts
Outside duct wall
Tumor in porta hepatis
Tumor in pancreas
Pancreatitis, acute or chronic

Source: Yamada T et al. (eds) *Principles of Clinical Gastroenterology*. Oxford: Blackwell Publishing Ltd, 2008.

Congenital forms

Rotor syndrome is a rare, asymptomatic, autosomal recessive disorder that manifests as mild conjugated hyperbilirubinemia (2–5 mg/dL) in childhood. It is unclear whether the primary defect involves impaired hepatocyte secretion or impaired storage of bilirubin; although oral cholecystograms appear normal, biliary scintigraphy shows absent or delayed secretion. Dubin–Johnson syndrome is an asymptomatic autosomal recessive disorder from the impaired secretion of bilirubin, which produces serum bilirubin levels of 2–5 mg/dL. The results of scintigraphy and oral cholecystography are abnormal, whereas histological examination of the liver reveals darkly pigmented tissue. Patients with progressive familial intrahepatic cholestasis (PFIC) present with watery diarrhea, cholestasis, fat-soluble vitamin deficiency, jaundice, and occasionally pancreatitis caused by defective hepatic secretion of bile acids at the canalicular membrane. PFIC exists in different forms; all are autosomal recessive disorders, which have been mapped to several cloned transporters (FIC1, BSEP, MDR3). Choledochal cysts and Caroli disease are congenital malformations of the bile ducts and can manifest as jaundice or cholangitis, and eventually, cholangiocarcinoma. Choledochal cysts often are resectable, whereas Caroli disease (type IV choledochal cyst) usually requires liver transplantation for cure because of its diffuse intrahepatic nature.

Familial forms

Benign recurrent intrahepatic cholestasis (BRIC) presents with intense pruritus and elevated alkaline phosphatase levels, with mild increases in levels of aminotransferases and serum bilirubin (<10 mg/dL). Attacks, which begin from age 8 to 30, can last weeks to months, only to recur every several months to years. Liver biopsies reveal centrilobular cholestasis, which appears to be related to altered bile acid transport and enterohepatic circulation. BRIC is a milder form of PFIC-1 and, similarly, is caused by mutations in the *FIC1* gene. Cholestasis of pregnancy is an autosomal dominant trait that manifests in the third trimester as pruritus. This benign condition must be distinguished from acute fatty liver of pregnancy, toxemia, acute cholecystitis, and acute or chronic hepatitis.

Acquired forms

Acquired disorders constitute the largest group of diseases that manifest conjugated hyperbilirubinemia. Many of these conditions are associated with cholestasis and can exhibit symptoms of pruritus, hypercholesterolemia, and steatorrhea. Intrahepatic cholestasis may result from liver disease (e.g. fulminant hepatitis, chronic hepatitis with significant hepatocellular dysfunction, and the recovery phase of acute hepatitis), infections, and medications. Hyperbilirubinemia occurs in alcoholic patients with acute fatty liver, alcoholic hepatitis, and cirrhosis. Of patients with alcoholic hepatitis, 10–20% present with a predominantly cholestatic condition, which may have a poor prognosis if bilirubin levels exceed 10 mg/dL or if encephalopathy, renal failure, or coagulopathy develop. Primary hepatic malignancy, lymphoma, and metastatic carcinoma cause hyperbilirubinemia late in their courses, whereas cholangiocarcinoma and other biliary obstructing lesions produce early jaundice. Bone marrow transplant patients may develop jaundice because of chemotherapy-induced veno-oclusive disease and acute or chronic graft-versus-host disease. Postoperative jaundice may result from anesthesia, intrahepatic cholestasis, transfusions, hypotension, hypoxia, and hemolysis.

Rheumatological disorders (e.g. rheumatoid arthritis, systemic lupus erythematosus, and scleroderma) elevate alkaline phosphatase levels but rarely produce jaundice. Sjögren syndrome has an increased occurrence of antimitochondrial antibodies and is associated with primary biliary cirrhosis, which produces jaundice late in its course. Congestive heart failure, shock, and trauma may produce hyperbilirubinemia, whereas renal failure can exacerbate hyperbilirubinemia from any cause. Furthermore, obstructive jaundice increases the risk of renal insufficiency, especially in the postoperative period.

Infections can cause jaundice by bile duct obstruction (e.g. ascariasis), cholestasis (e.g. tuberculosis), or by sepsis and endotoxemia. Infections with *Legionella*, *Escherichia coli*, *Klebsiella*, *Pseudomonas*, *Proteus*, *Bacteroides*, and *Streptococcus* produce conjugated hyperbilirubinemia. Two-thirds of patients with acquired immunodeficiency syndrome have elevated levels of aminotransferases or alkaline phosphatase because of hepatitis, infectious sclerosing cholangitis, papillary stenosis, acalculous cholecystitis, malignancy, or medication effects, and all of these disorders may elevate bilirubin levels.

Hepatotoxicity accounts for 3.5% of adverse drug effects. Oral contraceptives induce intrahepatic cholestasis that leads to jaundice in up to 4 of 10,000 patients. Nonsteroidal anti-inflammatory drugs can cause hepatitis, cholestasis, granulomatous liver disease, and hypersensitivity reactions. Acetaminophen can produce dose-dependent hepatotoxicity, a condition that occurs at lower doses in individuals who consume significant quantities of alcohol. Alcohol induces expression of cytochrome P450 and leads to increased metabolism of acetaminophen to its hepatotoxic metabolite. Alcoholic patients also may have reduced glutathione stores secondary to chronic malnutrition. Isoniazid produces jaundice in 1% of patients. Chemotherapeutic agents delivered into the hepatic arterial circulation may cause a syndrome similar to sclerosing cholangitis. Numerous other medications affect the liver; when identified, the offending medication should be discontinued. Total parenteral nutrition causes hyperbilirubinemia as a result of intrahepatic cholestasis, infection, and the development of gallstones.

The common extrahepatic obstructive causes of jaundice include stones, blood, and malignant and benign strictures. Gallstone disease represents the most common cause of obstructive jaundice in the United States, although biliary parasitic infection is a common problem in certain areas of the world. The most common malignant causes include pancreatic carcinoma, cholangiocarcinoma, and lymphoma. Pancreatitis may produce swelling of the pancreatic head, leading to common bile duct obstruction. Primary sclerosing cholangitis (PSC) is most commonly associated with inflammatory bowel disease. With obstructive jaundice, alkaline phosphatase levels are elevated concurrently. For hyperbilirubinemia to develop, the bile ducts must be largely obstructed. Ductal dilation may not be detectable on radiographs for 72 h or in chronic liver disease, such as PSC.

Unconjugated hyperbilirubinemia

Hemolysis and ineffective erythropoiesis
Hemolysis and ineffective erythropoiesis lead to overproduction of bilirubin that exceeds the conjugative capability of the liver. Hemolysis may result from sickle cell anemia, thalassemia, glucose-6-phosphate dehydrogenase deficiency, paroxysmal nocturnal hemoglobinuria, ABO blood group incompatibility, or medications. Severe hemolysis rarely elevates serum bilirubin levels above 5 mg/dL, although hepatocyte dysfunction or Gilbert syndrome can magnify the hyperbilirubinemia. Iron deficiency, vitamin B_{12} deficiency, lead toxicity, sideroblastic anemia, and dyserythropoietic porphyria produce unconjugated hyperbilirubinemia due to ineffective erythropoiesis. Resorption of large hematomas may also increase production of unconjugated bilirubin.

Neonatal jaundice
Physiological neonatal jaundice is noticed in the first 5 days of life in term infants; unconjugated bilirubin levels peak near 6 mg/dL by day 3 and then decrease to normal within 14 days because of the increased activity of uridine diphosphate glucuronosyltransferase (UGT), the hepatic enzyme responsible for bilirubin conjugation. Higher levels of unconjugated bilirubin may persist up to 1 month in preterm infants. Nonphysiological causes in neonates include ABO blood group incompatibility between mother and infant, glucose-6-phosphate dehydrogenase deficiency, pyruvate kinase deficiency, and hypothyroidism. Lucey–Driscoll syndrome is transient unconjugated hyperbilirubinemia resulting from a UGT inhibitor in the mother's blood. Breast milk jaundice, which may produce bilirubin levels up to 20 mg/dL, results from an inhibitor of UGT activity

in breast milk. Severe unconjugated hyperbilirubinemia produces kernicterus in infants, which manifests as lethargy, hypotonia, and seizures.

Uridine diphosphate glucuronosyltransferase deficiencies

Gilbert syndrome, which is inherited in an autosomal dominant manner, is the most common cause of unconjugated hyperbilirubinemia; it affects 3–8% of the population. One half of the patients have mild associated hemolysis, and some have splenomegaly. Gilbert syndrome results from a partial defect of bilirubin conjugation (50% of normal). However, affected patients are asymptomatic and occasionally exhibit jaundice (bilirubin levels up to 6 mg/dL) with intercurrent illness, fasting, stress, fatigue, and ethanol use, or during the premenstrual period. Type I Crigler–Najjar syndrome is an autosomal recessive disorder characterized by the absence of UGT activity. Untreated patients develop profound unconjugated hyperbilirubinemia and die by 18 months. Treatment consists of phototherapy, plasmapheresis, or liver transplantation, which is curative. Type II Crigler–Najjar syndrome (Arias disease) is an autosomal dominant condition characterized by 10% of normal UGT activity, which often leads to jaundice by age 1 year. Treatment of type II Crigler–Najjar usually is unnecessary unless it affects the very young who are at risk for developing kernicterus.

Other causes of unconjugated hyperbilirubinemia

Probenecid and rifampin decrease hepatic bilirubin uptake. Sulfonamides, aspirin, contrast dye, and some parenteral nutritional formulations displace bilirubin from albumin and thereby reduce its transport into the hepatocyte. Penicillin, quinine, and methyldopa induce hemolysis.

A summary of the approach to the differential diagnosis of jaundice is outlined in Figure 12.1.

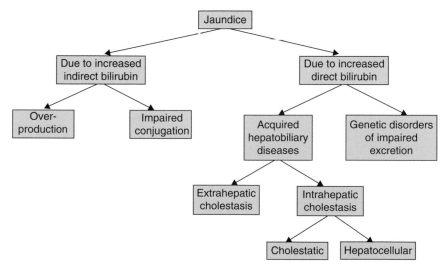

Figure 12.1 Differential diagnosis of the jaundiced patient. (Source: Yamada T et al. (eds) *Principles of Clinical Gastroenterology*. Oxford: Blackwell Publishing Ltd, 2008.)

Clinical presentation

History

The primary aim in evaluating a jaundiced patient is to determine if the hyperbilirubinemia is unconjugated or conjugated and if the process is acute or chronic. If it is unconjugated, the roles of increased production, decreased uptake, or impaired conjugation must be assessed. For conjugated hyperbilirubinemia, the process must be localized to an intrahepatic or extrahepatic site. Fever, abrupt-onset jaundice, right upper quadrant pain, and tender hepatomegaly suggest acute disease. Shaking chills and high fever suggest cholangitis or a bacterial infection, whereas low-grade fevers and flu-like symptoms are more common with viral hepatitis. Pain radiating to the back may indicate pancreatic disease. Pruritus is reported with obstructive jaundice of more than 3–4 weeks' duration, regardless of the cause. Weight loss, anorexia, nausea, and vomiting are seen nonspecifically in many hyperbilirubinemic disorders.

   Related historical features may provide etiological clues. Recent blood transfusions, intravenous drug abuse, and sexual exposure suggest possible viral hepatitis. Drugs, solvents, ethanol, or oral contraceptives produce jaundice by inducing cholestasis or hepatocellular damage. A history of gallstones, prior biliary surgery, and previous episodes of jaundice suggests bile duct disease. A family history of jaundice raises the possibility of a defect in bilirubin transport or conjugation or a heritable liver disease (e.g. Wilson disease, hemochromatosis, α_1-antitrypsin deficiency). Patients younger than age 30 are likely to present with acute parenchymal disease, whereas those older than age 65 are at risk for stones or malignancy. Conditions more common in men include alcoholic liver disease, pancreatic or hepatocellular carcinoma, and hemochromatosis. Disorders that are more prevalent in women include primary biliary cirrhosis, gallstones, and autoimmune hepatitis.

Physical examination

The examination can assess the cause, severity, and chronicity of jaundice. Fever may occur with acute or chronic disease, although high fever warrants a search for a bacterial process. Cachexia, muscle wasting, palmar erythema, a Dupuytren contracture, testicular atrophy, parotid enlargement, xanthelasma, gynecomastia, and spider angiomas suggest chronic liver disease. A shrunken, nodular liver with splenomegaly signals cirrhosis, whereas masses or lymphadenopathy raise the possibility of malignancy. A liver span of more than 15 cm suggests fatty infiltration, congestion, malignancy, or other infiltrative diseases. A friction rub may be found in malignancy. Ascites is found with cirrhosis, malignancy, and severe acute hepatitis. A palpable, distended gallbladder suggests malignant biliary obstruction. Asterixis and changes in mental status are noted with advanced liver disease.

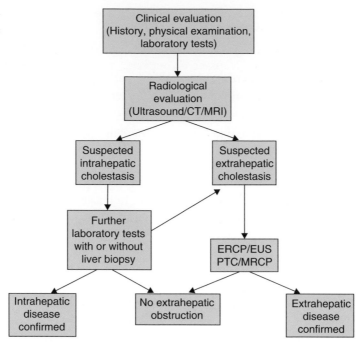

Figure 12.2 The evaluation of the jaundiced patient. CT, computed tomography; ERCP, endoscopic retrograde cholangiopancreatography; EUS, endoscopic ultrasound; MRCP, magnetic resonance cholangiopancreatography; MRI, magnetic resonance imaging; PTC, percutaneous transhepatic cholangiography. (Source: Yamada T et al. (eds) *Principles of Clinical Gastroenterology*. Oxford: Blackwell Publishing Ltd, 2008.)

Additional testing and diagnostic investigations

See Figure 12.2.

Laboratory studies

Laboratory tests can confirm suspicions raised by the history and physical examination. The reticulocyte count, lactate dehydrogenase and haptoglobin levels, and examination of the peripheral blood smear can provide evidence of hemolysis. If hemolysis is documented, specific testing of the immune mechanisms and tests for vitamin B_{12} deficiency, lead intoxication, thalassemia, and sideroblastic anemia can be performed. In the absence of hemolysis, most patients with pure, unconjugated hyperbilirubinemia are diagnosed with Gilbert syndrome. Initial tests for conjugated hyperbilirubinemia should distinguish hepatocellular causes from cholestatic causes and include determining the levels of aminotransferases, alkaline phosphatase, total protein, and albumin. If the alkaline phosphatase level is normal, then extrahepatic biliary obstruction is unlikely. Although neither aspartate nor alanine aminotransferase levels are specific for liver disease, levels higher than 300 IU/mL are uncommon in nonhepatobiliary disease. Aminotransferase elevations less than

300 IU/mL characterize alcoholic hepatitis and most drug-induced injury, whereas elevations more than 1000 IU/mL usually indicate acute hepatitis, certain drug responses (e.g. acetaminophen), or ischemic injury. Measurement of leucine aminopeptidase, 5′-nucleotidase, and γ-glutamyltransferase levels can help to distinguish alkaline phosphatase elevations caused by hepatobiliary disease from those of bony sources.

Specific liver diseases can be evaluated by blood testing (e.g. antimitochondrial antibody with primary biliary cirrhosis; hepatitis serological findings with viral hepatitis; α_1-antitrypsin levels, iron studies, and ceruloplasmin levels in hereditary liver disease; α-fetoprotein in malignancy; sedimentation rate, immunoglobulins, antinuclear and smooth muscle antibodies with autoimmune disease). Elevated globulin levels with hypoalbuminemia support the diagnosis of cirrhosis, as does failure of the prothrombin time to correct after administering vitamin K. Hypercholesterolemia often occurs with cholestasis.

Noninvasive imaging studies

Ultrasound, the initial test for detecting biliary obstruction, has an accuracy of 77–94%. With acute obstruction, biliary dilation may not be evident for 4 h to 4 days. Partial or intermittent obstruction may not produce dilation. Ultrasound is inconsistent in defining the site of obstruction because the distal common bile duct is difficult to visualize. Furthermore, 24–40% of patients with choledocholithiasis have bile ducts of normal diameters. Computed tomography (CT) may be performed if ultrasound findings are equivocal or nondiagnostic. CT scans may provide better definition of intrahepatic and extrahepatic mass lesions. Fine needle aspiration of mass lesions is possible with both modalities. Magnetic resonance imaging (MRI) is a sensitive method for detecting hepatic mass lesions. MR cholangiopancreatography (MRCP) has replaced invasive bile duct imaging with endoscopic retrograde cholangiopancreatography (ERCP) as a reliable diagnostic tool for many conditions.

Radionuclide imaging with ^{99m}Tc-labeled iminodiacetic acid derivatives is the procedure of choice for detecting cystic duct obstruction resulting from acute cholecystitis. The inability to visualize the gallbladder after 6 h is diagnostic of cystic duct obstruction, whereas common bile duct obstruction is reported if no contrast passes into the intestine within 60 min. False-positive test results (i.e. lack of gallbladder or duct filling) can occur with prolonged fasting, parenteral nutrition, and bilirubin levels higher than 5 mg/dL. Di-isopropyl and p-isopropyl iminodiacetic acid tracers allow biliary duct visualization with greater degrees of jaundice.

Invasive diagnostic studies

Percutaneous transhepatic cholangiography (PTC) and ERCP use cholecystographic dye and radiography to visualize the biliary tree. ERCP is successful in localizing the site of biliary obstruction in 90% of cases and is particularly useful for patients with choledocholithiasis because of the therapeutic capability of endoscopic sphincterotomy. The complications of ERCP include pancreatitis, cholangitis, bleeding, and perforation. Unsuccessful ERCP may result from the inability to cannulate the ampulla of Vater or to reach the ampulla (e.g. the patient with a Roux-en-Y gastrojejunostomy). PTC localizes the site of biliary obstruction in 90% of patients with dilated ducts, but it is less useful if the ductal diameter is normal. Contraindications to PTC include thrombocytopenia, severe coagulopathy, and ascites. PTC complications include infection, bleeding, pneumothorax, and peritonitis. Both ERCP and PTC afford the capability of obtaining biopsy or brushing specimens of suggestive biliary strictures and provide the possibility of stent placement for benign and malignant biliary strictures.

If obstruction has been excluded or hepatocellular disease is suspected, a liver biopsy should be performed. Specific findings from liver biopsy include hepatitis, cirrhosis, granulomas, infection, malignancy, certain autoimmune diseases, venous congestion, infiltrative processes, and hereditary liver disease. For 15% of cases, a liver biopsy is not helpful in determining the cause of hyperbilirubinemia. Dilated ducts are a relative contraindication to liver biopsy. Liver biopsy can be done percutaneously or using a transvenous approach. The transjugular approach is recommended for patients with ascites, thrombocytopenia, or coagulopathy.

Management

Management of a jaundiced patient depends on the underlying cause. In general, a patient with hereditary unconjugated hyperbilirubinemia does not need or does not respond to therapy, although phenobarbital may reduce bilirubin levels in type II Crigler–Najjar syndrome and Gilbert syndrome. Hemolysis may subside with discontinuation of an offending medication or with corticosteroid treatment of an underlying autoimmune process. Certain hepatocellular diseases may respond to specific therapies, for example, pegylated interferon and ribavirin for chronic active hepatitis C infection and therapeutic phlebotomy for hemochromatosis.

The goals for treating a patient with bile duct obstruction are to drain bile from above the blockage to provide relief of pruritus, to decrease the risk of complications, and to remove or bypass the cause of the obstruction. For an otherwise healthy patient with choledocholithiasis, laparoscopic cholecystectomy with common bile duct exploration and removal of the biliary stones is the standard of care, although some clinicians recommend preoperative or postoperative ERCP. For elderly or frail patients who cannot undergo surgery, ERCP with endoscopic sphincterotomy may represent the safest alternative. If a stone cannot be removed with standard endoscopic techniques, surgical extraction is indicated, and if surgery is associated with exceptional risk, endoscopic stenting

Table 12.2 Management of fat-soluble vitamin deficiency in prolonged cholestasis

Monitoring fat-soluble vitamins

25-OH vitamin D level (normal range 10–55 mg/mL). If renal disease, check 1,25-(OH)2 vitamin D

Vitamin A level (normal range 360–1200 μg/L)

Vitamin E level, with fasting total lipid profile (normal range 5.5–17.0 mg/L). Total lipids = cholesterol plus triglycerides (in grams). To calculate vitamin E level: serum vitamin E (mg)/total lipid (g). If ≥0.8, normal; if <0.6, supplement

Vitamin K: measure prothrombin time (normal range 11.4–13.2 sec)

Replacement

Vitamin D: calcium, 1–1.5 g po per day

Calcidiol (Calderol) 20–50 μg po, three times weekly, before transplantation. If coexistent renal disease, use calcitriol (Rocaltrol) 0.25–0.5 μg po daily

Vitamin A: β-carotene 15 mg (25,000 U vitamin A) po qid, or Aquasol A 50,000 U IM, daily for 2 weeks

Vitamin E: liquid E (D-α-tocopherol), water soluble, 100 IU po, daily

Vitamin K: 10 mg subcutaneously daily, for 3 days, then monthly if cholestatic

ADEK po 1–2 daily

Evaluation of therapy

After 3 months: 24-h urine calcium (normal range 50–250 mg/day)

Yearly: 25-OH vitamin D (1,25-(OH)2 vitamin D if renal disease), vitamins A and E, and prothrombin time

Source: Yamada T et al. (eds) *Principles of Clinical Gastroenterology*. Oxford: Blackwell Publishing Ltd, 2008.

or percutaneous transhepatic extraction is the alternative. If a malignant biliary obstruction cannot be drained endoscopically or radiographically, a surgical procedure (e.g. choledochojejunostomy or hepaticojejunostomy) may be necessary to bypass the obstructed segment.

Complications

The potential for complications depends on the cause and severity of the jaundice and on patient characteristics. Infants with unconjugated hyperbilirubinemia who have bilirubin levels higher than 20 mg/dL are at risk of kernicterus, in which bilirubin deposition in the thalamus, hypothalamus, and cerebellum produces irreversible impairment of motor and cortical function. Many hepatic diseases carry the risk of morbidity or death from the underlying disorder. Extrahepatic biliary obstruction may result in secondary biliary cirrhosis, bacterial cholangitis, or hepatic abscess formation; all are life threatening if the obstruction is not relieved. Pruritus, hepatic osteodystrophy, and fat-soluble vitamin deficiency are direct results of cholestasis and inadequate biliary secretion. Screening for fat-soluble vitamin deficiency and osteopenia and osteoporosis is recommended because effective therapy exists for these conditions (Table 12.2). Control of pruritus can be challenging, although several treatment options exist (Table 12.3).

Table 12.3 Management of pruritus of cholestasis

Topical therapy
Lower bathing water temperature and use fewer or lighter clothes and bed coverings
Minimize dry skin by using moisturizing soaps (e.g. Dove) and applying topical moisturizers liberally
(e.g. Eucerin cream)

Anion-exchange resins
Cholestyramine or colestipol: start with 4 g (one scoop or packet) po twice daily, before and after
breakfast, and increasing to six packets or scoops daily, separated from other medications by 2 h
(esp. ursodeoxycholic acid)

Bile salts
Ursodeoxycholic acid, 15 mg/kg/day po

Doxepin
25–50 mg po daily taken at night

Hepatic microsomal enzyme induction
Rifampin, 150 mg po, two to three times daily

Opioid receptor antagonists
Naltrexone, 12.5 mg po daily, increasing slowly to 50 mg po daily
Naloxone and nalmefene are only commonly available for parenteral use

Source: Yamada T et al. (eds) *Principles of Clinical Gastroenterology.* Oxford: Blackwell Publishing Ltd, 2008.

Case studies

Case 1

A 19-year-old male college student is seen in your outpatient hepatology clinic.
He was referred by the student health physician for evaluation of new-onset
jaundice. He has no significant past medical history and takes no medications.
He denies recreational drug use. The patient feels fairly well, although endorses
mild malaise. His main complaint is that of pruritus, which has been severe for
the past week. He denies any known history of liver disease, but recalls his liver
tests may have been abnormal years ago. On physical exam, his is a young, thin
male who is noticeably jaundiced. There is mild tenderness in the right upper
quadrant. His total bilirubin is 6.5, direct bilirubin is 3.4, and alkaline phosphatase is 842. The patient undergoes MRCP, which shows classic changes of PSC,
with a dominant stricture in the common hepatic duct. He subsequently
undergoes ERCP with balloon dilation and brushing of the dominant stricture.
Cytology is negative for malignancy and the patient's laboratory values show
significant improvement after the dilation.

Discussion and potential pitfalls

The patient's laboratory values are consistent with a direct hyperbilirubinemia. His marked alkaline phosphatase elevation suggests a hepatobiliary source. The patient's age and gender raise suspicion for PSC. MRCP allows for noninvasive evaluation for this diagnosis. All dominant strictures should be sampled for cytological and histological evaluation, to assess for cholangiocarcinoma. Because of the high suspicion for the disease, the patient was not subjected to a liver biopsy. Liver biopsies may show only nonspecific findings in PSC, and can incorrectly stage the disease, as fibrosis can be patchy in the liver.

Case 2

A 19-year-old man presents to your outpatient gastroenterology clinic for further evaluation of mild-to-moderate heartburn. He reports that his symptoms are fairly mild and sporadic, but his mother wanted him to be evaluated. She told the patient he might need an endoscopy, so he arrived to the appointment fasting. On physical exam, you notice that he appears mildly icteric, but the remainder of his exam is normal. You obtain laboratory values, and his total bilirubin is 2.8, direct bilirubin is 0.4, aspartate aminotransferase (AST) is 23, alanine aminotransferase (ALT) is 24, and alkaline phosphatase is 118. His blood counts are entirely normal, with a hematocrit of 41. You add on a reticulocyte count and lactate dehydrogenase (LDH) level to his labs, which return as normal. You request that the patient repeat labs in 4 weeks, and repeat values show a total bilirubin of 1.6, direct bilirubin of 0.2, AST 19, ALT 24, alkaline phosphatase 120, and hematocrit 40. You explain to the patient that he likely has Gilbert's syndrome. The patient is reassured that he has a benign condition but counseled that his lab tests are likely to be periodically abnormal in the future.

Discussion and potential pitfalls

This healthy individual has no symptoms or significant abnormalities on physical exam, and lab tests are consistent with an unconjugated hyperbilirubinemia. The remainder of his liver tests are entirely normal, arguing against hepatobiliary disease. His normal blood counts, reticulocyte count and LDH argue against significant hemolysis or hematological disease. It is important to make the diagnosis without subjecting the patient to unnecessary testing, including invasive testing. This diagnosis has a benign course, although patients with Gilbert's may be at increased risk for certain drug toxicities, especially with medications that require UGT1A1 for metabolism.

Key practice points

- Jaundice may be due to conjugated or unconjugated hyperbilirubinemia.

- Unconjugated hyperbilirubinemia may be due to overproduction of bilirubin (e.g. hemolysis) or defects in bilirubin conjugation (e.g. abnormal function or absence of UGT activity as seen in neonatal jaundice, Gilbert's, Crigler–Najjar).

- Conjugated hyperbilirubinemia has a broad differential, and can be rarely due to genetic disorders resulting in impaired excretion or transport of bilirubin. The typical causes are due to acquired hepatobiliary diseases, either extrahepatic (e.g. bile duct strictures or stones) or intrahepatic (e.g. viral, drug-induced or alcoholic hepatitis, infiltrative diseases, infections).

- The management of the jaundiced patient is dependent on the underlying cause.

CHAPTER 13

Approach to the Patient with Abnormal Liver Biochemical Tests

Introduction, background and pathogenesis

Evaluating suspected liver disease requires understanding the diverse tests of liver function and serum markers of hepatobiliary disease. Measurements of hepatic function evaluate the liver's ability to excrete substances and assess its synthetic and metabolic capacity.

Serum markers of hepatic function

Bilirubin

Serum bilirubin determination measures capabilities for hepatic conjugation and organic anion excretion. Hyperbilirubinemia can occur from increases in the unconjugated or conjugated bilirubin fractions. Increased production of bilirubin because of hemolysis and defective conjugation produces unconjugated hyperbilirubinemia, whereas hepatocellular disorders and extrahepatic obstruction cause conjugated hyperbilirubinemia. A third form of bilirubin, seen with prolonged cholestasis, is covalently bound to albumin. The presence of this albumin-bound bilirubin explains the slow resolution of jaundice in convalescing patients with resolving liver disease. The urine bilirubin level is elevated in conjugated, not unconjugated, hyperbilirubinemia.

Albumin

Total serum albumin is a useful measure of hepatic synthetic function. With a half-life of 20 days, albumin is a better index of disease severity in chronic rather than acute liver injury. Hypoalbuminemia may result from increased catabolism of albumin, decreased synthesis, dilution with plasma volume expansion, and increased protein loss from the gut or urinary tract. Prealbumin has a shorter half-life (1.9 days) than albumin and therefore has been proposed as a useful measure of hepatic synthetic capacity after acute injury (e.g. acetaminophen overdose).

Yamada's Handbook of Gastroenterology, Third Edition. Edited by Tadataka Yamada and John M. Inadomi.
© 2013 John Wiley & Sons, Ltd. Published 2013 by John Wiley & Sons, Ltd.

Clotting factors

Prothrombin time detects the activity of vitamin K-dependent coagulation factors (II, VII, IX, and X). Synthesis of these factors requires adequate intestinal vitamin K absorption and intact hepatic synthesis. Therefore, prolonged prothrombin times result from hepatocellular disorders that impair synthetic functions and from cholestatic syndromes that interfere with lipid absorption. Parenteral vitamin K administration distinguishes these possibilities. Improvement in prothrombin time by 30% within 24 h of vitamin K administration indicates that the synthetic function is intact and suggests vitamin K deficiency. Prolonged prothrombin time is a poor prognostic finding which signifies severe hepatocellular necrosis in acute hepatitis and the loss of functional hepatocytes in chronic liver disease. Individual clotting proteins have been proposed as useful clinical guides in severe acute hepatitis. Factor VII is the best indicator of liver disease severity and prognosis.

Miscellaneous tests of hepatic function

Serum bile acid determination has been advocated for assessing suspected liver disease, although poor diagnostic sensitivity in mild disease has prevented widespread application. However, the finding of normal levels of fasting serum bile acids in a patient with unconjugated hyperbilirubinemia supports a diagnosis of Gilbert syndrome in questionable cases. Plasma clearance of sulfobromophthalein, an organic anion, may help distinguish between Dubin–Johnson syndrome and Rotor syndrome. Serum globulin determinations can also give useful diagnostic information. Levels in excess of 3 g/dL are observed primarily in autoimmune liver disease, whereas selective increases in levels of immunoglobulin A (IgA) and IgM are noted in alcoholic cirrhosis and primary biliary cirrhosis (PBC), respectively. Elevated serum ammonia levels may be noted with severe acute or chronic liver disease and can correlate roughly with hepatic encephalopathy. Acute viral and alcoholic hepatitis decrease the α and pre-β bands in serum protein electrophoresis because of the reduced activity of lecithin-cholesterol acyltransferase, whereas the β band may be broad because of altered triglyceride lipase activity that results in elevated low-density lipoproteins. Breath tests of antipyrine clearance and aminopyrine demethylation measure impaired hepatic drug metabolism.

Serum markers of hepatobiliary dysfunction or necrosis
Aminotransferases

Aspartate aminotransferase (AST; serum glutamic oxaloacetic transaminase, SGOT) and alanine aminotransferase (ALT; serum glutamic pyruvic transaminase, SGPT) are markers of hepatocellular injury. Because AST is also found in muscle, kidney, heart, and brain, ALT elevations are more specific for liver processes. The highest elevations occur in viral, toxin-induced, and ischemic hepatitis, whereas smaller (<300 IU/mL) elevations are observed in alcoholic hepatitis and other hepatocellular disorders. An AST/ALT ratio greater than 2 suggests alcoholic liver disease, whereas a ratio less than 1 characterizes viral infection and biliary obstruction. When evaluating a patient with liver disease, decreases in AST and ALT levels usually suggest resolving injury, although decreasing aminotransferase levels may also be an ominous indicator of overwhelming hepatocyte death in fulminant liver failure, especially when associated with progressive increases in prothrombin time.

Alkaline phosphatase

Alkaline phosphatase originates in the bile canalicular membranes. Elevations of this enzyme are prominent in cholestasis and infiltrative liver disease; smaller increases are observed in other liver diseases. Alkaline phosphatase activity also occurs in bone, placenta, intestine, kidney, and some malignancies. Low levels of alkaline phosphatase may be observed in acute hemolysis complicating Wilson disease, as well as in hypothyroidism, pernicious anemia, and zinc deficiency.

Miscellaneous markers of hepatobiliary dysfunction

Serum levels of γ-glutamyltransferase (GGT), 5′-nucleotidase, and leucine aminopeptidase (LAP) are elevated in cholestatic syndromes and may help distinguish hepatobiliary from bony sources of alkaline phosphatase elevations. Levels of GGT are also elevated with pancreatic disease, myocardial infarction, uremia, lung disease, rheumatoid arthritis, nonalcoholic fatty liver disease, and diabetes. Alcohol, anticonvulsants, and warfarin induce hepatic microsomal enzymes, producing striking increases in GGT level. Levels of LAP may be elevated in normal pregnancy. The hepatic mitochondrial enzyme glutamate dehydrogenase is elevated in alcoholic patients and in patients with liver disease secondary to congestive heart failure. The lactate dehydrogenase concentration is frequently obtained as a "liver function test" but it has limited specificity for liver processes.

Consideration must always be given to potential nonhepatic causes of abnormal liver chemistries (Table 13.1).

Abnormalities in liver chemistry levels may result from cholestasis, hepatocellular injury, and infiltrative diseases of the liver (Table 13.2).

Cholestatic disorders

Cholestasis may result from intrahepatic or extrahepatic processes. Intrahepatic causes of cholestasis include PBC, sepsis, medications, postoperative cholestasis, familial conditions (e.g. benign recurrent intrahepatic cholestasis, cholestasis of pregnancy), and congenital disorders (e.g. Rotor syndrome, Dubin–Johnson syndrome, Byler disease). Extrahepatic biliary obstruction is caused by choledocholithiasis, benign and malignant strictures, extrinsic compression, and sclerosing cholangitis.

Table 13.1 Nonhepatic causes of abnormal liver chemistries

Test	Nonhepatic causes	Discriminating tests
Albumin	Protein-losing enteropathy	Serum globulins, α_1-antitrypsin clearance
	Nephrotic syndrome	Urinalysis, 24-h urinary protein
	Malnutrition	Clinical setting
	Congestive heart failure	Clinical setting
Alkaline phosphatase	Bone disease	GGT, SLAP, 5'-NT
	Pregnancy	GGT, 5'-NT
	Malignant disease	Alkaline phosphatase electrophoresis
Serum aspartate aminotransferase	Myocardial infarction	MB-CPK
	Muscle disorders	Creatine kinase, aldolase
Bilirubin	Hemolysis	Reticulocyte count, peripheral smear, urine bilirubin
	Sepsis	Clinical setting, cultures
	Ineffective erythropolesis	Peripheral smear, urine bilirubin, hemoglobin electrophoresis, bone marrow examination
	"Shunt" hyperbilirubinemia	Clinical setting
GGT	Alcohol, drugs	History
Ferritin	Systemic disease, chronic Inflammation	Clinical setting
Prothrombin time	Antibiotic and anticoagulant use, steatorrhea, dietary deficieny of vitamin K (rare)	Response to vitamin K, Clinical setting

GGT, γ-glutamyltransferase; MB-CPK, MB Isoenzyme of creatine phosphokinase; 5'-NT, 5'-nucleotidase; SLAP, serum leucine aminopeptidase.
Source: Yamada T et al. (eds) *Principles of Clinical Gastroenterology*. Oxford: Blackwell Publishing Ltd, 2008.

Table 13.2 Routine biochemical tests in the patient with idealized hepatobiliary disease

Test	Hepatocellular necrosis	Cholestasis	Infiltrative process
Aminotransferase	++ to +++	0 to +	0 to +
Alkaline phosphatase	0 to +	++ to +++	++ to +++
Total/direct bilirubin	0 to +++	0 to +++	0 to +
Prothrombin time	Prolonged	Prolonged; responsive to vitamin K	Normal
Albumin	Decreased in chronic disorders	Normal	Normal

0, normal; + to +++, Increasing degrees of abnormality.
Source: Yamada T et al. (eds) *Principles of Clinical Gastroenterology*. Oxford: Blackwell Publishing Ltd, 2008.

Disorders with hepatocellular injury

Hepatocellular injury may result from a diverse group of diseases. Acute viral hepatitis in the United States most commonly results from infection with hepatitis A or B, or, less commonly, C viruses. Hepatitis D complicates the course of infection in chronic hepatitis B carriers. Hepatitis E occurs primarily in developing countries, where it is well recognized as a cause of fulminant hepatic failure, particularly in pregnant women. Other viral causes of hepatitis include cytomegalovirus, herpes simplex virus, Epstein–Barr virus, and varicella zoster virus. Chronic infection with either hepatitis B or C viruses may also produce chronic hepatitis or cirrhosis. Chronic ethanol consumption produces a broad range of liver diseases, including fatty liver, alcoholic hepatitis, and cirrhosis. Hereditary liver diseases that produce hepatocellular injury are Wilson disease, hemochromatosis, and α_1-antitrypsin deficiency. Congestive and ischemic disease in the liver is caused by congestive heart failure, constrictive pericarditis, hypotension, portal vein thrombosis or hepatic vein outflow obstruction from Budd–Chiari syndrome, inferior vena cava occlusion, or veno-occlusive disease. Significant liver disease during pregnancy, such as acute fatty liver of pregnancy and hepatocellular damage secondary to toxemia, usually occurs in the third trimester. Medication-induced and toxin-induced causes of injury are very common and require a high index of suspicion and careful questioning.

Infiltrative diseases

Malignant diseases, including primary tumors (e.g. hepatocellular carcinoma, cholangiocarcinoma), metastases, lymphoma, and leukemia, may produce infiltrative liver disease. Granulomatous liver infiltration may result from infections (e.g. tuberculosis, histoplasmosis), sarcoidosis, and numerous medications.

Clinical presentation

History

An accurate history is critical for a patient whose laboratory studies provide evidence of liver disease. The presenting symptoms provide important diagnostic clues. Pruritus is a common and early symptom in patients with cholestasis. Although classically associated with PBC and primary sclerosing cholangitis, pruritus also is reported in extrahepatic biliary obstruction and hepatocellular disease. Many conditions that produce abnormal liver chemistry levels are painless, but acute biliary obstruction from stones can produce intense right upper quadrant pain. Concurrent high fever raises concern for cholangitis. Acute hepatitis produces less well-defined right upper quadrant discomfort with profound fatigue, whereas hepatic tumors may cause subcostal aching.

A family history is useful in diagnosing and evaluating hereditary hemolytic states, benign recurrent intrahepatic cholestasis, hemochromatosis, Wilson disease, and α_1-antitrypsin deficiency. Exposure to ethanol and industrial and environmental toxins should be identified. A detailed medication history, including over-the-counter and herbal remedies, is critical. In particular, the use of episodic or intermittent medications, such as steroid tapers for asthma or antibiotics, may require specific questioning. Alcoholic patients should be questioned about acetaminophen use because hepatotoxicity can occur in these persons with therapeutic dosing as a result of cytochrome P450 induction. Intravenous drug abuse, sexual contact, and blood transfusions are associated with a risk for viral hepatitis B or C, whereas sudden worsening of liver chemistry levels in a chronic hepatitis B carrier suggests possible hepatitis D superinfection. Waterborne outbreaks of viral hepatitis have been reported in South East Asia and India, underscoring the importance of obtaining a travel history. Risk factors for hepatitis A include recent ingestion of raw or undercooked oysters or clams, male homosexuality, or exposure through day care.

Other diseases associated with liver disorders should be ascertained. Right-sided congestive heart failure, hypotension, and shock are recognized causes of abnormal liver chemistry findings. Chronic pancreatitis may produce abnormal liver tests as a result of stenosis of the common bile duct. Primary sclerosing cholangitis affects 10% of patients with inflammatory bowel disease, in particular those with ulcerative colitis. Obesity, hyperlipidemia, diabetes, and corticosteroid use are risk factors for nonalcoholic fatty liver disease. Hematological disorders (e.g. polycythemia rubra vera, myeloproliferative disorders, and paroxysmal nocturnal hemoglobinuria) associated with hypercoagulable states predispose to hepatic vein thrombosis. Hemoglobinopathies (e.g. sickle cell anemia, thalassemia) lead to pigment stone formation. Rashes, arthritis, renal disease, and vasculitis may develop with viral hepatitis. The presence of hypogonadism, heart disease, and diabetes suggests possible hemochromatosis. Concurrent lung disease may occur with α_1-antitrypsin deficiency, and central nervous system findings are associated with Wilson disease. Patients with leptospirosis will present with hepatic and renal abnormalities. Renal cell carcinoma manifests as abnormal liver chemistry levels in the absence of metastases. Recent surgery should be noted because anesthetic exposure, perioperative hypotension, and blood transfusions all may affect the liver. Recent biliary tract surgery raises concern for bile duct stricture. Cirrhosis is a late complication of jejunoileal, but not gastric, bypass surgery for morbid obesity.

Physical examination

Physical findings are of discriminative value for a patient with abnormal liver chemistry findings. Fever suggests an infectious cause or hepatitis. Jaundice is visible when the serum bilirubin concentration exceeds 2.5–3.0 mg/dL. Spider angiomas, palmar erythema, parotid enlargement, gynecomastia, a Dupuytren contracture, and testicular atrophy are stigmata of chronic liver disease, usually cirrhosis, though many of these signs have low specificity. Hyperpigmentation is seen with hemochromatosis and PBC. Ichthyosis and koilonychia are manifestations of hemochromatosis. Xanthomas and xanthelasma appear in chronic cholestasis. Kayser–Fleischer rings and sunflower cataracts suggest Wilson disease. Conjunctival suffusion raises the possibility of leptospirosis. A liver span greater than 15 cm suggests passive congestion or liver infiltration. Splenomegaly is found with portal hypertension or infiltrative processes. Abdominal tenderness suggests an inflammatory process (e.g. cholecystitis, cholangitis, pancreatitis, hepatitis), whereas a palpable, nontender gallbladder (i.e. the Courvoisier sign) raises the possibility of an obstructive malignancy. A Murphy sign (i.e. inspiratory arrest during deep, right upper quadrant palpation) is highly suggestive of acute cholecystitis. A pulsatile liver suggests tricuspid insufficiency, and hepatic bruits or rubs raise the possibility of hepatocellular carcinoma. Occult or gross fecal blood on rectal examination suggests possible inflammatory bowel disease or neoplasm.

Additional testing and diagnostic investigations
Disease-specific markers
Viral serology

The hepatitis A IgM antibody (anti-HAV IgM) is initially detectable at the onset of clinical illness and persists for 120 days. Anti HAV IgG is a convalescent marker that may persist for life. Hepatitis B surface antigen (HBsAg) precedes aminotransferase elevations and symptom development and persists for 1–2 months in self-limited infections. The antibody to core antigen (anti-HBc) is detected 2 weeks after the appearance of HBsAg and initially is of the IgM class. The antibody to HBsAg (anti-HBs) appears some time after the disappearance of HBsAg and may persist for life. During the period between the disappearance of HBsAg and the appearance of anti-HBs, anti-HBc IgM may be the only marker of recent hepatitis B infection. Measurement of hepatitis B e antigen and antibody, as well as a polymerase chain reaction assay for serum hepatitis B DNA levels, can be used to quantify the degree of active viral replication in some patients with chronic hepatitis B infection. Enzyme-linked immunosorbent assays (ELISAs) are screening tests for detecting exposure to hepatitis C. Recombinant immunoblot assays can be used as supplements to ELISAs if a false-positive result with the ELISA is suspected. Both tests may produce negative findings for up to 6 months after acute infection; therefore, if hepatitis C is a diagnostic possibility, hepatitis C viremia should be determined by a polymerase chain reaction assay of hepatitis C RNA. Quantitative measurement of hepatitis C RNA levels as well as genotype should also be determined prior to therapy, and RNA levels should be followed serially during hepatitis C therapy. Hepatitis D infection occurs only in patients with HBsAg positivity and can be measured by hepatitis D viral RNA and antihepatitis D antibodies. Persistence of anti-HDV IgM predicts progression to chronic hepatitis D infection. Acute hepatitis E can be detected by ELISA for antihepatitis E. A subset of patients in whom the tests for the above viral markers have negative results will exhibit positive serological findings for cytomegalovirus, herpes simplex, coxsackievirus, or Epstein–Barr virus.

Immunological tests

Markers that may be detected in autoimmune liver disease include antinuclear antibody (ANA, homogeneous pattern) and the anti-smooth muscle antibodies (ASMAs). ASMAs are detected in 70% of patients with autoimmune chronic active hepatitis but may also be present in 50% of patients with PBC. The presence of anti-liver/kidney microsomal antibodies (anti-LKM1) with reduced titers of antiactin antibodies or ANAs identifies a subset of patients with autoimmune chronic active hepatitis, a disease that follows an aggressive course in young women. Antimitochondrial antibodies (AMAs) are present in 90% of patients with PBC and 25% of patients with chronic active hepatitis or drug-induced liver disease. Antibodies to the Ro antigen and to anticentromeric antibodies are observed with PBC, especially in patients with sicca syndrome or scleroderma.

Copper storage variables

Ceruloplasmin is a copper transport protein in the plasma that circulates in low concentrations in Wilson disease; low levels (<20 mg/dL) are measured in 90% of homozygotes and 10% of heterozygotes. Reduced levels may also occur with severely depressed synthetic function caused by other end-stage liver diseases. Alternative diagnostic tests for Wilson disease include urinary copper, which exceeds 100 mg per 24 h in nearly all patients, and free serum copper, which is markedly elevated. Urinary copper also is elevated in patients with cholestasis or cirrhosis. Although the gene for Wilson disease has been identified (*ATP7B*), the lack of a dominant mutation has prevented the development of genetic tests for the disease.

Iron storage variables

Serum iron level and total iron-binding capacity (transferrin) are useful measures in diagnosing hemochromatosis. Transferrin is normally 20–45% saturated. A transferrin saturation higher than 45% will identify more than 98% of patients with hemochromatosis. Elevations in serum iron with normal transferrin saturation occur in alcoholic liver disease. Serum ferritin more closely correlates with hepatic and total body iron stores, although ferritin may be elevated in inflammatory disease because it is an acute-phase reactant. The identification of a single recessive mutation in the *HFE* gene (*C282Y*), which is responsible for the majority of hemochromatosis, has eliminated the need for a liver biopsy in diagnosing many cases. A liver biopsy may be required for older patients with high ferritin levels to quantify tissue iron and to determine the extent of fibrosis, which will guide the need for screening for hepatocellular carcinoma.

α_1-Antitrypsin

α_1-Antitrypsin is a hepatic glycoprotein that migrates in the α_1-globulin fraction in serum protein electrophoresis. Homozygotes for the Pi ZZ variant of this protein (normal is Pi MM) exhibit decreased serum α_1-antitrypsin activity, which predisposes to development of chronic liver and pulmonary disease. Hepatocytes that cannot excrete the Z protein accumulate periodic acid-Schiff (PAS)-positive, diastase-resistant globules, as seen in liver biopsy specimens. Phenotyping is more accurate for diagnosis than determination of serum levels of the protein. Whether heterozygotes (Pi MZ) can develop liver disease in the absence of other hepatic insults remains controversial.

Percutaneous liver biopsy

As a general rule, direct forms of liver injury tend to cause predominant centrizonal necrosis; immunologically mediated forms of hepatocyte injury are localized to the periportal region; and cholestatic injury is recognized by the accumulation of canalicular bile and feathery degeneration of hepatocytes in the absence of a significant inflammatory infiltrate. Clinical applications of liver biopsy include evaluating persistently abnormal liver chemistry levels, establishing the diagnosis in unexplained hepatomegaly, and evaluating suspected systemic disease or carcinoma involving the liver. Contraindications to liver biopsy are an unco-operative or unstable patient, ascites, right-sided empyema, and suspected hemangioma. Impaired coagulation function is a relative contraindication. For patients with ascites or an increased risk of bleeding, a transjugular approach is an alternative to the percutaneous approach.

Management

Liver disease is classified into three groups: cholestatic, hepatocellular, and infiltrative. Screening the patient by determining levels of AST and ALT activity, serum alkaline phosphatase, serum total and direct bilirubin, serum protein and albumin, and prothrombin time can direct the subsequent evaluation into one of these groups.

Cholestatic liver disease usually results in increased serum bilirubin and alkaline phosphatase levels with normal to mildly elevated aminotransferase levels, although transient, profound, aminotransferase elevations may occur in early biliary obstruction. In extrahepatic cholestasis, the serum bilirubin level increases by 1.5 mg/dL per day and reaches a maximum of 35 mg/dL in the absence of renal dysfunction or hemolysis. In partial biliary obstruction, the bilirubin level may remain normal in the face of an elevated alkaline phosphatase concentration.

The most direct approach to evaluating suspected cholestasis is performing ultrasound to assess bile duct size. If malignancy or pancreatic disease is suspected, a computed tomography (CT) scan may provide better anatomical definition of

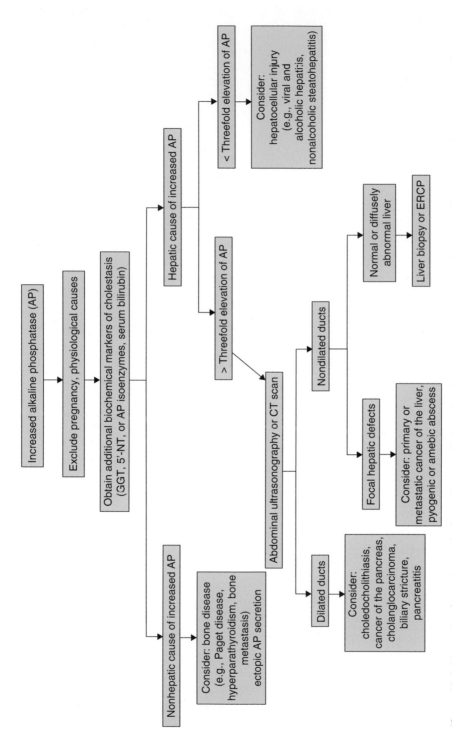

Figure 13.1 Diagnosing the patient with elevated serum alkaline phosphatase levels. CT, computed tomography; ERCP, endoscopic retrograde cholangiopancreatography; GGT, serum γ-glutamyltransferase; 5′-NT, 5′-nucleotidase. (Source: Yamada T et al. (eds) *Principles of Clinical Gastroenterology.* Oxford: Blackwell Publishing Ltd, 2008.)

the desired structures. If biliary dilation is detected, endoscopic retrograde cholangiopancreatography (ERCP) or percutaneous transhepatic cholangiography (PTC) can further define and potentially be used to treat the abnormality. In some cases of extrahepatic obstruction, bile duct size will be normal; in these cases, ERCP or PTC may still be indicated because of a high clinical suspicion. In questionable cases, percutaneous liver biopsy may provide a definitive diagnosis. However, intrahepatic cholestasis cannot always be distinguished from extrahepatic cholestasis on liver biopsy specimens. The approach to evaluation of a patient with elevated alkaline phosphatase is outlined in Figure 13.1.

Hepatocellular injury is suggested by aminotransferase levels higher than 400 IU/mL; levels less than 300 IU/mL are nonspecific and are observed with cholestasis as well as with hepatocellular disease. Alkaline phosphatase and bilirubin elevations are variable in hepatocellular disease, depending on the cause and severity of the clinical condition. Prolongation of prothrombin time and decreases in serum albumin levels indicate significant hepatic synthetic dysfunction. In patients with acute malaise, anorexia, nausea, jaundice, tender hepatomegaly, and elevated levels of aminotransferases, serum should be screened for viral markers to exclude hepatitis A, B, or C infection, depending on the patient risk factors. With disease duration of more than 6 months, additional studies (e.g. serum protein electrophoresis, ferritin or iron studies, and measurement of serum ceruloplasmin) should be added to the viral serological studies to exclude hereditary liver disease. Eosinophilia suggests possible drug hypersensitivity. For a patient with prominent systemic symptoms that suggest autoimmune disease, the clinician should determine the sedimentation rate; perform serum protein electrophoresis; measure quantitative immunoglobulins in the blood; and measure the presence of ANA, AMA, and ASMA. A hepatocellular pattern is observed with ischemic and congestive liver disease, but measures to improve hepatic blood flow in these conditions can produce brisk reductions in aminotransferases to near normal levels within 48–72 h. With congestive liver disease, the prothrombin time may be prolonged out of proportion to other signs of liver disease. Hepatic vein thrombosis (Budd–Chiari syndrome) may be suggested by increased caudate lobe size on CT scanning and usually is confirmed by Doppler ultrasound, CT, or magnetic resonance imaging that shows hepatic vein outflow obstruction and narrowing of the inferior vena cava.

Most acute elevations in aminotransferase levels do not require further evaluation unless they are severe or progressive. If aminotransferase levels remain high for longer than 6 months without an identifiable cause, a liver biopsy is indicated for diagnosis and to offer prognostic information about possible progression to cirrhosis. Many persons with persistently high aminotransferase levels are obese or use ethanol, and the usual finding on liver biopsy is fatty liver disease in the absence of serological diagnosis. However, the unexpected finding of chronic active hepatitis in a subset of these patients provides support for biopsy even in asymptomatic individuals.

Case studies

Case 1

A 65-year-old woman is referred to the hepatology clinic with concerns for possible cirrhosis due to a low serum albumin of 2.8g/dL, elevated INR of 1.8 and lower extremity edema. Upon review of her laboratory tests, it is noted that her ALT and AST are normal at 30 and 28, alkaline phosphatase is normal at 110. Bilirubin is normal at 1.1mg/dL. CBC is unremarkable, with platelets of 250,000/μL. On physical exam, there is no hepatosplenomegaly, but she has pitting edema of her lower extremities. On review of her medical history, you note she has long-standing diabetes complicated by severe gastroparesis. You suspect she may have protein in her urine, and urine tests confirm nephrotic range proteinuria for which she is started on an angiotensin-converting enzyme (ACE) inhibitor. You further suspect that she is malnourished as a result of her gastroparesis, and you provide her with vitamin K supplementation. Follow-up laboratory values after several months reveal improved serum albumin to 3.6 and INR of 1.1.

Discussion and potential pitfalls

While albumin and INR are the two most important measures of liver function, it is important to recognize that there are many alternative etiologies for abnormalities in these values. Protein losses due to proteinuria, protein-losing enteropathy and malnutrition can result in marked hypoalbuminemia. The use of antibiotics and anticoagulants can prolong the prothrombin time, as can persistent cholestasis, steatorrhea, and malnutrition.

Case 2

You are asked to see a 21-year-old man who has been diagnosed with Wilson disease and would like to transfer care to your medical center. He is being maintained on trientene. His diagnosis of Wilson disease was made in the setting of abnormal liver tests. Liver biopsy was nonspecific, but showed advanced fibrosis. The patient's ceruloplasmin was borderline low, and a subsequent 24-h urine showed a markedly elevated copper quantitation. Upon review of his labs, you note his alkaline phosphatase is elevated at 490 U/L. This raises your suspicion that the diagnosis of Wilson disease is incorrect. You obtain a magnetic resonance cholangiopancreatography scan, which shows classic changes of primary sclerosing cholangitis (PSC).

Discussion and potential pitfalls

The diagnosis of Wilson disease is challenging, and it is typically a combination of tests and a high level of suspicion that results in the diagnosis. Classic diagnostic features include low serum ceruloplasmin, high urinary copper, and elevated quantitative tissue copper. Kayser–Fleischer rings may be noted on ophthalmological exam. Less specific but more readily available diagnostic clues include elevated serum bilirubin, hemolytic anemia and low serum alkaline phosphatase. It is important to note that prolonged cholestasis, which often accompanies PBC and PSC, can result in significant elevations of urinary copper and hepatic copper quantitation.

Key practice points

- Liver chemistries provide information regarding liver function and serve as markers of hepatobiliary disease.
- The pattern of liver test abnormalities can direct the diagnosis towards a cholestatic, hepatocellular, or infiltrative process.
- Based on the pattern of laboratory test abnormality, additional serological, imaging, and biopsy studies can be obtained to clarify the diagnosis.

CHAPTER 14

Approach to the Patient with Ascites

Ascites is the pathological accumulation of fluid within the peritoneal cavity. It is important to establish a cause for its development and to initiate a rational treatment regimen to avoid some of the complications of ascites. Most cases of ascites in the United States result from liver disease, although disorders involving other organ systems may produce abdominal fluid accumulation in certain situations (Table 14.1).

Pathogenesis

Chronic parenchymal liver disease

Portal hypertension is a prerequisite for ascites formation in patients with liver disease. In general, ascites is a complication of chronic liver diseases (e.g. cirrhosis) but some acute diseases such as acute alcoholic hepatitis or fulminant hepatic failure may result in ascites. In this setting, a high (>1.1 g/dL) serum-ascites albumin gradient (SAAG) indicates acute portal hypertension and a mechanism of fluid formation similar to that in chronic liver disease.

Three theories have been proposed to explain fluid accumulation. The underfill theory postulates that an imbalance of Starling forces produces intravascular fluid loss into the peritoneum, with resultant hormonally mediated renal sodium retention. The overfill theory proposes that primary renal sodium retention produces intravascular hypervolemia that overflows into the peritoneum. The more recent peripheral arterial vasodilation theory proposes that portal hypertension leads to vasodilation and reduced effective arterial blood volume, which increases renal sodium retention and promotes fluid accumulation. In the vasodilation theory, the underfill mechanism is operative in early, compensated cirrhosis, whereas the overflow mechanism operates in advanced disease (Figure 14.1).

Yamada's Handbook of Gastroenterology, Third Edition. Edited by Tadataka Yamada and John M. Inadomi.
© 2013 John Wiley & Sons, Ltd. Published 2013 by John Wiley & Sons, Ltd.

Table 14.1 Causes of ascites

Chronic parenchymal liver disease (cirrhosis and alcoholic hepatitis)
"Mixed" (portal hypertension plus another cause, e.g. cirrhosis and peritoneal carcinomatosis)
Heart failure
Malignancy
Tuberculosis
Fulminant hepatic failure
Pancreatic
Nephrogenous ("dialysis ascites")
Miscellaneous*

*Includes biliary ascites and chylous ascites resulting from lymphatic tears, lymphoma, and cirrhosis.

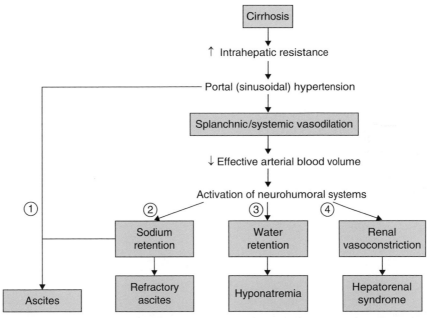

Figure 14.1 Common pathogenesis of ascites, hyponatremia and hepatorenal syndrome. Ascites (1) results from increased sinusoidal pressure and sodium retention. Sinusoidal pressure increases as a result of increased intrahepatic resistance. Sodium retention results from splanchnic and systemic vasodilation that leads to decreased effective arterial blood volume and subsequent upregulation of sodium-retaining hormones. With progression of cirrhosis and portal hypertension, vasodilation is more pronounced, leading to further activation of the renin–angiotensin–aldosterone and sympathetic nervous systems. The resulting increase in sodium and water retention can lead to refractory ascites (2) and hyponatremia (3), respectively, while the resulting increase in vasoconstrictors can lead to renal vasoconstriction and hepatorenal syndrome (4). (Source: Yamada T et al. (eds) *Principles of Clinical Gastroenterology*. Oxford: Blackwell Publishing Ltd, 2008.)

Cardiac disease

Ascites is an uncommon complication of both high-output and low-output heart failure. High-output failure is associated with decreased peripheral resistance; low-output disease is defined by reduced cardiac output. Both lead to decreased effective arterial blood volume and, subsequently, to renal sodium retention. Pericardial disease is a rare cardiac cause of ascites.

Renal disease

Nephrotic syndrome is a rare cause of ascites in adults. It results from protein loss in the urine, leading to decreased intravascular volume and increased renal sodium retention. Nephrogenous ascites is a poorly understood condition that develops with hemodialysis; its optimal treatment is undefined and its prognosis is poor. Continuous ambulatory peritoneal dialysis is an iatrogenic form of ascites that takes advantage of the rich vascularity of the parietal peritoneum to eliminate endogenous toxins and control fluid balance. Urine may accumulate in the peritoneum in newborns or as a result of trauma or renal transplantation in adults.

Pancreatic disease

Pancreatic ascites develops as a complication of severe acute pancreatitis, pancreatic duct rupture in acute or chronic pancreatitis, or leakage from a pancreatic pseudo-cyst. Many patients with pancreatic ascites have underlying cirrhosis. Pancreatic ascites may be complicated by infection or left-sided pleural effusion.

Biliary disease

Most cases of biliary ascites result from gallbladder rupture, which usually is a complication of gangrene of the gallbladder in elderly men. Bile also can accumulate in the peritoneal cavity after biliary surgery or biliary or intestinal perforation.

Malignancy

Malignancy-related ascites signifies advanced disease in most cases and has a dismal prognosis. Exceptions are ovarian carcinoma and lymphoma, which may respond to debulking surgery and chemotherapy, respectively. The mechanism of ascites formation depends on the location of the tumor. Peritoneal carcinomatosis produces exudation of proteinaceous fluid into the peritoneal cavity, whereas primary hepatic malignancy or liver metastases are likely to induce ascites by producing portal hypertension, either from vascular occlusion by the tumor or arteriovenous fistulae within the tumor. Chylous ascites can result from lymph node involvement with tumor.

Infectious disease

In the United States, tuberculous peritonitis is a disease of Asian, Mexican, and Central American immigrants, and it is a complication of the acquired immunodeficiency syndrome (AIDS). One half of patients with tuberculous peritonitis have underlying cirrhosis, usually secondary to ethanol abuse. Patients with liver disease tolerate antituberculous drug toxicity less well than patients with normal hepatic function. Exudation of proteinaceous fluid from the tubercles lining the peritoneum induces ascites formation. *Coccidioides* organisms cause infectious ascites formation by a similar mechanism. For sexually active women who have a fever and inflammatory ascites, chlamydia-induced, and the less common gonococcus-induced, Fitz-Hugh–Curtis syndrome should be considered.

Chylous ascites
Chylous ascites is a result of the obstruction of or damage to chyle-containing lymphatic channels. The most common causes are lymphatic malignancies (e.g. lymphomas, other malignancies), surgical tears, and infectious causes.

Other causes of ascites formation
Serositis with ascites formation may complicate systemic lupus erythematosus. Meigs syndrome (ascites and pleural effusion due to benign ovarian neoplasms) is a rare cause of ascites formation. Most cases of ascites caused by ovarian disease are from peritoneal carcinomatosis. Ascites with myxedema is secondary to hypothyroidism-related cardiac failure. Mixed ascites occurs in about 5% of cases when the patient has two or more separate causes of ascites formation, such as cirrhosis and infection or malignancy. A clue to the presence of a second cause is an inappropriately high white cell count in the ascitic fluid.

Clinical presentation

History
The history can help to elucidate the cause of ascites formation. Increasing abdominal girth from ascites may be part of the initial presentation of patients with alcoholic liver disease; however, the laxity of the abdominal wall and the severity of underlying liver disease suggest that the condition can be present for some time before it is recognized. Patients who consume ethanol only intermittently may report cyclic ascites, whereas patients with nonalcoholic disease usually have persistent ascites. Other risk factors for viral liver disease should be ascertained (i.e. drug abuse, sexual exposure, blood transfusions, and tattoos). A positive family history of liver disease raises the possibility of a heritable condition (e.g. Wilson disease, hemochromatosis, or α_1-antitrypsin deficiency) that might also present with symptoms referable to other organ systems (diabetes, cardiac disease, joint problems, and hyperpigmentation with hemochromatosis; neurological disease with Wilson disease; pulmonary complaints with α_1-antitrypsin deficiency). Patients with cirrhotic ascites may report other complications of liver disease, including jaundice, pedal edema, gastrointestinal hemorrhage,

or encephalopathy. The patient with long-standing, stable cirrhosis who abruptly develops ascites should be evaluated for possible hepatocellular carcinoma.

Information concerning possible nonhepatic disease should be obtained. Weight loss or a prior history of cancer suggests possible malignant ascites, which may be painful and produce rapid increases in abdominal girth. A history of heart disease raises the possibility of cardiac causes of ascites. Some alcoholics with ascites have alcoholic cardiomyopathy rather than liver dysfunction. Obesity, diabetes, and hyperlipidemia are risk factors for nonalcoholic fatty liver disease, which can cause cirrhosis on its own or can act synergistically with other insults (e.g. alcohol, hepatitis C). Tuberculous peritonitis usually presents with fever and abdominal discomfort. Patients with nephrotic syndrome usually have anasarca. Patients with rheumatological disease may have serositis. Patients with ascites associated with lethargy, cold intolerance, and voice and skin changes should be evaluated for hypothyroidism.

Physical examination

Ascites should be distinguished from panniculus, massive hepatomegaly, gaseous overdistension, intra-abdominal masses, and pregnancy. Percussion of the flanks can be used to determine rapidly if a patient has ascites. The absence of flank dullness excludes ascites with 90% accuracy. If dullness is found, the patient should be rolled into a partial decubitus position to test whether there is a shift in the air–fluid interface determined by percussion (shifting dullness). The fluid wave has less value in detecting ascites. The puddle sign detects as little as 120 mL of ascitic fluid but it requires the patient to assume a hands-and-knees position for several minutes and is a less useful test than flank dullness.

The physical examination can help to determine the cause of ascites. Palmar erythema, abdominal wall collateral veins, spider angiomas, splenomegaly, and jaundice are consistent with liver disease. Large veins on the flanks and back indicate blockage of the inferior vena cava that is caused by webs or malignancy. Masses or lymphadenopathy (e.g. Sister Mary Joseph nodule, Virchow node) suggest underlying malignancy. Distended neck veins, cardiomegaly, and auscultation of an S_3 or pericardial rub suggest cardiac causes of ascites, whereas anasarca may be observed with nephrotic syndrome.

Additional testing and diagnostic investigations
Blood and urine studies

Laboratory blood studies can provide clues to the cause of ascites. Abnormal levels of aminotransferases, alkaline phosphatase, and bilirubin are seen with liver disease. Prolonged prothrombin time and hypoalbuminemia are also observed with hepatic synthetic dysfunction, although low albumin levels are noted with renal disease, protein-losing enteropathy, and malnutrition. Hematological abnormalities, especially thrombocytopenia, suggest liver disease. Renal disease may be suggested by electrolyte abnormalities or elevations in blood urea nitrogen and creatinine. Urinalysis may reveal protein loss with nephrotic syndrome or bilirubinuria with jaundice. Specific tests (e.g. α-fetoprotein) or serological tests (e.g. antinuclear antibody) may be ordered for suspected hepatocellular carcinoma or immune-mediated disease, respectively.

Ascitic fluid analysis

Abdominal paracentesis is the most important means of diagnosing the cause of ascites formation. It is appropriate to sample ascitic fluid in all patients with new-onset ascites, as well as in all those admitted to hospital with ascites, because there is a 10–27% prevalence of ascitic fluid infection in the latter group. Paracentesis is performed in an area of dullness either in the midline between the umbilicus and symphysis pubis, because this area is avascular, or in one of the lower quadrants. Needles should not be inserted close to abdominal wall scars with either approach because of the high risk for bowel perforation; puncture sites too near the liver or spleen should be avoided as well. In 3% of cases, ultrasound guidance may be needed. The needle is inserted using a Z-track insertion technique to minimize postprocedure leakage, and 25 mL or more of ascitic fluid is removed for analysis.

Analysis of ascitic fluid should begin with gross inspection. Most ascitic fluid from portal hypertension is yellow and clear. Cloudiness raises the possibility of infectious processes, whereas a milky appearance is seen with chylous ascites. A minimum density of 10,000 erythrocytes per μL is required to provide a red tint to the fluid, which raises the possibility of malignancy if the paracentesis is atraumatic. Pancreatic ascitic fluid is tea colored or black. The ascitic fluid cell count is the most useful test. The upper limit of the neutrophil cell count is 250 cells per μL, even in patients who have undergone diuresis. If paracentesis is traumatic, only 1 neutrophil per 250 erythrocytes and 1 lymphocyte per 750 erythrocytes can be attributed to blood contamination. With spontaneous bacterial peritonitis (SBP), the neutrophil count exceeds 250 cells per μL and represents more than 50% of the total white cell count in the ascitic fluid. Chylous ascites may produce increases in ascitic lymphocyte counts. If infection is suspected, ascitic fluid should be inoculated into blood culture bottles at the bedside and sent for bacterial culture. Gram stain is insensitive for detecting bacterial infection, and results should not be considered reliable if negative because 10,000 organisms per milliliter are needed for a positive Gram stain, whereas spontaneous peritonitis may occur with only 1 organism per milliliter. Similarly, the direct smear has only 0–2% sensitivity for detecting tuberculosis. Ascites fluid culture for tuberculosis is only 40% sensitive and the sensitivity of peritoneal biopsy is 64–83%. If tuberculosis is strongly suspected, laparoscopic rather than blind biopsy of the peritoneum is indicated, because it requires direct visualization of the peritoneal surface with a laparoscope and is almost 100% sensitive. Certain infections can reduce ascitic fluid glucose levels (usually related to perforation of the gastrointestinal tract) but because glucose concentrations usually are normal with SBP, this measure has limited utility. Similarly,

Table 14.2 Etiology of ascites and classification by SAAG and ascites protein level

	SAAG	Ascites protein
Main etiological factors of ascites		
Cirrhosis or alcoholic hepatitis	High	Low
Congestive heart failure	High	High
Peritoneal malignancy	Low	High
Peritoneal tuberculosis	Low	High
Other etiologies of cirrhosis (account for <2% of all cases)		
Massive hepatic metastases	High	Low
Nodular regenerative hyperplasia	High	Low
Fulminant liver failure	High	Low?
Budd-Chiarl syndrome (late)	High	Low
Budd-Chiarl syndrome (early)	High	Low
Constrictive pericarditis	High	High
Veno-occlusive disease	High	High
Myxedema	High	High
Nephrogenous (dialysis) ascites	High	High
Mixed ascites (cirrhosis + peritoneal malignancy)	High	Variable
Pancreatic ascites	low	High
Serositis (connective tissue disease)	Low	High
Chlamydial/gonococcal	Low	High
Biliary	Low	High?
Ovarian hyperstimulation syndrome	Low?	High
Nephrotic syndrome	Low	Low

Those assessments followed by a question mark are theoretical and have not been confirmed by data in the literature.
Source: Yamada T et al. (eds) *Principles of Clinical Gastroenterology*. Oxford: Blackwell Publishing Ltd, 2008.

testing of ascitic fluid pH and lactate levels has been proposed to evaluate for infected fluid; however, their sensitivities are low.

The serum-ascites albumin gradient provides important information about the cause of ascites (Table 14.2). Calculating the gradient involves subtracting the albumin concentration in the ascitic fluid from the serum value. A patient can be diagnosed with portal hypertension with 97% accuracy if the serum albumin minus ascitic albumin concentration is 1.1 g/dL or higher. Causes of high-gradient ascites include cirrhosis, alcoholic hepatitis, cardiac ascites, massive liver metastases, Budd–Chiari syndrome, portal vein thrombosis, veno-occlusive disease, acute fatty liver of pregnancy, myxedema, and some mixed ascites. Conversely, a gradient less than 1.1 g/dL signifies ascites that is not caused by portal hypertension. Low-albumin gradient ascites may result from peritoneal carcinomatosis, tuberculosis, pancreatic or biliary disease, nephrotic syndrome, or connective tissue disease. Previous means of assessing the cause included measuring total ascitic fluid protein and ascitic fluid-to-serum lactate dehydrogenase ratios. Although sometimes still used to distinguish "exudative" from "transudative," the accuracy of these measures is only 55–60%.

Detecting malignancy in ascitic fluid can be a diagnostic challenge. Although nearly 100% of patients with peritoneal carcinomatosis have positive results on cytological analysis of the peritoneal fluid, patients with liver metastases, lymphoma, and hepatocellular carcinoma usually have negative cytological results. Peritoneal biopsy is rarely needed for peritoneal carcinomatosis. The value of ascitic fluid levels of carcinoembryonic antigen and humoral tests of malignancy in detecting malignant ascites is undefined. Other ascitic fluid tests may be ordered, depending on the clinical scenario. In uncomplicated cirrhotic ascites, the ascitic fluid amylase level is low with an ascitic fluid-to-serum ratio of 0.4. With pancreatic ascites, the levels may exceed 2000 IU/L and amylase ratios may increase to 6. With milky ascitic fluid, a triglyceride level is obtained. Chylous ascites triglyceride levels exceed 200 mg/dL versus 20 mg/dL in cirrhotic ascites. Brown ascitic fluid and a bilirubin level higher in the ascitic fluid than in the serum suggest a biliary or bowel perforation.

Management

Initial management of ascites involves diagnostic evaluation to confirm the etiology. Sampling and analysis of the ascitic fluid for cell count, total protein, albumin and cytology can lead to the appropriate diagnosis (Table 14.3). Subsequent testing and management hinges on initial fluid results (Figure 14.2).

Table 14.3 Tests performed in diagnostic paracentesis

Routine analysis of ascitic fluid
Gross appearance
Total protein
Albumin (with simultaneous estimation of serum albumin) so that the ascities–serum albumin gradient can be calculated by subtracting the ascetic fluid value from the serum value
White blood cell count and differential
Bacteriological cultures

Focused analysis of ascetic fluid
Cytology (to exclude malignant ascites)
Amylase (if pancreatic ascites is suspected)
Acid-fast bacilli smear and culture and adenosine deaminase determination (if peritoneal tuberculosis is suspected)
Glucose and lactic dehydrogenase (if secondary peritonitis is suspected in a patient with ascites PMN > 250/mm³)
Triglycerides (if the fluid has a milky appearance, i.e., chylous ascites)
Red blood cell count (if the fluid is bloody)

PMN, polymorphonuclear leukocytes.
Source: Yamada T et al. (eds) *Textbook of Gastroenterology*. Oxford: Blackwell Publishing Ltd, 2009.

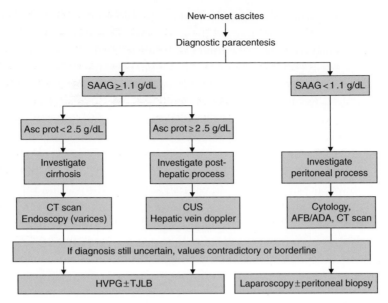

Figure 14.2 Approach to the patient with new-onset ascites. ADA, adenosine deaminase; AFB, acid-fast bacilli; Asc prot, ascites total protein levels; CT, computed tomography; CUS, cardiac echosonography; HVPG, hepatic venous pressure gradient; SAAG, serum–ascites albumin gradient; TJLB, transjugular liver biopsy. (Source: Yamada T et al. (eds) *Textbook of Gastroenterology*. Oxford: Blackwell Publishing Ltd, 2009.)

Ascites unrelated to portal hypertension

In patients with peritoneal carcinomatosis, peripheral edema responds to diuretic administration but the ascites does not. The mainstay for treating these patients is periodic therapeutic paracentesis. Peritoneovenous shunts may be used in selected cases but in most instances, the short life expectancy does not warrant this aggressive intervention. Nephrotic ascites will respond to sodium restriction and diuretics. Tuberculous peritonitis requires specific antituberculosis agents. Pancreatic ascites may resolve spontaneously, respond to octreotide therapy, or require endoscopic stenting or surgery if a ductal leak is present. Postoperative lymphatic leaks may require surgical intervention or peritoneovenous shunting. Nephrogenous ascites may respond to vigorous dialysis.

Ascites related to portal hypertension

For patients with ascites secondary to portal hypertension, restricting dietary sodium to a daily intake of 2g is essential. Fluids do not need to be restricted unless the serum sodium is less than 120 mEq/L. If single-agent diuretic therapy is planned, a daily dose of 100 mg spironolactone is the best choice. For patients who experience spironolactone side-effects (e.g. painful gynecomastia), 10 mg/d of amiloride may be given. The physician should expect a slow response to spironolactone because of its long half-life; weight loss may not be evident for 2 weeks. It is often reasonable to add a loop diuretic (e.g. furosemide) at 40 mg/d to maximize natriuresis. Doses may be increased slowly to maxima of 400 mg/d of spironolactone and 160 mg/d of furosemide. If diuresis is still suboptimal, metolazone or hydrochlorothiazide may be added, although the hyponatremic and hypovolemic effects of such triple-drug regimens mandate close physician follow-up, often on an inpatient basis.

There should be no limit to the amount of weight that can be diuresed daily if pedal edema is present. Once the dependent edema has resolved, diuretics should be adjusted to achieve a daily weight loss of 0.5 kg. Urine sodium levels may be used to direct diuretic therapy. Patients with urine sodium excretion less than potassium excretion are likely to require higher diuretic doses. If urine sodium excretion exceeds potassium excretion, the total daily sodium excretion is likely to be adequate (i.e. >78 mmol/d) in 95% of circumstances. Development of encephalopathy, a serum sodium level less than 120 mEq/L that does not respond to fluid restriction, or serum creatinine higher than 2 mg/dL are relative indicators for discontinuing diuretic therapy. Because concurrent use of nonsteroidal anti-inflammatory drugs promotes renal failure, inhibits the efficacy of diuretics, and may cause gastrointestinal hemorrhage, their use is discouraged.

Various nonmedical means to treat refractory ascites are available. Large-volume paracentesis, with removal of 5 L of fluid, can be performed in 20 min. If greater than 5 L of ascites fluid is removed, it is generally recommended that the patient receive intravenous albumin (8 g/L ascites removed) to prevent paracentesis-induced changes in electrolytes and creatinine. Transjugular intrahepatic portosystemic shunts (TIPSs) are effective in many patients with diuretic-resistant ascites. Peritoneovenous shunts (e.g. Denver and LeVeen) drain ascitic fluid into the central venous circulation; however, they have not achieved widespread use because of a lack of efficacy, shunt occlusion, and side-effects (e.g. pulmonary edema, variceal hemorrhage, diffuse intravascular coagulation, and thromboembolism). Surgical portocaval shunt procedures were used in the past but frequent postoperative complications (e.g. encephalopathy) have tempered enthusiasm for the techniques. Liver transplantation cures both refractory ascites and underlying cirrhosis and should be considered for patients without contraindications. The management of simple and refractory ascites is outlined in Figures 14.3 and 14.4.

Complications

Infection

Spontaneous bacterial peritonitis is defined as ascitic fluid infection with pure growth of a single organism and an ascitic fluid neutrophil count higher than 250 cells per μL without evidence of a surgically remediable intra-abdominal cause. SBP occurs only in the setting of liver disease, for all practical

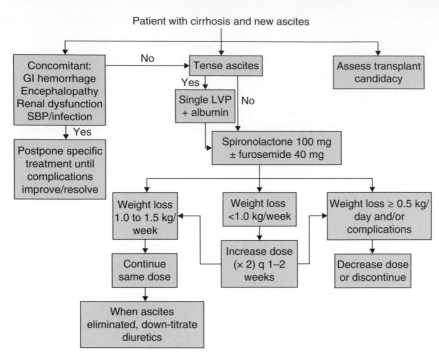

Figure 14.3 Approach to the patient with cirrhosis and uncomplicated ascites. GI, gastrointestinal; LVP, large-volume paracentesis; SBP, spontaneous peritonitis. (Source: Yamada T et al. (eds) *Textbook of Gastroenterology*. Oxford: Blackwell Publishing Ltd, 2009.)

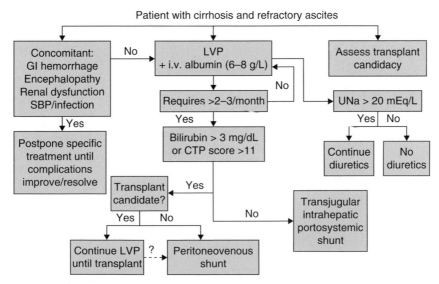

Figure 14.4 Approach to the patient with cirrhosis and refractory ascites. CTP, Child–Turcotte–Pugh; GI, gastrointestinal; IV, intravenous; LVP, large-volume paracentesis; SBP, spontaneous bacterial peritonitis; UNa, urine sodium concentration. (Source: Yamada T et al. (eds) *Textbook of Gastroenterology*. Oxford: Blackwell Publishing Ltd, 2009.)

purposes, although it has been reported with nephrotic syndrome. Ascites is a prerequisite for SBP but it may not be detectable on physical examination. Infection usually occurs with maximal fluid accumulation. *Escherichia coli*, *Klebsiella pneumoniae*, and *Pneumococcus* organisms are the most common isolates in SBP; anaerobes are the causative organism in 1% of cases. Eighty-seven percent of patients with SBP present with symptoms, most commonly fever, abdominal pain, and changes in mental status, although the clinical manifestations may be subtle.

Antibiotics should be initiated when an ascitic fluid neutrophil count higher than 250 cells per μL is documented before obtaining formal culture results. The most accepted antibiotic for SBP is cefotaxime, the third-generation cephalosporin to which 98% of offending bacteria are sensitive, though ceftriaxone, amoxicillin-clavulanic acid, and fluoroquinolones have been used in trials with seemingly equivalent results. When susceptibility testing is available, a drug with a narrower spectrum may be substituted. A randomized trial comparing 5–10 days of therapy showed no difference, supporting a shorter antibiotic course. The treatment course generally is 5–7 days. A repeat paracentesis that demonstrates a reduction in neutrophil counts 48 h after initiating antibiotic treatment indicates that the antibiotic choice was appropriate. If the correct antibiotics are given in a timely manner, the mortality rate of SBP should not exceed 5%; however, many patients succumb to other complications of the underlying liver disease. Renal function is a major cause of death in patients with SBP. It is therefore recommended to give intravenous albumin (1.5 g/kg on day 1, 1 g/kg on day 3), which is of greatest benefit in patients with a bilirubin >4 and creatinine >1. Oral quinolones and trimethoprim-sulfamethoxazole are given as prophylactic agents after an initial episode of SBP because of a reported 1-year recurrence rate of 69% in the absence of prophylaxis.

Spontaneous bacterial peritonitis is not the only infectious complication of ascites. Monomicrobial bacterascites is defined as the presence of a positive result from ascitic fluid culture of a single organism with a concurrent fluid neutrophil count lower than 250 cells per μL. One series of patients with bacterascites demonstrated a predominance of Gram-positive organisms, whereas another showed flora similar to SBP. Because of the high mortality rate of untreated bacterascites (22–43%), antibiotic treatment is warranted for many patients. Alternatively, paracentesis may be repeated for cell count and culture. Culture-negative neutrocytic ascites is defined as ascitic fluid with a neutrophil count higher than or equal to 250 cells per μL with negative fluid culture results in patients who have received no prior antibiotics. Spontaneously resolving SBP is the likely explanation of culture-negative neutrocytic ascites; however, empirical antibiotics generally are given. A decline in ascitic neutrophil counts on repeat paracentesis indicates an appropriate response to therapy.

If there is no response to antibiotics, cytological analysis and culture of the ascitic fluid for tuberculosis may be indicated. Secondary bacterial peritonitis manifests as a polymicrobial infection with a very high ascitic fluid neutrophil count from an identified intra-abdominal source such as appendicitis, diverticulitis, or intra-abdominal abscess. In contrast to SBP, secondary peritonitis usually requires surgical intervention. Gut perforation is suspected with two of the following three criteria: ascitic protein concentration higher than 1 g/dL, glucose level lower than 50 mg/dL, and lactate dehydrogenase level higher than 225 mU/mL. In patients with secondary peritonitis but no perforation, repeat paracentesis 48 h after initiating antibiotic treatment will usually demonstrate increasing neutrophil counts. Polymicrobial bacterascites with an ascitic neutrophil count less than or equal to 250 cells per μL is suggestive of inadvertent gut perforation by the paracentesis needle. It is usually treated with broad-spectrum antibiotics that include coverage for anaerobes. Alternatively, the decision to treat may be deferred until the results of a repeat paracentesis are obtained.

Tense ascites

Some patients develop tense ascites with abdominal discomfort or dyspnea with as little as 2 L of ascitic fluid, whereas others may accumulate 20 L or more before becoming tense. Therapy for tense ascites relies on large-volume paracentesis, which may have the added benefit of increasing the venous return to the heart with resultant improvement in cardiac output and stroke volume.

Abdominal wall hernias

Umbilical and inguinal hernias are common in patients with ascites. These hernias may produce skin ulceration or rupture (Flood syndrome) or they may become incarcerated. More than half of these patients will need surgery. If the patient is a candidate for liver transplantation, hernia repair should be delayed until the time of transplant. A more aggressive surgical approach is needed for ulceration, rupture, or incarceration because of the risk for systemic infection but surgery should be performed after preoperative paracentesis or TIPS to control the ascites. The mortality of rupture is significant (11–43%), and it increases in patients with jaundice or coagulopathy.

Hepatic hydrothorax

Pleural effusions (usually right-sided) are prevalent in patients with cirrhotic ascites. Left-sided effusions are more common with tuberculosis or pancreatic disease. Hepatic hydrothorax is postulated to result from a defect in the diaphragm, which preferentially permits fluid passage into the thorax when negative pressure is generated by normal inspiration. Infection of this fluid is unusual, except in a patient with concurrent SBP. Treatment of hepatic hydrothorax is often challenging because it often does not respond to diuretics. TIPS placement is often successful, whereas pleurodesis and peritoneovenous shunts often lead to complications.

Hepatorenal syndrome

Hepatorenal syndrome is the final stage of functional renal impairment in patients with cirrhosis and portal hypertension; it occurs almost exclusively in patients with refractory ascites. It is characterized by peripheral vasodilation and a creatinine clearance less than 40 mL/min (or serum creatinine level higher than 1.5 mg/dL) with normal intravascular volume and the absence of intrinsic renal disease or other renal insults. Urine sodium content is typically less than 10 mmol/L. Treatment initially involves withdrawing diuretics and nephrotoxins, followed by infusing saline and/or albumin. Vasoactive agents, octreotide, midodrine, and vasopressin, as well as TIPS, have been used with some encouraging results in largely uncontrolled studies. Liver transplantation is the only definitive cure and should be undertaken for all appropriate candidates.

Case studies

Case 1

A 56-year-old male patient with chronic hepatitis C and cirrhosis presents with new-onset, tense ascites resulting in abdominal discomfort and shortness of breath. A 6 L paracentesis is performed, with infusion of 50 g of intravenous albumin. Fluid analysis reveals a SAAG of >1.1, total protein of 1.7 and <100 white blood cells. The patient is counseled regarding dietary sodium restriction, and started on Lasix 40 mg daily plus spironolactone 100 mg daily. Over a 3-month period, the patient's diuretics are gradually increased but he requires repeat paracentesis every 3 weeks. In addition, he develops a right-sided pleural effusion which does not respond to diuretic increases. Laboratory tests reveal a serum bilirubin of 1.8 mg/dL and a MELD score of 9. After obtaining an echocardiogram with normal results, the patient undergoes TIPS and within 3 months has significant improvement in ascites and hydrothorax.

> ### Discussion and potential pitfalls
>
> Portal hypertensive ascites is characterized by a SAAG >1.1. Management consists of sodium restriction, diuretics, and paracentesis. The use of intravenous albumin (8 g/L ascites removed) is recommended for paracentesis >5 L. In patients with refractory ascites and/or hepatic hydrothorax, consideration can be given to placement of a TIPS. This is typically reserved for patients with adequately preserved liver function (MELD <12, bilirubin <3).

Case 2

A 58-year-old woman presents to your clinic with lower extremity edema and significant ascites, requesting a paracentesis. Her ascites has developed over the course of several months. Her medical history is notable for a history of breast cancer, for which she underwent mastectomy followed by radiation therapy.

You are concerned that her ascites represents peritoneal or liver involvement with recurrent metastatic breast cancer. A CT abdomen is obtained which shows mild hepatomegaly, otherwise unremarkable. A diagnostic paracentesis is performed revealing <100 white blood cells, negative cytology, SAAG >1.1, and total protein of 2.9. You pursue a transjugular liver biopsy in view of the high SAAG, and during that procedure it is noted that she has a markedly elevated right atrial pressure. Referral to cardiology with subsequent echocardiogram and right heart catheterization confirms the diagnosis of constrictive pericarditis.

Discussion and potential pitfalls

Ascites can be due to cardiac disease, including congestive heart failure and pericardial disease. Typically the ascites in these cases has a high SAAG, with a high total protein in the fluid. Management is focused on treatment of the underlying cardiac disease.

Key practice points

- Ascites can be due to hepatic and nonhepatic causes.

- Etiology of ascites can be determined based on clinical history and examination of ascites fluid. Serum to ascites albumin gradient (SAAG) >1.1 is suggestive of portal hypertension.

- Initial management of portal hypertensive ascites includes dietary sodium restriction, diuretics, and potentially paracentesis. If ascites is refractory to this management, consider TIPS or liver transplantation.

- It is recommended that intravenous albumin be given for large-volume paracentesis to prevent postparacentesis circulatory dysfunction with renal failure.

CHAPTER 15

Approach to the Patient Requiring Nutritional Support

Most people can ingest the necessary fluids, nutrients, vitamins, and minerals to maintain health. However, certain patients cannot satisfy their nutritional requirements with oral intake alone because of disease or surgical procedures. It is possible to supplement or provide the complete fluid and nutrition needs of these patients with enteral or intravenous solutions. In healthy adults, 30–35 mL of fluid is required for each kilogram of body weight. An additional 360 mL per day is required for each degree centigrade of fever. In anabolic conditions, 300–400 mL more water is needed. Fluids may need to be restricted with volume overload or hyponatremia. Electrolyte requirements are affected by renal and gastrointestinal disease. Potassium and phosphate supplementation is required for diarrhea or vomiting and to compensate for intracellular shifts during intravenous nutrition. Sodium is restricted for heart failure, renal disease, and portal hypertension, whereas potassium, phosphate, and magnesium are reduced with renal failure. Levels of magnesium, iron, copper, selenium, and zinc should be monitored and supplemented as indicated.

Healthy adults require 20–25 kcal per kilogram of body weight to satisfy daily caloric requirements. With the stress of disease or surgery, this need increases to 30–40 kcal per kilogram per day. For nonstressed patients, the recommended dietary protein allowance is 0.8 g per kilogram daily. This increases to 1.5–2.0 g per kilogram daily for catabolic patients. There are nine amino acids that cannot be synthesized by human tissues and must be part of any protein-calorie supplement. Sufficient carbohydrates and fats must be provided to ensure that oral or intravenous proteins or amino acids are used for protein synthesis and not for energy from gluconeogenesis. For patients requiring long-term nutritional support, multivitamin supplementation may be necessary to prevent deficiency syndromes.

Yamada's Handbook of Gastroenterology, Third Edition. Edited by Tadataka Yamada and John M. Inadomi.
© 2013 John Wiley & Sons, Ltd. Published 2013 by John Wiley & Sons, Ltd.

Clinical presentation

History and physical examination

Patients with conditions such as Crohn's disease or pancreatitis exhibit historical features and physical findings characteristic of the illnesses. Persons with protein-calorie malnutrition have weight loss and clinical evidence of deficiencies of essential nutrients, vitamins, and minerals. Loss of greater than 15% of body weight usually indicates significant malnutrition. Development of dependent edema may cause the clinician to underestimate the amount of muscle mass lost. Affected patients may report fatigue resulting from anemia, neuropathy secondary to vitamin B_{12} deficiency, impaired night vision with vitamin A deficiency, or easy bruising resulting from decreased vitamin K levels. The physical examination may detect muscle wasting and edema, as well as signs specific for nutritional deficiencies. Pallor indicates anemia, whereas cheilosis and stomatitis are observed with B vitamin deficiencies.

Additional testing

Laboratory tests are important in assessing nutritional status and also are used during nutritional replenishment to test for the adequacy of supplementation and for complications of nutritional support. Low albumin, prealbumin, and transferrin levels are observed with malnutrition. Electrolyte abnormalities such as hypokalemia and alkalosis are consequences of chronic vomiting or diarrhea, whereas prerenal azotemia or renal failure may result from chronic fluid loss. Electrolytes (including magnesium, calcium, and phosphate), renal function, and albumin are monitored during enteral or parenteral supplementation. Because many regimens produce hyperglycemia or liver injury, serum glucose levels and liver chemistries are monitored during nutritional support.

Management

Implementation of nutritional support

The goal of nutritional support is to decrease morbidity and mortality by providing nutrients or modifying nutrient metabolism. A calorie count by the dietary staff may provide an assessment of nutrient intake. Allowance must be made for fecal losses in patients with malabsorption. Next, nutrient expenditure must be determined. The resting energy expenditure may double in highly catabolic conditions (e.g. burns). Finally, the degree of protein and calorie malnutrition is estimated using objective variables, including serum albumin, Creatinine-Height Index, serum transferrin, total circulating lymphocyte counts, delayed cutaneous hypersensitivity skin testing, serum transthyretin, Body Mass Index, and skinfold thickness. However, none of these measures is reliable by itself and there is no gold standard for determining nutritional status. Scales based on weight, dietary intake, symptoms, and functional capacity have been devised to correlate nutritional status with clinical outcome after surgery.

General rules of nutritional supplementation have been proposed. For patients who are not eating, enteral feeding is provided within 7–10 days for well-nourished, noncatabolic patients; in 1–5 days for catabolic or malnourished patients; and in 1–3 days for catabolic and malnourished patients. If parenteral nutrition is required, this should be initiated in 14–21 days, 1–10 days, and 1–7 days for each category of patients, respectively.

When initiating a nutritional program, energy and protein goals must be set. For patients who are not critically ill, optimal calorie support is obtained if energy equal to 100–120% of the total daily energy expenditure is received. A crude calculation of the energy goal for a given patient is to estimate the basal energy expenditure (20 kcal per kg per day) and multiply by a stress factor for the severity of illness, which ranges from 1.0 for mild disease to 2.0 for severe burns. An additional 0–20% of the basal energy expenditure is added for activity level, and if weight gain is desired, an additional 500–1000 kcal per day is included. A positive nitrogen balance is desired to incorporate amino acids into new protein. To achieve this goal, ingesting 25–35 kcal/g of protein is required. Individuals with renal or liver failure may require less protein, whereas highly catabolic patients, such as those with burns, may require more.

Oral rehydration therapy

Prolonged vomiting or diarrhea can result in loss of excessive amounts of fluid and electrolytes. Oral rehydration therapy enhances sodium and water absorption by stimulating intestinal sodium/glucose cotransport. Various solutions are currently available and include a glucose component (70–150 mmol/L) with variable concentrations of sodium and other electrolytes. In some severe diarrheal conditions, making the solution hypotonic by replacing the glucose with rice solids or other polymeric forms can decrease stool output. In a patient with short bowel syndrome, sodium concentrations greater than 90 mEq/L produce a net sodium and fluid balance.

Enteral nutrition

Enteral nutrition may be administered by several routes. Oral supplementation can be provided by increasing meal portions, adding high-calorie foods, or giving commercial nutritional supplements. Whole foods may include a standard diet or diets modified in consistency (liquid, pureed, or soft) or content (low residue, low fat, low sodium, low protein, high fiber). Nasogastric or nasoenteric formulas may be provided for patients who require short-term nutritional support (<6 weeks) and who cannot eat.

If nutritional support is required for more than 6 weeks, a gastrostomy or jejunostomy is indicated and may be placed endoscopically, radiographically, or surgically. Gastrostomy feedings generally are delivered in bolus fashion 4–6 times daily, although they may be given continuously if there is esophageal reflux of feedings or if gastric emptying is delayed. Jejunostomy feedings are indicated for patients undergoing gastric surgery, who have duodenal obstruction or in whom pulmonary aspiration is a significant risk. Jejunostomy feedings require continuous infusion to prevent diarrhea and abdominal pain and to ensure adequate nutrient absorption.

Standard formulas are appropriate for most patients, although high-protein formulas may be needed for those with extensive trauma or healing wounds. Formulas containing fiber can be given if diarrhea is a problem. Disease-specific preparations are available for patients with renal, hepatic, or pulmonary disease. Renal formulas are low in protein, high in essential amino acids, and low in electrolytes, whereas hepatic formulas are low in sodium, low in aromatic amino acids, and high in branched-chain amino acids. Pulmonary preparations are high in fat and low in carbohydrates because metabolism of carbohydrate generates carbon dioxide. Elemental formulas contain nitrogen as free amino acids and have very little fat. Such preparations are best for those with pancreatic insufficiency or for individuals who require an extremely low-fat diet.

Parenteral nutrition

Intravenous nutritional supplementation is provided by a peripheral (peripheral parenteral nutrition [PPN]) or central (total parenteral nutrition [TPN]) vein. PPN is reserved for patients whose nutritional status is nearly normal and in whom the goal of nutritional supplementation is to maintain lean body mass for a relatively short period of time. Such patients include those undergoing elective surgery who will not be given oral nutrition for 3–7 days. PPN also benefits inpatients who ingest inadequate nutrients or calories, by preventing a negative nitrogen balance during their hospitalization. The limiting factor for PPN is phlebitis induced by hypertonic solutions. Successful PPN mandates solutions with osmolarity less than 900 mOsm and glucose concentrations less than 10%. To meet the nutritional needs of most patients, combinations of hypertonic glucose, amino acids, and lipid emulsions are given with vitamins, minerals, and trace elements. These solutions provide the best nutritional support, if half of the caloric needs are met by the lipid infusion.

For patients who require long-term intravenous nutritional support (>10 days), TPN is preferred. TPN requires the central venous placement of a large-bore catheter, which permits rapid dilution of the hypertonic TPN formulation to prevent phlebitis or hemolysis. Temporary central venous access may be provided by peripherally inserted central catheter (PICC) lines or catheters aseptically placed into the subclavian or internal jugular veins. In patients who need TPN beyond their inpatient stay, permanent catheters (e.g. Hickman, Broviac) are surgically or radiographically placed for home TPN administration. TPN solutions are tailored to the specific needs of the patient. Standard TPN formulations provide 510–1020 kcal/L depending on the glucose concentration. Emulsified lipids are given 2–3 times weekly to prevent essential fatty acid deficiency in patients requiring TPN for more than 1 week. Commercially available multiple vitamin supplements are included that contain all the water-soluble and fat-soluble vitamins except vitamin K, which must be given separately.

Mineral and trace elements usually are included in standard TPN solutions but also may be given as additives. Iodine may be included if TPN is to be given long term. Iron is not routinely included because it is incompatible with the lipid emulsion. Medications including acid-suppressive agents can be included in TPN formulations, as clinically indicated. Patients with renal disease can receive TPN formulations rich in essential amino acids and with few or no nonessential amino acids to minimize the nitrogen load. Formulas for hepatic encephalopathy are high in branched-chain amino acids (leucine, isovaline, valine), which are oxidized outside the liver and block hepatic and muscle protein breakdown.

Total parenteral nutrition has been beneficial in several clinical settings. The most unequivocal indication for home TPN is intestinal failure from any cause. TPN is also the primary therapeutic modality that leads to closure of enterocutaneous fistulae in 30–50% of patients. If spontaneous closure does not occur after 30–60 days, continuation of TPN is unlikely to be successful. TPN is commonly used in managing inflammatory bowel disease, although bowel rest with TPN does not represent primary therapy nor does it decrease the need for surgery in patients with colitis. TPN corrects disease-associated vitamin, mineral, and nutrient deficiencies in severe Crohn's ileitis. It is indicated for patients with complicated acute pancreatitis, if enteral feeding exacerbates abdominal pain or if ascites, fistulae, or pseudocysts are present. Lipid emulsions are given cautiously and should be reduced if serum triglyceride levels exceed 400 mg/dL.

Differential diagnosis

Causes of nutrient deficiency

A variety of clinical conditions mandate nutritional support (Table 15.1). Many patients have diminished nutritional intake as a consequence of oral and upper gastrointestinal problems such as poorly fitting dentures, esophagitis, ulcer disease, or neoplasm of the head and neck. Medications can induce dyspepsia or suppress appetite. Similarly, anorexia is common in depression. Neurological disease, as with a stroke, can produce dysphagia or aspiration that prevents adequate oral intake. Volitional food consumption is impossible with obtundation from any cause. Decreased intake is most likely to affect nutrients that have small body stores, such as folate, water-soluble vitamins, and protein.

Table 15.1 Physical signs of deficiencies of specific nutrients

Hair
Thin, sparse (protein, zinc, biotin)
Flag sign (transverse pigmentation) (protein, copper)
Easy pluckability (protein)

Nails
Spoon-shaped (i.e. koilonychia) (iron)
No luster, transverse ridging (protein, energy)

Skin
Dry, scaling (i.e. xerosis) (vitamin A, zinc)
Seborrheic dermatitis (essential fatty acids, zinc, pyridoxine, biotin)
Flaky paint dermatosis (protein)
Follicular hyperkeratosis (vitamin A, vitamin C, essential fatty acids)
Nasolabial seborrhea (niacin, pyridoxine, riboflavin)
Petechiae, purpura (vitamins C, K, A)
Pigmentation, desquamation (niacin)
Pallor (folate, iron, cobalamin, copper, biotin)

Eyes
Angular palpebritis (riboflavin)
Blepharitis (B vitamins)
Corneal vascularization (riboflavin)
Dull, dry conjunctiva (vitamin A)
Bitot spot (vitamin A)
Keratomalacia (vitamin A)
Fundal capillary microaneurysms (vitamin C)
Ophthalmoplegia (Wernicke encephalopathy) (thiamine)

Mouth
Angular stomatitis (B vitamins, iron, protein)
Cheilosis (riboflavin, niacin, pyridoxine, protein)
Atrophic lingual papillae (niacin, iron, riboflavin, folate, cobalamin)
Glossitis (niacin, pyridoxine, riboflavin, folate, cobalamin)
Decreased taste and smell (vitamin A, zinc)
Swollen, bleeding gums (vitamin C)

Glands
Parotid enlargement (protein)
Sicca syndrome (vitamin C)
Thyroid enlargement (iodine)

Heart
Enlargement, tachycardia, high-output failure (i.e. beriberi) (thiamine)
Small heart, decreased output (protein, energy)
Cardiomyopathy (selenium)
Cardiac arrhythmias (magnesium, potassium)

Extremities
Edema (protein, thiamine)
Muscle weakness (protein, energy, selenium)

Table 15.1 (*cont'd*)

Bone and joint tenderness (vitamins C, A)
Osteopenia, bone pain (vitamin D, calcium, phosphorus, vitamin C)

Neurological
Confabulation, disorientation (i.e. Korsakoff psychosis) (thiamine)
Decreased position and vibration sense, ataxia (cobalamin, thiamine)
Decreased tendon reflexes (thiamine)
Weakness, paresthesias (cobalamin, pyridoxine, thiamine)
Mental disorders (cobalamin, niacin, thiamine, magnesium)

Other
Delayed wound healing (vitamin C, protein, zinc, essential fatty acids)
Hypogonadism, delayed puberty (zinc)
Glucose intolerance (chromium)

All of these patient subsets exhibit normal gut absorptive function and can be supplemented with oral or enteral formulas.

Other clinical conditions without impairment of food intake are associated with nutrient deficiencies. Malabsorptive conditions may produce profound nutrient deficiency, especially those that impair the effective small intestinal mucosal absorptive surface area (e.g. celiac disease, short bowel syndrome, Whipple disease). Affected patients also lose endogenous stores of minerals, vitamins, and proteins that are not reabsorbed from gastric, pancreaticobiliary, and small intestinal secretions. When steatorrhea is present, divalent cations (calcium, magnesium, zinc) are lost because they combine with unabsorbed fatty acids to form nonabsorbable soaps.

Drugs may induce malabsorption by several mechanisms. Cholestyramine binds fats and fat-soluble vitamins, whereas neomycin precipitates bile salts. Sulfasalazine inhibits folate absorption and colchicine inhibits enterocyte release of fat-soluble vitamins. In addition to suppressing appetite, chronic ingestion of large amounts of ethanol is toxic to intestinal enterocytes, causing decreased transport of glucose, amino acids, folate, and thiamine.

Protein-calorie malnutrition occurs in conditions with increased catabolism, such as Crohn's disease or high-dose corticosteroid use. Likewise, increased caloric and fluid needs are observed with pregnancy, lactation, sepsis, trauma, and burns. Additional deficiencies in Crohn's disease include those of calcium, vitamin D, iron, vitamin B_{12}, zinc, and potassium. Other causes of intestinal failure that result in malabsorption include radiation enteritis, intestinal pseudo-obstruction with bacterial overgrowth, chronic adhesive peritonitis, and mucosal diseases without effective treatment (collagenous sprue). Advanced liver disease may alter the plasma amino acid profile. Increased fluid and electrolyte losses occur in the absence of malabsorption in patients with diarrhea, vomiting, enterocutaneous fistulae, gastric suctioning, and renal wasting.

Mineral deficiency states

Major mineral deficiencies elicit a range of clinical manifestations. Sodium deficiency results from increased losses caused by vomiting, diarrhea, diuresis, salt-wasting renal disease, fistulae, or adrenal insufficiency. Among hospitalized patients, hyponatremia commonly results from excess free water caused by cardiac, renal, or hepatic insufficiency. Severe sodium depletion with dehydration produces nausea and vomiting, exhaustion, cramps, seizures, and cardiorespiratory collapse.

Pseudohyponatremia results from excess lipid, glucose, blood urea nitrogen, mannitol, or glycerin in the serum. Potassium depletion results from gastrointestinal or urinary losses (diuretics, alkalosis, mineralocorticoid excess, renal tubular acidosis). Hypokalemia also results from potassium shifts from the extracellular to the intracellular compartment during alkalosis, after insulin or glucose administration, or periodic paralysis. Symptoms of potassium depletion include confusion, lethargy, weakness, cramps, myalgias, cardiac arrhythmias, glucose intolerance, nausea, vomiting, diarrhea, ileus, and gastroparesis. Hypocalcemia is caused by vitamin D deficiency, failed vitamin D synthesis or action, hypoparathyroidism, hypomagnesemia, acute pancreatitis, osteoblastic malignancies, malabsorption, and medications (e.g. aminoglycosides, cisplatin, calcitonin, furosemide, phosphates, and anticonvulsants). Manifestations of hypocalcemia include a positive Chvostek or Trousseau sign, tetany, hyperreflexia, paresthesias, seizures, mental status changes, increased intracranial pressure, bradycardia, heart block, and choreoathetotic movements. Chronic calcium deficiency causes rickets in children and osteomalacia in adults. Eighty percent to 85% of phosphorus stores are in bone.

Hypophosphatemia occurs in 2–3% of hospitalized patients because of decreased intestinal absorption (antacids, malabsorption, vitamin D deficiency, hypoparathyroidism), increased renal excretion (proximal tubule disease, alkalosis, diuretics, hyperparathyroidism, burns, corticosteroids), and intracellular shifts (respiratory alkalosis, carbohydrate administration). Severe hypophosphatemia produces hemolysis, encephalopathy, seizures, paresthesias, muscle weakness, rhabdomyolysis, decreased glucose utilization, and reduced oxygen delivery. Similarly, 70% of magnesium stores are in bone. Magnesium absorption decreases in malabsorption syndromes. Excessive urinary loss results from hypercalcemia, volume expansion, tubular dysfunction, alcoholism, diabetes, hyperparathyroidism, hypophosphatemia, and medications (e.g. diuretics, aminoglycosides, cyclosporine, amphotericin, cisplatin, digoxin). Shifts into the intracellular space result from refeeding, treating diabetic ketoacidosis, pancreatitis, and correcting acidosis in renal failure. Patients with hypomagnesemia present with tremors, myoclonic jerks, ataxia, tetany, psychiatric disturbances, coma, ventricular arrhythmias, hypotension, or cardiac arrest.

Trace mineral deficiencies also are prevalent. Iron deficiency results from gastrointestinal bleeding, excessive menstrual loss, and malabsorption (e.g. celiac sprue, achlorhydria). Clinical manifestations of iron deficiency stem from anemia and include weakness, light-headedness, decreased exercise tolerance, and tachycardia. Zinc deficiency results from malabsorption, cirrhosis, alcoholism, nephrotic syndrome, sickle cell anemia, pregnancy, pica, pancreatic insufficiency, use of penicillamine, and chronic diarrhea of any cause. Clinical manifestations of zinc deficiency include growth retardation, scaling skin, alopecia, diarrhea, apathy, night blindness, poor wound healing, and dysgeusia. Copper deficiency in adults is rare and occurs with parenteral nutrition without copper supplements and during penicillamine therapy. Clinical manifestations of copper deficiency include microcytic anemia, leukopenia, neutropenia, and skeletal abnormalities. Selenium deficiency occurs with small bowel causes of malabsorption, fistulae, alcoholism, cirrhosis, acquired immunodeficiency syndrome, cancer, and with parenteral nutritional formulas without supplemental selenium. Symptoms of selenium deficiency include myositis, weakness, and cardiomyopathy.

Only 2% of dietary chromium is absorbed. Chromium deficiency occurs with short bowel syndrome and in patients who receive poorly supplemented parenteral nutritional formulas. Clinical manifestations include hyperglycemia, insulin insensitivity, encephalopathy, peripheral neuropathy, and weight loss. Iodine deficiency usually is caused by inadequate intake and results in hypothyroidism, thyroid hyperplasia, and hypertrophy. Iodine supplements are rarely needed in parenteral nutritional solutions, presumably because sufficient iodine is present as a contaminant or is absorbed from the skin.

Several minerals are considered essential but deficiency syndromes have not been reported. Fluoride is essential for growth, reproduction, and iron absorption. Molybdenum is needed to metabolize purines and sulfur-containing compounds. Manganese is a cofactor for pyruvate carboxylase and manganese superoxide dismutase. Vanadium, nickel, cobalt, tin, and silicon also are considered essential in mammals. Cadmium, lead, boron, aluminum, arsenic, mercury, strontium, and lithium eventually may prove to be essential.

Vitamin deficiency states

In general, deficiencies of fat-soluble vitamins (A, D, E, and K) take years to develop because large stores are present in adipose tissue. Vitamin D is made endogenously in sun-exposed skin. Vitamins that undergo enterohepatic circulation (e.g. A and D) may be lost in malabsorptive conditions. Blood values for fat-soluble vitamins are difficult to interpret because of adipose stores and plasma-binding proteins. Vitamin A or its carotenoid precursors are present in animal products (e.g. liver, kidney, dairy products, eggs) and in green and yellow vegetables. Vitamin A deficiency results from decreased intake and fat malabsorption, although impaired carotenoid conversion in mucosal disease, inability to store the vitamin in liver disease, and increased urinary losses (e.g. as from tuberculosis, cancer, pneumonia, urinary tract infection) may contribute.

Vitamin A deficiency produces night blindness, xerophthalmia, follicular hyperkeratosis, altered taste and smell, increased cerebrospinal fluid pressure, and increased infections.

Vitamin D from fish liver oils, eggs, liver, and dairy products is absorbed by the small intestine. Cholecalciferol (vitamin D_3) is synthesized on ultraviolet exposure of the skin. Vitamin D deficiency results from inadequate exposure to the sun, steatorrhea, severe liver or kidney disease, Crohn's disease, or small bowel resection. Manifestations of deficiency include hypocalcemia, hypophosphatemia, bone demineralization, osteomalacia in adults, rickets in children, and bony fractures. Vitamin E is a fat-soluble antioxidant and a free radical scavenger found in plants and vegetable oils. Deficiency is rare in humans but may occur with malabsorption in $\alpha\beta$-lipoproteinemia, cystic fibrosis, cirrhosis, malabsorption, and from ingesting excess mineral oil. Vitamin E deficiency elicits hemolysis and a progressive neurological syndrome (areflexia, gait disturbance, decreased vibratory and proprioceptive sensation, and gaze paresis). Vitamin K is abundant in the diet and is synthesized by intestinal bacteria. Deficiency results from malabsorption of fat, diminished liver function or bile secretion, or antibiotic inhibition of bacterial production. Vitamin K deficiency prolongs prothrombin time and increases the risk of hemorrhage.

In contrast to fat-soluble vitamins, water-soluble vitamins are not stored in large quantities in the body. Blood levels of water-soluble vitamins reflect body stores and fall before clinical manifestations of vitamin deficiency develop. Thiamine (vitamin B_1) is readily available in the diet, and deficiency presents in alcoholics or in patients with malabsorption, severe malnutrition, prolonged fever, or on chronic hemodialysis. Thiamine deficiency causes beriberi, which is characterized by easy fatigability, weakness, paresthesias, and high-output congestive heart failure. Other manifestations include peripheral neuropathy, cerebellar dysfunction, subacute necrotizing encephalomyelopathy, and Wernicke encephalopathy (with mental changes, ataxia, nystagmus, paresis of upward gaze). Thiamine deficiency may also play a role in Korsakoff syndrome. Riboflavin (vitamin B_2) is present in milk, eggs, and leafy green vegetables. Deficiency occurs in conjunction with other B vitamin deficiencies in alcoholism and malabsorption. Riboflavin deficiency produces angular stomatitis, cheilosis, glossitis, seborrhea-like dermatitis, pruritus, photophobia, and visual impairment.

Niacin (vitamin B_3) and its precursor, tryptophan, are found in animal proteins, beans, nuts, whole grains, and enriched breads and cereals. Niacin deficiency occurs rarely as a complication of alcoholism, malabsorption, carcinoid syndrome, or Hartnup disease. Niacin deficiency causes pellagra, which presents with a scaly, hyperpigmented dermatitis localized to sun-exposed surfaces, diarrhea, and central nervous system dysfunction (irritability and headache progressing to psychosis, hallucinations, and seizures). Pyridoxine (vitamin B_6) is present in animal protein and whole-grain cereals. Pyridoxine deficiency most commonly occurs during treatment with pyridoxine antagonists (isoniazid, hydralazine, and penicillamine) but also occurs in alcoholics and malabsorption. Pyridoxine deficiency produces peripheral neuropathy, seborrheic dermatitis, glossitis, angular stomatitis, cheilosis, seizures, and sideroblastic anemia. Folate is abundant in vegetables, legumes, kidney, liver, and nuts. Folate deficiency is caused by poor intake or altered small bowel mucosal function in alcoholics, by malabsorption, and during use of sulfasalazine or anticonvulsants. Folate deficiency elicits macrocytic anemia, thrombocytopenia, leukopenia, glossitis, diarrhea, fatigue, and possibly neurological findings. Cobalamin (vitamin B_{12}) is found in animal tissues. Cobalamin deficiency occurs in some vegetarians and also is caused by pernicious anemia, gastrectomy, ileal disease or resection, or bacterial overgrowth, in which bacteria bind dietary cobalamin so that it cannot be absorbed. Clinical findings of deficiency include macrocytic anemia, anorexia, loss of taste, glossitis, diarrhea, dyspepsia, hair loss, impotence, and neurological disease (i.e. peripheral neuropathy, loss of vibratory sensation, inco-ordination, muscle weakness and atrophy, irritability, and memory loss).

Ascorbic acid (vitamin C) is present in fruits (especially citrus) and vegetables. Scurvy develops after 2–3 months of a diet deficient in ascorbic acid. Other causes of deficiency include alcoholism, malabsorption, and Crohn's disease. Vitamin C deficiency produces weakness, irritability, aching joints and muscles, and weight loss, which progress to perifollicular hyperkeratotic papules, petechiae, and swollen, hemorrhagic gums. Biotin deficiency occurs in persons whose diet is high in egg whites, which contain a biotin-binding glycoprotein, and in patients who take hyperalimentation solutions without biotin supplements. Biotin deficiency produces anorexia, nausea, dermatitis, alopecia, mental depression, and organic aciduria.

Essential fatty acid deficiency

Essential fatty acids are long-chain compounds that cannot be synthesized by mammals (i.e. linoleic, linolenic, and arachidonic acids). Because humans synthesize arachidonic acid from exogenous linoleic acid, only linoleic acid (and, to a lesser degree, linolenic) is required in the diet. Vegetable oils are rich dietary sources. Parenteral nutritional lipid emulsions consist of soybean or safflower oil, which are predominantly linoleic acid. Essential fatty acid deficiency, caused by fat-free hyperalimentation, appears within 3–6 weeks as scaly dermatitis, alopecia, coarse hair, hepatomegaly, thrombocytopenia, diarrhea, and growth retardation.

Protein-calorie malnutrition

From 20% to 60% of inpatients may have protein-calorie malnutrition. Healthy adults die of starvation after 60–90 days if no proteins or calories are provided, which may decrease to 14 days in hypermetabolic conditions. Protein-calorie malnutrition produces weakness, impaired immune responses, skin breakdown, infection, apathy, and irritability. If malnutrition is severe, full recovery of cardiac and skeletal muscle function may not occur.

Complications

Enteral nutrition

The major complications of enteral feedings are pulmonary aspiration, nausea and vomiting, abdominal pain, diarrhea, metabolic abnormalities, and infection (pneumonia, gut infections). Aspiration is rare if feedings are delivered distal to the ligament of Treitz. During gastric feedings, the upper body should be elevated at least 30° above the horizontal. Residual volumes of 200 mL after nasogastric feeding or 100 mL after gastrostomy feeding predispose to aspiration. Diarrhea results from excessive infusion rates, concurrent use of antibiotics and antacids, sorbitol-containing elixir, inadequate fiber supplementation, too much lipid with fat malabsorption, hypertonic formulations, vitamin or mineral deficiency, or hypoalbuminemia. If no remediable cause of diarrhea is found, loperamide elixir, diphenoxylate with atropine, or tincture of opium may be given. Complications of gastrostomies and jejunostomies include wound infections, leakage, tube migration, ileus, fever, peritonitis, and necrotizing fasciitis.

Parenteral nutrition

Potential complications of intravenous nutrition include mechanical, infectious, and metabolic problems. Pneumothorax, hemorrhage, brachial plexus injury, air or guidewire embolism, cardiac tamponade, and death may result from inserting a central venous catheter. Catheters can become occluded by blood, fibrin, intravenous lipid, or precipitated drugs. Vascular catheters are responsible for one-third of nosocomial bacteremias and half of candidemias. Skin flora are the most common pathogens and include *Staphylococcus aureus*, *Staphylococcus epidermidis*, *Klebsiella pneumoniae*, *Pseudomonas aeruginosa*, *Enterobacter* species, and *Candida albicans*. Early metabolic complications of TPN include electrolyte abnormalities, hyperglycemia or hypoglycemia, hyperlipidemia, acid–base disturbances, hypercapnia, and fluid overload (Table 15.2). Lipid emulsions can cause pulmonary dysfunction, impaired function of the immune system, pancreatitis, delayed platelet aggregation, and hypersensitivity reactions. Delayed metabolic consequences include liver dysfunction, bone demineralization, essential fatty acid deficiency, and mineral deficiency or excess. Liver abnormalities occur frequently with long-term TPN, including calculous and acalculous cholecystitis, hepatic steatosis, steatohepatitis, fibrosis, and cirrhosis. TPN-induced liver abnormalities may be minimized by not exceeding the caloric needs of the patient, especially the glucose component.

Table 15.2 Metabolic complications associated with total parenteral nutrition

Early
Electrolyte abnormalities
   Sodium
   Potassium
   Calcium
   Magnesium
   Phosphate
Refeeding syndrome
Hyperglycemia
Hypoglycemia
Elevated urea nitrogen
Adverse reactions to lipid emulsions
   Hyperlipidemia
   Poor lipid clearance
   Thrombocytopenia
Hypercapnia
Hyperammonemia
Fluid overload
Hyperosmolar nonketotic hyperglycemic coma
Acidosis
Alkalosis

Delayed
Lipid overload syndrome
Essential fatty acid deficiency
Metabolic bone disease
Liver dysfunction
Gallbladder disease
Mineral deficiency or excess
   Zinc
   Copper
   Chromium
   Selenium
   Molybdenum
   Iron
   Manganese

Case studies

Case 1

A 27-year-old man with refractory Crohn's disease is admitted to the hospital due to a partial small bowel obstruction. The patient has been experiencing severe diffuse abdominal pain, nausea, and vomiting for the past 48 h. He vomits immediately after any attempt at oral intake. The patient has a history of a stricture involving the terminal ileum that required resection 2 years before. He has had multiple small bowel strictures requiring surgical intervention. The patient is currently being treated with adalimumab and azathioprine for his Crohn's disease. He is noted to have an albumin of 2.4 g/dL and a sedimentation rate of 94 mm/h. Physical exam demonstrates a diffusely tender abdomen and multiple surgical scars across the abdomen. CT scan demonstrates a small bowel obstruction with dilated loops of small bowel. Surgery has evaluated the patient and is recommending conservative management with placement of a nasogastric tube for decompression, IV hydration, and TPN given the low albumin, active inflammation, and likelihood that the patient will not receive any enteral nutrition while the small bowel obstruction is being monitored.

Discussion and potential pitfalls

Total parenteral nutrition in Crohn's disease patients admitted to hospital who either require bowel rest or are unable to tolerate oral intake should be considered early. Due to the catabolic state of inflammation in Crohn's disease and the fact that many Crohn's patients have nutritional deficiencies, TPN should be initiated within 1–5 days. Furthermore, TPN can also be used to correct nutritional deficiencies prior to surgery. Once TPN is initiated, routine monitoring should include fluid intake and output measurements, serum electrolytes, aminotransferases, bilirubin, and triglycerides. Patients receiving TPN are at increased risk of bloodstream infection and patients with Crohn's disease on immunosuppressive therapies are at even greater risk and should be monitored carefully for signs of infection.

Case 2

A 50-year-old man presents to the emergency department with a 1-day history of sudden-onset severe periumbilical pain, nausea, and vomiting. He admits to heavy alcohol consumption prior to the onset of abdominal pain. On physical examination, he is afebrile, pulse is 120 bpm, respiratory rate is 22. He is tachypneic and anxious. His abdomen is tender to palpation with no bowel sounds appreciated. His labs are notable for a WBC of 22 K cells/mL, hematocrit of 56%, BUN of 26 mg/dL, amylase 2000 U/L, and lipase of 1947 U/L. The patient is diagnosed with acute pancreatitis. He is aggressively hydrated with normal saline. A CT scan performed 48 h after admission demonstrates significant necrosis of the pancreatic gland with absence of perfusion in 70% of the gland. He is determined to have severe acute pancreatitis and early enteral nutrition is initiated through a nasojejunal feeding tube.

Discussion and potential pitfalls

Enteral feeding should be initiated as soon as severe acute pancreatitis has been diagnosed as this has demonstrated reduced infectious complications, decreased hospital days, and a trend toward improving mortality. Benefit has been demonstrated when enteral nutrition is initiated within 36–48 h of presentation. Enteral nutrition should be performed through a nasojejunal feeding tube.

Key practice points

- Healthy adults require 20–25 kcal per kilogram of body weight to satisfy daily caloric requirements.
- Loss of greater than 15% of body weight usually indicates significant malnutrition.
- Laboratory tests are important in assessing nutritional status and also are used during nutritional replenishment to test for the adequacy of supplementation and for complications of nutritional support.
- When initiating a nutritional program, energy and protein goals must be set.
- Jejunostomy feedings require continuous infusion to prevent diarrhea and abdominal pain and to ensure adequate nutrient absorption.
- Blood values for fat-soluble vitamins are difficult to interpret because of adipose stores and plasma-binding proteins.

CHAPTER 16

Approach to the Patient Requiring Endoscopic Procedures

Introduction and background

Utility of endoscopy

Gastrointestinal endoscopy has transformed all aspects of diagnosing and treating patients with diseases of the gastrointestinal tract. Each endoscopic procedure has a specific set of indications and contraindications. In general, an endoscopic procedure is indicated only when the results are expected to influence the course of patient management. In some cases, however, the attendant risks of endoscopy may outweigh the benefits. Before proceeding with endoscopic intervention, a patient should give a complete history and have a complete physical examination to establish the indication for the study and exclude the presence of any contraindications. Many procedures require bowel cleansing or prolonged fasting; therefore, the clinician must be aware of comorbid conditions, such as diabetes, heart failure, or renal dysfunction, which may require adjusting the instructions for patient preparation. All patients should be counseled on the risks and benefits of endoscopy; written and verbal informed consent are mandatory.

Principles of conscious sedation

Most endoscopic procedures require conscious sedation to permit a safe and complete examination. The optimal agents and dosages vary but all carry the risk of cardiopulmonary complications. All patients should be monitored for changes in blood pressure, heart rate, and respiratory rate throughout the course of sedation. Many centers use pulse oximetry and electrocardiographic monitoring but it is uncertain if routine use of these more expensive monitoring procedures improves treatment outcomes. No electronic monitoring can replace clinical judgment. Therefore, if significant cardiopulmonary signs or symptoms arise, the procedure should be aborted. The benzodiazepine antagonist flumazenil and the opiate antagonist naloxone can be used to reverse the effects of benzodiazepines and narcotics, respectively, in patients with complications of oversedation but

Yamada's Handbook of Gastroenterology, Third Edition. Edited by Tadataka Yamada and John M. Inadomi.
© 2013 John Wiley & Sons, Ltd. Published 2013 by John Wiley & Sons, Ltd.

Table 16.1 Recommendations for antibiotic prophylaxis

Risk group	Procedure	Antibiotic prophylaxis
High risk of endocarditis (prosthetic valve, prior endocarditis, systemic pulmonary shunt, or synthetic vascular graft <1 y old)	Stricture dilation, sclerotherapy	Recommended
	Esophagogastroduodenoscopy or colonoscopy	Insufficient data (endoscopist's discretion)
Moderate risk of endocarditis (rheumatic valvular disease, mitral valve prolapse with insufficiency, hypertrophic cardiomyopathy, and most congenital malformations)	Stricture dilation, sclerotherapy	Insufficient data (endoscopist's discretion)
	Esophagogastroduodenoscopy or colonoscopy	Not recommended
Low risk of endocarditis (coronary bypass surgery, pacemakers, and implantable defibrillators)	All endoscopic procedures	Not recommended
Prosthetic joints	All endoscopic procedures	Not recommended
Obstructed biliary system or pancreatic pseudocyst	Endoscopic retrograde cholangiopancreatography	Recommended
Cirrhosis and ascites	Stricture dilation, sclerotherapy	Insufficient data (endoscopist's discretion)
	Esophagogastroduodenoscopy or colonoscopy	Not recommended
All patients	Percutaneous gastrostomy	Recommended

they should not be used routinely to reverse sedation. Slow titration of the initial dose of the sedative agent is the best way to avoid oversedation.

Antibiotic prophylaxis

The role of preprocedure antibiotics to prevent endocarditis or bacteremia in patients with vascular or other prostheses is undefined. Based on the documented risks of bacteremia with given procedures and the risks of establishing an infection in certain pre-existing conditions, the American Society of Gastrointestinal Endoscopy promotes guidelines for antibiotic prophylaxis before endoscopic procedures (Table 16.1). In many circumstances, no definitive recommendations can be made and the decision is made at the clinician's discretion. Antibiotics can be costly, and many have a substantial risk of allergic reactions. These issues must be considered when contemplating the use of prophylactic antibiotics.

Coagulation disorders

Although coagulation abnormalities are not absolute contraindications to endoscopy, the use of endoscopic biopsy can be associated with an increased risk of bleeding. Before any therapeutic intervention, including percutaneous gastrostomy tube placement and electrocoagulation for polypectomy or hemostasis, attempts should be made to correct coagulation disorders. Prolongation of prothrombin time unrelated to the administration of warfarin may require parenteral vitamin K therapy. If there is no response to vitamin K or if emergency therapy is necessary, coagulation factors should be supplemented with fresh-frozen plasma. Antiplatelet agents (e.g. aspirin) should ideally be withheld for 7–10 days before and after these therapeutic measures, although there is no evidence that routine endoscopy including polypectomy is associated with an increased risk of bleeding complications in patients using daily aspirin. Depending on the underlying medical condition, warfarin can often be withheld for 5–7 days before the procedure and reinstituted 1–2 days after therapy.

If medical conditions prohibit discontinuation, one of two potential management pathways can be used. In the first, the patient is hospitalized, warfarin is discontinued, and heparin is initiated. When the prothrombin time normalizes, the patient is prepared for the procedure, and heparin is discontinued 4 h before the intervention. Heparin can be restarted 4 h after the procedure, and warfarin can be reinstituted 12–24 h after heparin if no procedure-related hemorrhage occurs. Alternatively, warfarin may be stopped 5 days prior to the procedure and subcutaneous low molecular weight heparin (e.g. dalteparin) initiated, once or twice daily, according to the patient's weight. The last low molecular weight heparin dose is given the night before the procedure and then restarted the evening of the procedure and continued for 5 days, whereas warfarin is restarted the evening of the procedure and continued as previously taken. This second approach avoids hospitalization because the subcutaneous low molecular weight heparin is self-administered in an outpatient setting.

Upper gastrointestinal endoscopy

Indications and contraindications

Many symptoms attributable to diseases of the esophagus, stomach, and duodenum are best assessed by esophagogastroduodenoscopy (EGD) or upper gastrointestinal endoscopy. The American Society of Gastrointestinal Endoscopy has established consensus guidelines for the appropriate use of EGD (Table 16.2). Therapeutic endoscopy is often indicated for control of variceal and nonvariceal bleeding, dilation of strictures, removal of some foreign bodies, palliation of advanced malignancies with stents or tumor ablation, and placement of a percutaneous gastrostomy tube. The advent of longer endoscopes has expanded the capability of upper gastrointestinal endoscopy in diagnosing and potentially treating diseases of the small intestine. Enteroscopy is indicated when investigating chronic bleeding presumed secondary to a source in the small intestine or if visualization or sampling the small intestine is warranted by radiological abnormalities.

Table 16.2 Indications for upper gastrointestinal endoscopy

Diagnostic

Upper abdominal distress despite an appropriate trial of therapy

Upper abdominal distress associated with signs or symptoms of organic disease (weight loss, anorexia)

Refractory vomiting of unknown cause

Dysphagia or odynophagia

Esophageal reflux symptoms unresponsive to therapy

Upper gastrointestinal bleeding

When sampling of duodenal or jejunal tissue or fluid is indicated

To obtain a histological diagnosis for radiographically demonstrated gastric or esophageal ulcers, upper intestinal tract strictures, or suspected neoplasms

To screen for varices so that patients with cirrhosis can be identified as possible candidates for prophylactic medical or endoscopic therapy

To assess acute injury after caustic ingestion

When management of other disease processes is affected by the presence of upper gastrointestinal pathological conditions (e.g. use of anticoagulants)

Therapeutic

Treatment of variceal and nonvariceal upper gastrointestinal bleeding

Removal of foreign bodies

Removal of selected polypoid lesions

Dilation of symptomatic strictures

Palliative treatment of stenosing neoplasms

Placement of percutaneous feeding gastrostomy tube

Surveillance

Follow-up of selected gastric, esophageal, or stomal ulcers to document healing

Barrett esophagus

Familial adenomatous polyposis

Adenomatous gastric polyps

Follow-up of varices eradicated by endoscopic therapy

The major contraindications to upper gastrointestinal endoscopy include perforation, hemodynamic instability, cardiopulmonary distress, and inadequate patient co-operation. Coagulation disorders are relative contraindications to therapeutic intervention. Percutaneous gastrostomy tube placement is contraindicated if the stomach is inaccessible because of a prior gastrectomy or interposed bowel, liver, or spleen.

Patient preparation and monitoring

Patients should not ingest solid food for 6–8 h or liquids for 4 h before elective upper gastrointestinal endoscopy. If delayed gastric emptying is suspected, a liquid diet can be instituted 24 h before the procedure and the fasting interval increased to 8–12 h. For complete gastric outlet obstruction, evacuation of the stomach with a nasogastric tube is usually necessary. If an emergency endoscopic procedure is required for gastrointestinal bleeding, measures should be taken to avoid aspiration. Evacuation of the stomach with an orogastric tube before the procedure, attentiveness to oral suction during the procedure, and prophylactic endotracheal intubation in an obtunded patient protect the patient's airway.

Conscious sedation is typically performed using a combination of a short-acting benzodiazepine (e.g. midazolam) along with a short-acting opiate (e.g. fentanyl), although the synergistic cardiopulmonary depressant effects of this combination may increase the rate of cardiopulmonary complications. Throughout the procedure, a trained assistant should work together with the endoscopist to monitor the oral secretions as well as the overall clinical condition of the patient.

Performance of the procedure

The endoscope is introduced blindly or under direct visualization by passing the instrument into the posterior pharynx and instructing the patient to swallow. Direct visualization is preferred because it is less traumatic and provides a view of the larynx. A standard EGD involves a complete inspection of the esophagus, stomach, and the first two portions of the duodenum. A pediatric colonoscope or push enteroscope can be advanced into the proximal jejunum. Enteroscopy can also be performed with the sonde enteroscope, which relies on peristaltic movement to propel the instrument into the distal jejunum or ileum, but this instrument does not provide biopsy or therapeutic capabilities.

Endoscopic biopsy or brush cytology studies may provide a pathological diagnosis. For some disease processes (e.g. infections caused by *Helicobacter pylori* and causes of malabsorption in the small intestine), random biopsies of normal-appearing mucosa may be indicated. Upper gastrointestinal endoscopy also provides the capability of therapeutic intervention. Dysphagia from esophageal strictures or achalasia can be relieved with endoscopic dilation using pneumatic balloon or sequential bougienage techniques. The safest means of bougienage dilation involves passage of the dilator over a guidewire placed endoscopically into the distal stomach. Although fluoroscopy reduces the complication rate of dilation, radiation exposure and resource limitations have precluded its routine use in many centers. Acute or chronic nonvariceal hemorrhage can be controlled with electrocoagulation, heater probe application, injection therapy, or laser photocoagulation. Large or bleeding esophageal varices may be treated with injection sclerotherapy or band ligation. Mucosal polyps can be excised with electrocoagulation using hot biopsy forceps or with snare polypectomy. Deep tissue sampling and excision of mucosal lesions may be accomplished with submucosal injection and endoscopic mucosal resection (EMR). Large stenosing esophageal or gastric malignancies can be ablated with laser photocoagulation or electrocoagulation. Esophageal malignancies can also be palliated by deploying metallic expandable stents.

Complications

Diagnostic upper gastrointestinal endoscopy is usually very safe, and rates of serious complications are low. Most complications are related to oversedation, emphasizing the need for preprocedural patient assessment and vigilant patient monitoring throughout the period of sedation. The high rate of wound infections associated with gastrostomy tube placement can be substantially reduced by prophylactic anti-biotics. The benefit of prophylactic antibiotics for other indications remains unproven.

Video capsule endoscopy

Indications and contraindications

Wireless capsule endoscopy or video capsule endoscopy (VCE) uses a wireless, short focal length lens to capture two images per second as the capsule traverses the gastrointestinal tract. The video images are transmitted by radiotelemetry to an array of aerials attached to the body via a recording belt. The primary indication for VCE is for evaluating obscure gastrointestinal bleeding. However, indications continue to evolve, and it has been used for evaluating small bowel tumors and small intestinal Crohn's disease. Contraindications to VCE include esophageal stricture and intermittent or partial small bowel obstruction. Relative contraindications include dementia, gastroparesis, and the presence of a pacemaker because of potential interference as the capsule traverses the chest. No cases of complications in patients with pacemakers who have undergone VCE have been reported.

Performance of the procedure

The procedure is generally performed in ambulatory patients after an overnight fast with or without a polyethylene glycol preparation. An eight-lead sensor array is fastened to the abdomen in a designated pattern that allows image capture and continuous triangulation of the capsule location in the abdomen. The images are stored on a small portable recorder carried on the belt and are subsequently downloaded for interpretation. Patients may proceed with normal activities and can consume clear liquids 2 h after capsule ingestion and food 4 h after capsule ingestion. The capsule itself is disposable and is passed by normal excretion.

Complications

The primary risk of VCE is capsule retention, which occurs in up to 25% of patients but requires surgical intervention in less than 1%. Retained capsules rarely cause obstructive symptoms, and most cases can be observed for extended periods during which most capsules will pass spontaneously, thereby avoiding surgery.

Lower gastrointestinal endoscopy

Indications and contraindications

Diseases or symptoms referable to the colon and rectum are best evaluated by colonoscopy or flexible sigmoidoscopy. The American Gastroenterology Association, the American Cancer Society, and the American Medical Association

Table 16.3 Indications for colonoscopy

Diagnostic
Fecal occult blood
Hematochezia in the absence of a convincing anorectal source
Melena, if an upper intestinal source is excluded
Unexplained iron deficiency
Abnormality on barium enema that is probably significant (filling defect, stricture)
To exclude the presence of synchronous cancer or polyps in a patient with confirmed colorectal neoplasia
Chronic, unexplained diarrhea
Selected patients with altered bowel habits at risk of colonic neoplasia
Inflammatory bowel disease, if establishing a diagnosis or determining the extent of disease will alter management decisions

Therapeutic
Excision of polyps
Bleeding from vascular ectasias, neoplasia, polypectomy site, or ulceration
Foreign body removal
Decompression of acute colonic pseudo-obstruction or volvulus
Balloon dilation of stenotic lesions
Palliative treatment of inoperable stenosing or bleeding neoplasms

Surveillance
Prior history of colorectal cancer or adenomatous polyps
Family history of hereditary nonpolyposis colon cancer
Family history of colorectal cancer in a first-degree relative (<age 55) or in several family members
Long-standing (>7–10 y) chronic ulcerative pancolitis with biopsies to detect dysplasia; colitis limited to the left side may require less intensive surveillance

have deemed colonoscopy superior to flexible sigmoidoscopy for detecting colonic lesions (even within the limited area seen on sigmoidoscopy) but recognize sigmoidoscopy with or without barium enema as an acceptable alternative to colonoscopy (in average risk individuals) when patient preference or local expertise limits the use of full colonoscopy. Patients with increased risk because of personal or family history of previous colon cancer or colon polyps or with a genetic syndrome predisposing to colon cancer should undergo full colonoscopy for colon cancer screening. Sigmoidoscopy is used to complete the examination of the colon in conjunction with barium enema radiography and to investigate rectosigmoid symptoms in young persons who are at extremely low risk of colorectal neoplasia. All patients older than 40 years with symptoms referable to any portion of the colon are best evaluated by total colonoscopy. The American Society of Gastrointestinal Endoscopy has established recommendations for using colonoscopy (Table 16.3) that are intended as guidelines. They should not replace the clinical judgment of the clinician.

As with any endoscopic procedure, colonoscopy is contraindicated if a perforation is suspected or if the patient is unco-operative. Lower gastrointestinal endoscopy is specifically contraindicated in fulminant colitis and the suppurative phase of acute diverticulitis. Recent myocardial infarction is a relative contraindication to colonoscopy and should delay elective procedures for several weeks.

Patient preparation and monitoring

Most lower gastrointestinal endoscopic procedures require cleansing the colon. Limited preparation of the left colon is usually sufficient for flexible sigmoidoscopy and can be achieved with two tap water or small-volume sodium phosphate enemas administered 1 h before the examination. This limited preparation precludes the use of electrocautery because of the hazard of residual explosive gases. Colonoscopy or any lower gastrointestinal endoscopic procedure using electrocautery requires full preparation of the colon. This is achieved using a balanced electrolyte solution containing polyethylene glycol (PEG). PEG solutions are administered in 0.5 gallon to 1 gallon volumes, often in split doses with half the solution being taken the night prior to the procedure and the remaining half being taken the morning of the procedure and completed at least 4 h prior to the scheduled procedure. Mannitol and other carbohydrate purgatives should be avoided if electrocoagulation is anticipated because bacterial fermentation produces explosive hydrogen gas. In the past sodium phosphate solutions were used for bowel clensing; however, sodium phosphate may lead to dangerous fluid and electrolyte shifts in patients with heart failure or renal insufficiency and its use has been associated with acute renal failure. Therefore, sodium phosphate solutions are typically no longer used for bowel clensing.

Sedation and monitoring are similar to the practices used for upper gastrointestinal endoscopy. Unlike colonoscopy, flexible sigmoidoscopy to the splenic flexure is often accomplished without sedation. A skilled endoscopist can often perform this procedure with minimal discomfort to the patient.

Performance of the procedure

Flexible sigmoidoscopy involves introducing the instrument to the descending colon or splenic flexure, whereas total colonoscopy involves passing the instrument to the cecum. Although experienced endoscopists may reach the cecum in 90–98% of examinations, a significant number of patients have colonic anatomies that preclude safe completion of the procedure. Therefore, the well-trained endoscopist should be willing to abandon a colonoscopic study that appears unreasonably traumatic.

As with upper gastrointestinal endoscopy, colonoscopy provides the capability of obtaining biopsy specimens to establish the diagnosis of endoscopic abnormalities and to sample normal-appearing mucosa if occult conditions (e.g. microscopic colitis) are suspected. Therapeutic colonoscopic techniques include polypectomy with hot biopsy forceps or with snare polypectomy using electrocoagulation to promote hemostasis. Acute and chronic bleeding from angiodysplasias can be treated with electrocoagulation, heater probe application, and laser photocoagulation. Less common procedures include through-the-scope pneumatic balloon dilation of discrete benign strictures, decompressive colonoscopy with tube placement for acute pseudo-obstruction, and palliative laser ablation of inoperable neoplasms.

Complications

The overall risk of serious complications, including perforation and uncontrolled hemorrhage, is approximately 1 in 500 for diagnostic colonoscopy. Therapeutic maneuvers increase the risk of complications, although there are wide variations in reported rates. Hemorrhage after polypectomy is common. It may occur in up to 1–2% of patients and often occurs up to 7–10 days after the procedure when residual necrotic tissue and scar tissue are sloughed. The risk of perforation is also increased in therapeutic maneuvers. The transmural burn syndrome represents a localized, contained perforation that may be associated with localized pain, fever, and leukocytosis 6–24 h after polypectomy or after any therapy that uses electrocoagulation. Many patients can be treated conservatively with parenteral broad-spectrum antibiotics but any patient with signs of frank perforation should undergo surgical exploration.

Endoscopic retrograde cholangiopancreatography

Indications and contraindications

Endoscopic retrograde cholangiopancreatography (ERCP) is indicated for evaluating patients with suspected biliary or pancreatic disorders when noninvasive imaging with ultrasonography or computed tomographic (CT) scanning is equivocal and when therapeutic intervention is necessary (Table 16.4). Various abdominal symptoms can be attributed to the pancreaticobiliary system, and the decision to proceed with ERCP should be made by a clinician experienced in caring for patients with these disorders. ERCP has a role in the preoperative evaluation of selected patients undergoing laparoscopic cholecystectomy, pancreatic resection, or surgical pseudocyst drainage. Many of the available therapeutic options, including endoscopic sphincterotomy, stone extraction, endoscopic cystgastrostomy, and biliary or pancreatic stent placement, also require the availability of surgical support. Thus, the treatment of patients undergoing ERCP often requires the combined expertise of the endoscopist and a surgeon.

In addition to the standard contraindications for all endoscopic procedures, ERCP is relatively contraindicated in the presence of an obstructed biliary system or a documented pancreatic pseudocyst, unless immediate endoscopic or surgical drainage is planned. Any procedure performed under these conditions should be accompanied by administration of prophylactic antibiotics (see Table 16.1). Therapeutic interventions, particularly endoscopic sphincterotomy, are contraindicated in patients with severe coagulopathy.

Table 16.4 Indications for endoscopic retrograde cholangiopancreatography

Suspected biliary disorders
Unexplained jaundice or cholestasis
Postcholecystectomy complaints
Postbiliary surgery complaints
Acute cholangitis
Acute gallstone pancreatitis
Evaluation of bile duct abnormalities in other imaging studies
Sphincter of Oddi manometry

Suspected pancreatic disorders
Chronic upper abdominal pain consistent with pancreatic origin
Unexplained weight loss
Steatorrhea
Unexplained recurrent pancreatitis
Evaluation of pancreatic abnormalities in other imaging studies
To obtain pancreatic duct brushings or pure pancreatic juice

Before therapeutic intervention
Endoscopic sphincterotomy
Endoscopic biliary drainage
Endoscopic pancreatic drainage
Endoscopic cystgastrostomy
Balloon dilation of pancreaticobiliary strictures
Preoperative mapping for pancreatic or biliary resections

Patient preparation and monitoring

All patients undergoing ERCP should be prepared in the same manner as patients undergoing EGD. Attention should be given to several factors specific to ERCP. First, because the endoscope used for ERCP is equipped with side-viewing rather than with forward-viewing optics, special attention should be given to patients with dysphagia. Passing the instrument through the esophagus is done blindly, increasing the risk of perforation if there is a Zenker diverticulum or esophageal stricture. The ductal injection of contrast material can result in significant systemic absorption, as demonstrated occasionally by the appearance of a post-injection nephrogram. Although anaphylactic reactions have not been reported, erythema and rash can occur, and some clinicians choose to pretreat patients who have histories of reactions to contrast agents with antihistamines and corticosteroids 12 and 2 h before the procedure. Because ERCP involves radiographic imaging of the upper abdomen, any residual gastrointestinal contrast agent should be evacuated with purgatives. Immediately before sedating the patient, abdominal radiographs should be obtained to ensure that all contrast material is gone and to establish the location of soft tissue shadows and calcifications.

The sedation of patients undergoing ERCP is similar to the procedure for patients undergoing upper gastrointestinal endoscopy. Patient movement should be minimized to obtain optimal imaging. Because the patient is in the prone position on the fluoroscopic table rather than in the left decubitus position used for upper gastrointestinal endoscopy, special attention should be given to removing oral secretions.

Performance of the procedure

Endoscopic retrograde cholangiopancreatography involves passing a side-viewing endoscope into the second portion of the duodenum and visualizing the major papilla. Both the pancreatic and biliary system can be cannulated with specialized catheters that are advanced through the duodenoscope. After selective cannulation of the pancreatic or biliary system, radiological contrast dye is injected under fluoroscopic guidance until the entire ductal system is visualized. Care should be taken to avoid injecting air because bubbles may be mistaken for biliary or pancreatic stones. Overinjection of dye into the pancreas leads to staining of the parenchyma, a pattern termed *acinarization*, which is associated with an increased risk of ERCP-induced pancreatitis. Abdominal radiographs are obtained during the injection and periodically as the contrast dye drains from the duct. After one ductal system is examined, the alternate system is cannulated and injected. For some disorders, only cholangiography or pancreatography is necessary. Biliary manometry can be performed in specialized centers as part of the ERCP examination with a specialized water-perfused manometry catheter positioned across the sphincter of Oddi. The ampulla of Vater may not be easily accessible in patients whose anatomy has been altered by a Billroth II or Roux-en-Y gastrojejunostomy.

Endoscopic retrograde cholangiopancreatography is a nonoperative method of treating many pancreaticobiliary disorders. Endoscopic sphincterotomy is often performed to facilitate biliary stone extraction. The procedure involves cannulation of the common bile duct with a papillotome, a specialized catheter with an exposed wire that extends across the most distal portion of the catheter. Positioning the wire across the papilla and applying electrical current produces a cut through the papilla. After sphincterotomy, stones may pass spontaneously but extraction with balloon catheters or baskets placed through the endoscope and into the bile duct is often necessary. If endoscopic stone extraction fails, a nasobiliary tube or endoscopic stent can be placed while the patient awaits definitive surgical therapy. Sphincterotomy also relieves obstruction caused by sphincter of Oddi dyskinesia or papillary stenosis. Specialized centers may perform sphincterotomy of the minor papilla to treat pancreas divisum.

Biliary or pancreatic strictures can also be treated with ERCP. Inoperable, malignant obstruction of the extrahepatic bile ducts is best relieved by endoscopic placement of a plastic or metallic stent, in many cases after sphincterotomy. Occasionally, patients with primary sclerosing cholangitis will have dominant strictures of the extrahepatic bile ducts, which are amenable to pneumatic balloon dilation followed by stent placement. For most benign biliary strictures, however, surgical therapy is preferred because of superior long-term patency.

Transpapillary placement of a pancreatic stent has been used to treat symptomatic pancreatic ductal strictures and pseudocysts in patients with chronic pancreatitis.

Complications

Acute pancreatitis is the most common complication of ERCP. Sixty percent to 80% of patients undergoing ERCP develop asymptomatic elevations in serum amylase and lipase levels but clinically overt pancreatitis is much less common. Retrospective series report an incidence of 1–2% but prospective series suggest that symptomatic acute pancreatitis occurs in 4–7% of patients undergoing ERCP. The risk is increased by acinarization of the pancreas, repeated attempts at cannulation, and sphincter of Oddi manometry. Conservative management leads to resolution for most patients but severe necrotizing pancreatitis occurs in a small subset of patients. Placement of a temporary pancreatic duct stent following free-cut sphincterotomy or sphincterotomy for sphincter of Oddi dysfunction reduces the risk of ERCP-induced pancreatitis.

Endoscopic sphincterotomy has an overall complication rate of 5–8%, equally divided among bleeding, perforation, cholangitis, and pancreatitis. One percent to 2% of patients undergoing sphincterotomy require surgical intervention for related complications; the mortality rate for sphincterotomy is 0.5–1%. Attempted biliary drainage with endoprosthesis placement has an 8% risk of cholangitis but most of these episodes occur when drainage is unsuccessful or incomplete. Stent occlusion and cholangitis are delayed complications that occur in 40% of patients in a mean of 5–6 months after endoprosthetic insertion.

Endoscopic ultrasound

Indications and contraindications

Endoscopic ultrasound (EUS) provides the capability of obtaining high-resolution ultrasound images within the upper and lower gastrointestinal tracts. Specialized endoscopes with ultrasound probes at the tips and oblique-viewing optics can generate acoustic images of gastrointestinal wall layers and surrounding strictures. The increased availability of the instruments and clinical experience with the technique have expanded the list of clinical indications for EUS (Table 16.5). Focal intramural and extramural mass lesions and wall thickening are easily identified by EUS. Localization to a specific wall layer (i.e. mucosa, submucosa, muscularis, serosa, extralumenal) often helps to identify the histological origin of the lesion. EUS is useful in detecting anal sphincter defects in patients with incontinence and has been used to localize enterocutaneous fistulae in Crohn's disease. EUS is also of value in identifying and staging several tumors, including esophageal carcinoma, gastric carcinoma, gastric lymphoma, ampullary carcinoma, distal bile duct carcinoma, pancreatic carcinoma, and rectal carcinoma. It is both sensitive and specific in determining the local extent of the tumor (T stage) and the presence of

Table 16.5 Indications for endoscopic ultrasound

Tumor staging (esophageal, gastric, pancreatic, ampullary, distal bile duct, rectal, non-small cell lung)
Neuroendocrine tumor localization
Evaluation of submucosal mass lesions
Suspected chronic pancreatitis
Detection of distal bile duct stones
Fine needle aspiration of adjacent lymph nodes or mass lesions
Evaluation of anal sphincters
Suspected enterocutaneous fistula
Direct endoscopic cystgastrostomy for pancreatic pseudocysts

regional lymph nodes (N stage) but it is not a reliable means of establishing distant metastatic disease (M stage). EUS is superior to CT and magnetic resonance imaging studies and to transabdominal ultrasound for pancreatic imaging, and it is the most accurate means for defining vascular invasion by tumors in the peripancreatic bed. Similarly, EUS can localize pancreatic islet cell tumors not detected by conventional imaging studies. Evidence suggests that the sensitivity of EUS is equivalent to that of ERCP for detecting common bile duct stones and chronic pancreatitis.

The introduction of instruments to obtain ultrasound-directed fine needle aspiration has further expanded the role of EUS. Sampling of pancreatic mass lesions has proved useful, particularly in patients with unresectable disease who are candidates for palliative radiation therapy or chemotherapy. EUS-directed transesophageal aspiration of mediastinal lymph nodes has proved superior to other nonsurgical methods of staging non-small cell lung cancer and often provides information critical to the decision to pursue surgical or nonsurgical therapy in these patients. The same instrumentation used in tissue sampling has launched EUS into therapeutics. EUS-guided needle injection of the celiac ganglia has been used to control chronic pain caused by chronic pancreatitis or pancreatic cancer. Endoscopic ultrasound can direct needle placement and detect pericystic blood vessels in patients undergoing endoscopic cystgastrostomy, thereby improving the safety profile of the procedure. Future refinements in endosonographic image quality and performance will probably expand the diagnostic and therapeutic capabilities of EUS.

Because EUS is a specialized form of upper and lower gastrointestinal endoscopy, contraindications are identical to those for diagnostic endoscopy in their respective locations in the gastrointestinal tract.

Patient preparation and monitoring

Preparation of the patient for EUS of the upper gastrointestinal tract is identical to that for EGD. Similarly, EUS of the rectum or colon requires bowel cleansing in accordance with the techniques used for flexible sigmoidoscopy or colonoscopy, respectively. The principles of sedation and monitoring are also based on the standard practices for upper and lower gastrointestinal endoscopy.

Performance of the procedure

There are two principal types of echoendoscopes. The linear or curved array instruments provide 100° sector images parallel to the longitudinal axis of the endoscope, whereas radial scanning instruments provide 360° images perpendicular to the longitudinal axis of the endoscope. Although upper echo-endoscopes usually have oblique-viewing optics, echocolonoscopes are also available with forward-viewing optics. The ultrasound frequency can be altered on most of the available instruments. Higher frequency imaging (12–20 MHz) provides increased resolution, and lower frequency imaging (5.0–7.5 MHz) provides increased depth of penetration. Because images from linear or curved array instruments are oriented along the axis of the endoscope, specialized needles can be advanced through the working channel and directed under real-time ultrasound guidance into a lesion for tissue aspiration.

Endoscopic ultrasound provides high-resolution images of the bowel wall and, in most structures, identifies five echolayers that correlate with the mucosa, muscularis mucosae, submucosa, muscularis propria, and serosa or adventitia. Directing the instrument to a focal submucosal mass or to an area of wall thickening can identify the layer from which the abnormality originates. The pancreas can be visualized from the duodenum or posterior wall of the stomach, whereas the bile duct and gallbladder can be identified from the duodenum. The major vascular structures of the splanchnic circulation can also be identified from the duodenum or stomach. Flow within these structures can be assessed by the color flow and pulse Doppler modes available on curved array instruments.

Complications

Endoscopic ultrasound has a safety profile similar to that of diagnostic upper and lower gastrointestinal endoscopy. The larger diameter of the echoendoscope makes traversing lumenal strictures more hazardous, which is problematic for esophageal tumors. Patients with significant dysphagia should undergo prelimi-nary forward-viewing endoscopy or barium swallow radiography, so that the severity of lumenal narrowing can be assessed. Although pancreatitis following EUS fine needle aspiration has been reported, EUS-directed biopsy is relatively safe, with a complication rate of 1–2%.

Key practice points

- Conscious sedation requires careful monitoring by an assistant to assess for any cardiopulmonary complications.
- AGA position statements related to the use of endoscopy and conscious sedation can be found at: www.gastro.org/practice/medical-position-statements.
- ASGE practice guidelines on endoscopy (EGD, colonoscopy, ERCP, EUS, and capsule endoscopy), conscious sedation, antibiotic prophylaxis, and management of anticoagulation can be found at: www.asge.org.

PART 2

Specific Gastrointestinal Diseases

CHAPTER 17
Motor Disorders of the Esophagus

Introduction

Clinically, motor disorders of the esophagus can be divided into oropharyngeal dysphagia, which includes abnormalities of the upper esophageal sphincter and proximal esophagus, and esophageal dysphagia, which results from achalasia and other distal esophageal disorders.

Oropharyngeal Dysphagia

Clinical presentation

Neuromuscular diseases of the hypopharynx and upper esophagus produce a form of dysphagia in which the patient cannot initiate swallowing or propel the food bolus from the hypopharynx into the esophageal body. The patient can usually localize symptoms to the cervical region. Patients may also describe nasal regurgitation, tracheal aspiration, drooling, or the need to dislodge impacted food manually. Gurgling, halitosis, and a neck mass suggest a Zenker diverticulum, whereas hoarseness may reflect nerve dysfunction or intrinsic vocal cord muscular disease. Dysarthria and nasal speech suggest muscle weakness of the soft palate and pharyngeal constrictors. Physical examination may demonstrate focal neurological deficits with cerebrovascular accidents, a palpable neck mass with a hypopharyngeal diverticulum, ptosis and end-of-day weakness with myasthenia gravis, and paucity of movement with Parkinson disease.

Yamada's Handbook of Gastroenterology, Third Edition. Edited by Tadataka Yamada and John M. Inadomi.
© 2013 John Wiley & Sons, Ltd. Published 2013 by John Wiley & Sons, Ltd.

Differential diagnosis

Hypopharyngeal diverticula and cricopharyngeal bars

Acquired hypopharyngeal (Zenker) diverticula occur between the fibers of the inferior pharyngeal constrictor and the cricopharyngeus muscle. Hypopharyngeal diverticula may result from delayed or failed upper esophageal sphincter (UES) relaxation, premature UES contraction, or restrictive UES myopathy with poor compliance. Such impaired compliance also gives the radiographic appearance of a cricopharyngeal bar on barium swallow in some patients with oropharyngeal dysphagia.

Neurological disorders

The most common causes of acute oropharyngeal dysphagia are cerebrovascular accidents. Symptoms usually appear abruptly and are associated with other neurological deficits. Degenerative neuronal changes with progressive bulbar palsy and pseudobulbar palsy produce tongue and pharyngeal paralysis. Polio and the postpolio syndrome alter pharyngeal function, as does amyotrophic lateral sclerosis. Patients with amyotrophic lateral sclerosis present with choking attacks and aspiration pneumonias secondary to dysfunction of the tongue as well as the pharyngeal and laryngeal musculature. Hypopharyngeal stasis, aspiration, and UES dysfunction are prevalent in Parkinson disease. Swallowing abnormalities, including difficult initiation, and UES abnormalities occur in patients with multiple sclerosis. Rare neurological causes of oropharyngeal dysphagia include brainstem tumors, syringobulbia, tetanus, botulism, lead poisoning, alcoholic neuropathy, carcinoma, chemotherapy, and radiation therapy.

Primary muscle disorders

Polymyositis and dermatomyositis produce poor pharyngeal and proximal esophageal contraction, barium pooling in the valleculae, and decreased UES tone. Myotonic and oculopharyngeal dystrophy are the two forms of muscular dystrophy that affect the swallowing mechanism. Myotonic dystrophy presents with myopathic facies, swan neck, myotonia, muscle wasting, frontal baldness, testicular atrophy, and cataracts. Oculopharyngeal dystrophy presents with ptosis and dysphagia but does not have other gastrointestinal manifestations. Myasthenia gravis affects striated esophageal musculature, producing dysphagia in two-thirds of patients that worsens with the duration of a meal. Hyperthyroidism and hypothyroidism affect swallowing, as do sarcoidosis, systemic lupus erythematosus, and the stiff man syndrome.

Diagnostic investigation

Video-esophagography

Videofluoroscopy records the complex and rapid sequence of events in the mouth, pharynx, and upper esophagus during a swallow. Dynamic recordings of the barium swallow include lateral and posteroanterior views after ingesting thin and thick liquid barium and barium-labeled solids. Motility disturbances manifest as delayed initiation and prolonged duration of swallowing or a disturbance in the sequence of muscle movements. Barium retention in the pharyngeal recesses is caused by altered mucosal sensitivity, decreased muscle tone, or alterations in recess shape or size. Pharyngeal stasis is another sign of altered motility. Misdirected swallows with laryngeal penetration or aspiration are striking abnormalities. Delayed UES opening and cricopharyngeal bars also may be noted.

Manometry

Intralumenal manometry obtains measurements from the oropharynx and proximal esophagus, including the strength of pharyngeal contraction, the completeness of UES relaxation, and the timing of these events.

Other modalities

Scintigraphic studies can demonstrate hypopharyngeal stasis, regurgitation, and tracheal aspiration. Brain images can be obtained from computed tomographic or magnetic resonance imaging studies. Testing with the anticholinesterase agent edrophonium is useful in diagnosing myasthenia gravis.

Management

The first step in managing a patient with oropharyngeal dysphagia is to recognize and correct reversible causes of symptoms, including Parkinson disease, myasthenia gravis, hyperthyroidism or hypothyroidism, and polymyositis. The treatment for hypopharyngeal diverticula is cricopharyngeal myotomy with or without diverticulectomy. Myotomy reduces resting UES tone and resistance to UES flow. Endoscopic dilation with a large-caliber bougie may be effective for a cricopharyngeal bar but the role of myotomy in this condition is less clear. The results of videofluoroscopy can be used to modify the properties of meals and the mechanics of food ingestion in some patients with neuromuscular etiologies of oropharyngeal dysphagia. In patients who cannot safely obtain adequate nutrition, enteral feedings through a nasoenteric tube or gastrostomy may be necessary.

Achalasia

Achalasia is characterized by aperistalsis of the smooth muscle esophagus and failure of the lower esophageal sphincter (LES) to relax completely with swallowing.

Clinical presentation

Patients with achalasia report solid food dysphagia and most also have liquid dysphagia. Many complain of regurgitation of undigested food eaten hours or days previously. Symptoms may be intermittent and insidious in onset, and the duration of symptoms prior to diagnosis averages 2 years. The patient may have learned special maneuvers such as throwing the shoulders back, lifting the neck, performing a Valsalva maneuver, and drinking carbonated beverages to promote swallowing. Chest pain is reported by two-thirds of patients and may be so severe as to cause decreased food intake and weight loss, but tends to improve as the disease progresses.

Differential diagnosis

Pseudoachalasia, caused by neoplasia, presents with manometric findings identical to those in primary achalasia. The most common is adenocarcinoma of the gastroesophageal junction; however, pancreatic carcinoma, small cell and squamous cell lung carcinoma, prostate carcinoma, and lymphoma may also cause secondary achalasia either by direct compression of the distal esophagus or by malignant cell infiltration of the esophageal myenteric plexus. Other tumors (e.g. Hodgkin disease, lung carcinoma, and hepatocellular carcinoma) produce achalasia by a paraneoplastic mechanism.

Infectious causes of secondary achalasia include Chagas disease, which is caused by the protozoan *Trypanosoma cruzi* that is transmitted by the reduviid (kissing) bug, endemic in Brazil, Venezuela, and Argentina. After an acute septic phase, chronic destruction of ganglion cells in the gut, urinary tract, heart, and respiratory tract develops over years. The presence of megaureter, megaduodenum, megacolon, or megarectum is helpful in distinguishing Chagas disease from primary achalasia. Complement fixation and polymerase chain reaction tests are available to confirm the diagnosis. Other causes of secondary achalasia include infiltrative diseases (with amyloid, sphingolipids, eosinophils, or sarcoid), diabetes, intestinal pseudo-obstruction, pancreatic pseudocysts, von Recklinghausen disease, multiple endocrine neoplasia type IIB, juvenile Sjögren syndrome, post-fundoplication dysphagia, and familial adrenal insufficiency with alacrima.

Diagnostic investigation

Radiographic studies
Barium swallow radiography is the initial screening test for achalasia and may show a dilated intrathoracic esophagus with impaired contrast transit, a loss of peristalsis, impaired LES relaxation, and a characteristic tapering of the distal esophagus ("bird's beak").

Esophageal manometry
The defining manometric features of achalasia are aperistalsis and incomplete LES relaxation. Incomplete LES relaxation with swallowing is usually (>80%

of cases) but not always observed in patients with achalasia because early in the course of disease, some patients exhibit complete LES relaxations of very short duration, and some individuals have short segments of aperistalsis. Sixty percent of patients have elevated LES pressure (>35 mmHg). The advent of high-resolution manometry with topographic analysis allows calculation of the transphincteric pressure gradient during the 2–6-second postswallow interval, with gradients exceeding 5 mmHg defining achalasia with a sensitivity of 94% and specificity of 98%.

Discussion and potential pitfalls

The advent of high-resolution manometry with esophageal pressure topography has revolutionized the categorization of achalasia by differentiating the contractile function of the esophageal body. All forms have an "integrated relaxation pressure" or mean esophagogastric junction pressure persisting for 4 sec after a swallow that is greater than 15 mmHg; however, classic achalasia requires absent peristalsis, while achalasia with esophageal compression includes at least 20% of swallows associated with panesophageal pressurization to >30 mmHg, while spastic achalasia has spastic contractions with >20% of swallows.

Source: Kahrilas PJ. Esophageal Motor Disorders in Terms of High-Resolution Esophageal Pressure Topography: What Has Changed? Am J Gastroenterol 2010;105:981–987.

Upper gastrointestinal endoscopy

Upper gastrointestinal endoscopy often misses achalasia but is necessary to exclude malignancy after the diagnosis is made. Typically, endoscopy reveals esophageal dilation, atony, and erythema, friability, and ulcerations from chronic stasis. The LES may be puckered but passage of the endoscope into the stomach should not be difficult in the absence of malignancy. Careful examination of the gastric cardia is mandatory to rule out secondary causes of achalasia.

Key practice points: manometric findings in achalasia

- Absence of peristalsis in esophageal body
- Incomplete relaxation of lower esophageal sphincter (complete relaxation of short duration may be seen in early achalasia)
- Elevated resting pressure of lower esophageal sphincter (common, not required)
- Elevated intraesophageal pressure relative to gastric pressures (common, not required)

Management

Achalasia is not curable, and no treatment can restore normal esophageal body peristalsis or complete LES relaxation. Treatment therefore rests with measures to reduce LES pressure sufficiently to enhance gravity-assisted esophageal emptying.

Medication therapy

Nitrates and calcium channel antagonists are the most common medical therapies for achalasia. Sublingual isosorbide dinitrate reduces LES pressures by 66% for 90 min. Sublingual nifedipine 30–40 mg per day is significantly better than placebo in symptom relief and lowers LES pressure by 30–40% for an hour or more. Sildenafil transiently decreases LES pressure in achalasia. Any medication therapy has significant limitations, such as duration of action and tachyphylaxis. However, elderly patients, patients who refuse more invasive therapy, patients who cannot give consent, and patients with very mild symptoms may benefit from these relaxant drugs.

Injection therapy

Botulinum toxin, a potent inhibitor of neural acetylcholine release, reduces LES pressure and relieves symptoms for up to 6 months in patients with achalasia when directly injected into the LES during endoscopy (80 units total divided into four-quadrant injections). Because of incomplete symptom control and the requirements for costly repeat injections, botulinum toxin is best reserved for elderly or frail patients who are poor risks for more definitive therapy.

Pneumatic dilation

Bougienage with a standard dilator (up to 20 mm diameter) usually produces only transient symptomatic relief. In contrast, pneumatic dilation to >30 mm diameter that forcefully disrupts the LES circular muscle produces long-lasting reductions in LES pressure. Balloons are inflated for several seconds to 5 min at pressures ranging from 360 to 775 mmHg, which produce responses in 32–98% of cases. A postdilation LES pressure of less than 10 mmHg predicts sustained remission to 2 years. Approximately 20–40% of patients require further dilation several years later. The most common complication of pneumatic dilation is perforation (1–5% of cases). It is common to obtain a water-soluble radiographic swallow film followed by barium swallow radiography (if no perforation is detected).

Surgery

Surgical therapy of achalasia usually involves a longitudinal incision of the muscle layers of the LES (i.e. Heller myotomy). Good to excellent responses to myotomy occur in 62–100% of patients. Thoracoscopic and laparoscopic procedures are associated with similar benefits and less morbidity than open approaches.

Complications and their management

Achalasia is associated with squamous cell carcinoma, which results from chronic stasis and occurs in 2–7% of patients, usually those who have had unsatisfactory treatment or no treatment. Surgery may be associated with symptomatic gastroesophageal reflux that occurs in 10% of cases, which may be further complicated by strictures. Rarely, refractory cases mandate more aggressive operations, including esophageal resection with gastric pull-up or colonic interposition.

Key practice points: achalasia treatment

- Surgical myotomy provides long-standing relief from dysphagia.
- Pneumatic dilation has proven efficacy but substantial risk of perforation.
- Patients in whom surgery or dilation is not performed can be treated using endoscopic injection of botulin toxin but the effect is transient.

Other Motor Disorders of the Distal Esophagus

Specific spastic disorders of the esophagus have been characterized on the basis of manometric criteria (Table 17.1). The required manometric feature of diffuse esophageal spasm (DES) is the presence of simultaneous esophageal body contractions with greater than 30% of water swallows. Other findings that

Table 17.1 Manometric criteria for spastic esophageal motor disorders

Disorder	Required findings	Associated findings
Diffuse esophageal spasm	Simultaneous contractions with >30% of water swallows	Repetitive contractions Prolonged contractions High-amplitude contractions Spontaneous relaxations Incomplete LES relaxation Increased LES pressure
Nutcracker esophagus	High-amplitude contractions (>180 mmHg on average)	Repetitive contractions Prolonged contractions Increased LES pressure
Hypertensive LES	Increased LES pressure (>40 mmHg) Normal LES relaxation	
Nonspecific esophageal motor disorder	Findings insufficient for other diagnoses	Frequent aperistaltic contractions Retrograde contractions Repetitive contractions Low-amplitude contractions Prolonged contractions High-amplitude contractions Spontaneous relaxations Incomplete LES relaxation

may be present include repetitive or prolonged contractions, high-amplitude contractions (>180 mmHg), spontaneous contractions, and rarely incomplete LES relaxation. Other conditions that produce similar findings include diabetic neuropathy, rheumatological disease, alcoholism, and pseudo-obstruction. Some cases of DES progress to achalasia, suggesting that these disorders represent a spectrum of a single encompassing disease in some patients.

Hypertensive LES is defined by a pressure higher than 45 mmHg with normal relaxation and esophageal body peristalsis. Radiographic and scintigraphic transit tests usually show no delay in bolus passage into the stomach, raising questions about the importance of this condition.

Nonspecific esophageal motor disorders do not satisfy manometric criteria for any other condition and are of uncertain relevance. Manometric findings include frequent simultaneous contractions, retrograde contractions, low-amplitude contractions, prolonged contractions, and isolated incomplete LES relaxation.

Clinical presentation

The major symptoms of spastic disorders are dysphagia and chest pain. Intermittent dysphagia for solids and liquids is present in 30–60% of patients with spastic disorders and may be exacerbated by large boluses of food, medications, or foods of extreme temperatures. Dysphagia is usually not severe enough to produce weight loss. Intermittent substernal chest discomfort with radiation to the back, neck, jaw, or arms lasting minutes to hours is reported by 80–90% of patients. Features that suggest an esophageal rather than a cardiac cause include pain that is nonexertional, continues for hours, interrupts sleep, is meal related, and is relieved by antacids. Associated heartburn, dysphagia, or regurgitation may favor an esophageal cause. Heartburn may not reflect excessive acid reflux into the esophagus but rather may result from hypersensitivity to normal amounts of esophageal acid.

Diagnostic investigation

Endoscopic and radiographic studies

Upper endoscopy is useful in evaluating patients with dysphagia or suspected esophageal pain to exclude structural lesions or esophagitis. Barium swallow radiography may define corkscrew esophagus, rosary bead esophagus, pseudodiverticula, or curling in some patients with DES. Unlike achalasia, "bird's beak" deformities are not observed.

Manometry and ambulatory pH monitoring

Ambulatory pH testing is probably the most useful functional test in patients with unexplained chest pain of presumed esophageal origin. Conversely, abnormal motor events are intermittent and may not be associated with symptoms. In unequivocal cases, nonperistaltic, high-amplitude, prolonged contractions seen during esophageal manometry are associated with the patient's report of chest pain. These unequivocal cases probably result from a myenteric neuronal defect that places the affected individuals along the continuum of achalasia.

Management

Spastic motor disorders of the esophagus are not life-threatening or progressive in most cases. Treatment should attempt to reduce symptoms without exposing the patient to potential therapeutic complications. If symptoms suggest gastro-esophageal acid reflux, ambulatory pH monitoring or antisecretory treatment with proton pump inhibitors should be used. If reflux is not a consideration, the most important step is to reassure the patient that there is no serious heart condition or other disease. When reassurance fails, medical, mechanical, and surgical treatment options are available. Behavioral modification and biofeed-back have shown some efficacy in selected refractory cases.

Medications
Small trials suggest that some DES patients experience relief with smooth muscle relaxants such as nitrates, calcium channel blockers, and hydralazine. One double-blind, placebo-controlled trial of the antidepressant trazodone reported improvements in global well-being as well as esophageal symptoms, possibly secondary to effects on visceral pain perception. Botulinum toxin injected at the gastroesophageal junction reduced symptoms in one investigation of patients with nonachalasic esophageal spasm.

Mechanical dilation
Therapeutic bougienage probably does not produce symptomatic benefits greater than sham dilation. However, pneumatic dilation has reduced symptoms in some patients with DES and hypertensive LES, especially if dysphagia is prominent.

Surgery
For patients with dysphagia or intractable pain caused by spastic motor esophageal dysfunction, a Heller myotomy to include the LES and the spastic portions of the esophageal body may reduce symptoms in more than 50% of cases. However, the risk of the procedure coupled with the uncertain therapeutic response mandates a cautious approach to surgery.

> **Key practice points**
> - Videofluoroscopy and manometry are key tests for evaluating motor disorders of the esophagus.
> - Upper endoscopy is indicated to exclude secondary causes of achalasia.
> - Ambulatory pH testing is most helpful in patients with noncardiac chest pain syndrome.

CHAPTER 18

Gastroesophageal Reflux Disease

The passage of gastric contents retrograde into the esophagus is a normal physiological event. The development of symptoms, signs, or complications of this process is termed gastroesophageal reflux disease (GERD). In addition to the esophagus, other structures affected by GERD include the pharynx, larynx, and respiratory tract. A minority of patients with GERD have reflux esophagitis, a term used to describe mucosal damage and inflammation.

Clinical presentation

The most common symptom of GERD is heartburn, which is described as substernal burning that moves orad from the xiphoid. Heartburn generally occurs after meals and may be relieved by acid-neutralizing agents. The frequency and severity of heartburn correlate poorly with endoscopically defined esophagitis. Patients with GERD may also present with substernal chest discomfort that mimics cardiac-related angina pectoris. Regurgitation of bitter or acid-tasting liquid is common. Water brash is the spontaneous appearance of salty fluid in the mouth from reflex salivary secretion in response to esophageal acid. Solid food dysphagia in a patient with GERD may be caused by either peptic strictures or adenocarcinoma from Barrett mctaplasia. Note that odynophagia is not a common symptom associated with erosive esophagitis.

Extraesophageal manifestations of GERD include otolaryngological and pulmonary complications. Acid damage to the oropharynx may produce sore throat, earache, gingivitis, poor dentition, and globus, whereas reflux damage to the larynx and respiratory tract causes hoarseness, wheezing, bronchitis, asthma, and pneumonia. Vagally mediated bronchospasm may be initiated by acidification of the esophagus alone; thus, tracheal penetration by the refluxate is not required for the development of asthma with GERD.

Yamada's Handbook of Gastroenterology, Third Edition. Edited by Tadataka Yamada and John M. Inadomi.
© 2013 John Wiley & Sons, Ltd. Published 2013 by John Wiley & Sons, Ltd.

Diagnostic investigation

A history of classic heartburn is sufficient for diagnosing GERD and provides an adequate rationale for initiating therapy. The proton pump inhibitor (PPI) test, which evaluates symptom response to proton pump inhibition, is likewise as sensitive and specific as more invasive tests for diagnosing GERD. Diagnostic studies should be considered for patients with atypical symptoms, symptoms unresponsive to therapy, or warning signs of GERD complications or malignancy (e.g. dysphagia, gastrointestinal hemorrhage, weight loss, and anemia).

Upper gastrointestinal endoscopy

Upper gastrointestinal endoscopy is used to document reflux-induced mucosal injury and complications of GERD. Endoscopic findings in patients with GERD include normal mucosa, erythema, edema, friability, exudate, erosions, ulcers, strictures, and Barrett metaplasia. Histological hallmarks of esophagitis are increased height of the esophageal papillae and basal cell hyperplasia. Acute injury to the vascular bed, edema, and neutrophilic (and sometimes eosinophilic) infiltration indicate esophageal damage. Chronic inflammation is characterized by the presence of macrophages and granulation tissue. With severe injury, fibroblasts may deposit enough collagen to form a stricture. Long-standing acid damage also promotes aberrant repair of the mucosa by specialized columnar epithelium that contains goblet cells (i.e. Barrett metaplasia).

Ambulatory esophageal pH monitoring

Traditionally, ambulatory 24-h pH monitoring is performed with a nasally inserted pH probe positioned 5 cm above the lower esophageal sphincter (LES). The patient is given an event marker to use with a recording device that is triggered to correlate symptoms with changes in esophageal pH. Maximal sensitivity (93%) and specificity (93%) are obtained by quantitating the percentage of time during which the pH is less than 4, using threshold values of 10.5% in the upright position and 6% in the supine position. Patients who exihibit esophageal acid exposure within physiological limits but have heartburn that correlates with acid reflux events may have a hypersensitive esophagus. Esophageal pH monitoring also can be used to correlate atypical symptoms, such as chest pain with acid reflux.

The advent of wireless pH monitoring has largely replaced catheter-based methods. A miniature probe that is attached to the esophageal mucosa transmits data to a receiver worn by the patient. This system affords the ability to study the patient under conditions of more normal eating and physical activity, and to record esophageal pH over several days.

Impedance

Intralumenal electrical impedance is a technique that measures the conductance of the esophageal contents. This test relies on the electrical properties of liquids (low impedance and high conductance) and gases (high impedance and low conductance) to differentiate between liquid and gas reflux (belching). More importantly, impedance allows detection of nonacidic reflux that would otherwise not be detectable by esophageal pH monitoring, thereby allowing characterization of esophageal reflux as either acid or nonacid in content.

Provocative tests

Provocative tests are sometimes requested as part of a manometric examination to establish the diagnosis of GERD. The Bernstein test determines whether symptoms are reproduced with esophageal acidification. It has a sensitivity of 7–27% and a specificity of 83–94% for diagnosing GERD. Initially, normal saline is infused into the middle esophagus for 5–15 min followed by infusion of 0.1 N hydrochloric acid. If symptoms are reproduced within 30 min of acid infusion, saline is reinfused to relieve symptoms and symptoms are again provoked by acid delivery. The appearance of symptoms with acid infusion in a patient who is blinded to the infusion sequence constitutes a positive test result. Complete symptom relief by saline infusion is not essential.

Esophageal manometry

Esophageal manometry generally is reserved for patients being considered for surgery. Although GERD is a condition of disordered motility, the major finding is increased transient LES relaxation (TLESR). Manometric assessment of esophageal body peristalsis also is important preoperatively because documentation of abnormal peristalsis may influence the type of antireflux surgery chosen.

Key practice point

Tests that quantify the amount of acid refluxing into the esophagus are often inaccurate in classifying abnormal from normal (physiological) reflux. For this reason, a classic symptom of heartburn, especially with response to acid suppression with a proton pump inhibitor, is as reliable a test as pH monitoring. Esophageal manometry does not improve the accuracy since substantial variation in the frequency of TLESRs occurs between asymptomatic individuals, and 30–50% of patients with documented GERD have normal LES pressures.

Management

The course of GERD is highly variable; most patients require medical therapy continuously but some respond to intermittent (medication used continuously for a predetermined duration) or on-demand (medication taken when symptoms occur) strategies of medication and others can discontinue medical therapy altogether.

Lifestyle modification

The modification of lifestyle is an integral part of the initial management of GERD. The head of the bed should be elevated to enhance nocturnal esophageal acid clearance. Smoking and alcohol, which have deleterious effects on LES pressure, acid clearance, and epithelial function, should be avoided. Reducing meal size and limiting the intake of fat, carminatives, and chocolate limit gastric distension, lower TLESR incidence, and prevent LES pressure reductions. Caffeinated and decaffeinated coffee, tea, and carbonated beverages should be avoided because they stimulate acid production. Tomato juice and citrus products may exacerbate symptoms because of osmotic effects. Medications that reduce LES pressure should be limited whenever possible.

Key practice points: lifestyle modifications for patients with gastroesophageal reflux

Elevate the head of the bed 6 inches
Stop smoking
Stop excessive ethanol consumption
Reduce dietary fat
Reduce meal size
Avoid bedtime snacks
Reduce weight (if overweight)
Avoid specific foods
   Chocolate
   Carminatives (e.g. spearmint, peppermint)
   Coffee (caffeinated, decaffeinated)
   Tea
   Cola beverages
   Tomato juice
   Citrus fruit juices
Avoid specific medications (if possible)
   Anticholinergics
   Theophylline
   Benzodiazepines
   Opiates
   Calcium channel antagonists
   β-Adrenergic agonists
   Progesterone (some contraceptives)
   α-Adrenergic antagonists

Medication therapy

Proton pump inhibitors are the drugs of choice for endoscopically proven erosive esophagitis and symptomatic GERD. These agents, which are H^+, K^+-adenosine triphosphatase antagonists, produce superior acid suppression compared with H_2 receptor antagonists. Recent concerns about adverse events associated with PPIs (*C. difficile* infection, pneumonia, bone fracture, drug interaction, magnesium deficiency) illustrate the need to use the lowest dose necessary to achieve therapeutic goals; however, the risk of adverse events is very low so appropriate use of PPIs to treat GERD is encouraged.

For patients with intermittent, mild symptoms, antacids and H_2 receptor antagonists provide rapid, safe, and effective relief from GERD symptoms. High-dose regimens may heal erosive disease; however, the required doses often induce significant side-effects (e.g. diarrhea with magnesium antacids and constipation with aluminum antacids) that make compliance difficult. Gaviscon (aluminum hydroxide and magnesium carbonate), an antacid-alginate combination, decreases reflux by producing a viscous mechanical barrier but it may also adversely affect bowel function. Sucralfate, the basic salt of aluminum hydroxide and sucrose octasulfate, acts topically to increase tissue resistance, buffer acid, and bind pepsin and bile salts, but its efficacy in treating patients with GERD is limited. H_2 receptor antagonists (e.g. cimetidine, ranitidine, famotidine, and nizatidine) are safe and effective for treating mild disease.

Prokinetic agents have been used as primary or adjunctive therapy for GERD. Cisapride, an agent that acts on serotonin 5-HT_4 receptors to facilitate myenteric acetylcholine release, promotes gastric emptying and increases LES pressure and was approved for treating GERD. However, it has been withdrawn from the market because of increased risk of cardiac arrhythmias. Emerging motility therapies include γ-aminobutyric acid (GABA) B agonists and mGluR5-negative allosteric modulators (inhibitors). These drugs have been shown in clinical trials to reduce TLESRs and reduce GERD symptoms; however, none is available at the time of this printing.

Treatment strategy

Most patients with heartburn self-medicate with over-the-counter antacids, H_2 receptor antagonists, or PPIs. Those who do not respond to therapy or those who initially respond but relapse may seek medical attention. In such individuals, the clinician should consider alternative causes of heartburn, including nonacid reflux, functional heartburn, and malignancy (Figure 18.1). The first step is to determine the presence of "alarm" symptoms or signs such as bleeding, anemia, dysphagia, or weight loss that may suggest the presence of upper gastrointestinal malignancy. Upper endoscopy is indicated if any of these factors is present. In the absence of alarm features, it is reasonable to assess whether an adequate trial of acid suppression has been attempted because most other disorders respond variably to acid suppression. PPIs are the most potent class of medications used to treat GERD; therefore, the use of these drugs is advocated. Note that most PPIs reduce symptoms of GERD most effectively if taken 30–60 min before ingesting a meal. Failure to respond to PPI therapy is an indication for upper endoscopy.

If symptoms are not relieved, ambulatory esophageal pH monitoring may differentiate between those individuals with persistent acid reflux (requiring higher doses of acid suppression) and those without abnormal esophageal acid exposure (Figure 18.2). The latter group comprises patients with nonacid

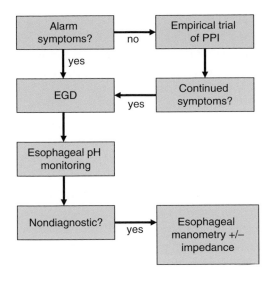

Figure 18.1 Evaluation of heartburn. EGD, esophagogastroduodenoscopy; PPI, proton pump inhibitor.

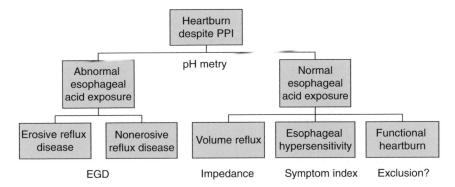

Figure 18.2 Evaluation of heartburn refractory to acid suppression. EGD, esophagogastroduodenoscopy; PPI, proton pump inhibitor.

reflux, which can be diagnosed by esophageal impedance testing, patients with hypersensitivity (pH within physiological limits but positive symptom index) and patients who have functional heartburn (normal acid exposure, poor correlation between symptoms and reflux [symptom index], and absence of nonacid reflux).

Potential pitfalls

Dyspepsia (discomfort in the upper abdomen) without heartburn or acid regurgitation should be managed differently from GERD and generally requires upper gastrointestinal endoscopy to examine the disorders under this differential diagnosis.

Evaluation for the presence of *H. pylori* is reasonable for patients presenting with dyspepsia; however, *H. pylori* is not a cause of GERD and eradication will not alleviate heartburn.

Baclofen and other agents that reduce TLESRs may be a reasonable therapy for nonacid reflux. Hypersensitivity may respond to greater acid suppression. Functional heartburn management remains problematic but therapy aimed at decreasing esophageal sensation may be useful (e.g. trazodone, tricyclics).

Surgical treatment

Antireflux surgery remains a viable option for treatment of GERD. However, failure of medical therapy predicts poor response to surgery. Patients who respond to medication but wish to consider surgical intervention to avoid drugs should be counseled about the potential for relapse requiring reinstitution of drugs after surgery. Appropriate candidates include patients intolerant or allergic to medical therapy and patients with symptoms associated with nonacid reflux. The Nissen (360° wrap) and Belsey (270° wrap) fundoplications and the Hill gastropexy produce an initial 85% success rate in relieving symptoms and healing lesions. Postoperative dysphagia or gas-bloat syndrome (i.e. the inability to belch or vomit) affects 2–8%. The operative mortality for these procedures is 1%.

Fundoplications reduce hiatal hernias and enhance LES competency, whereas a gastropexy anchors the gastroesophageal junction to the median arcuate ligament. The Belsey procedure is chosen for patients with impaired esophageal peristalsis to reduce the likelihood of postoperative dysphagia. The Hill operation is used for patients with prior gastric resection.

Endoscopic therapy

Several endoscopic technologies have been approved for treating GERD but none has achieved widespread use. Application of radiofrequency energy to the distal esophagus and proximal stomach (Stretta) illustrated efficacy in a sham-controlled clinical study. Although associated with symptom control and quality of life parameters superior to those of sham-treated patients, the rate of GERD medication use between groups did not differ and the device is no longer clinically available. Full-thickness plication is currently under study but no products are available at the time of this printing.

Complications and their management

Strictures are characterized by progressive dysphagia over months to years. Although strictures may be defined radiographically, endoscopy is required in all cases to exclude malignancy. Esophageal bougienage dilation may be performed without (Maloney, Hurst) or with (Savary) endoscopic guidance, or may be accomplished using through-the-scope balloon dilation. Hemorrhage may occasionally develop from esophageal erosions and ulcers. Perforation of an esophageal ulcer is a serious complication that may cause life-threatening mediastinitis.

Barrett esophagus is an acquired condition in which squamous epithelium is replaced by specialized columnar epithelium in response to chronic acid exposure. The clinical consequence of intestinal metaplasia is the development of esophageal adenocarcinoma. Barrett metaplasia is present in 5–15% of patients with GERD who undergo endoscopy. The management of patients with Barrett's esophagus is described in detail in Chapter 19. Hemorrhage may occasionally develop from esophageal erosions and ulcers. It may be chronic, with production of iron deficiency anemia, or acute. Perforation of an esophageal ulcer is a serious complication that may cause life-threatening mediastinitis.

Alkaline reflux esophagitis

Alkaline reflux esophagitis develops from prolonged contact of esophageal epithelium with nonacidic gastric or intestinal contents, usually in patients who have undergone ulcer surgery with vagotomy or, less commonly, in patients with achlorhydria who have not undergone surgery. Factors responsible for mucosal damage include deconjugated bile salts and pancreatic enzymes. Medications that may be effective include bile salt-binding agents (e.g. cholestyramine, colestipol, sucralfate) and mucosal coating agents (e.g. antacids). When medications fail, a Roux-en-Y gastrojejunostomy may divert intestinal contents away from the esophagus. Alternatively, fundoplication may be performed in patients with intact stomachs or adequate gastric remnants.

Guidelines on GERD

American Gastroenterological Association. Medical position statement on the management of gastroesophageal reflux disease. Gastroenterology 2008;135:1383–1391.

CHAPTER 19
Esophageal Tumors

Adenocarcinoma

The presence of Barrett esophagus (intestinal metaplasia with specialized columnar epithelium) is the most important risk factor for developing esophageal adenocarcinoma (EAC), and it is believed that EACs arise in areas of Barrett esophagus. The mechanism by which reflux of gastric contents into the esophagus induces the metaplastic response is unknown. The annual rate of cancer development among patients with Barrett esophagus is about 0.12–0.5%.

Genomic instability is common in dysplastic Barrett mucosa. Aneuploid cell populations and deletions or alterations of tumor suppressor genes, particularly chromosomal regions 17p (*p53*), 5q (*APC,MCC*), 18q (*DCC*), and 13q (*RB1*), are often observed in the mucosa of patients who develop carcinoma. Abnormalities of cell proliferation, as evidenced by the expression of proliferating cell nuclear antigen (PCNA) and Ki-67, are noted in Barrett tissue and EAC. Microsatellite instability, a marker of defective mismatch repair, has also been detected in patients with Barrett esophagus and EAC.

Clinical presentation

Barrett metaplasia does not produce symptoms and the endoscopic appearance of Barrett mucosa correlates poorly with the severity of reflux symptoms, which is why screening to detect Barrett metaplasia is difficult. The clinical manifestations of EAC include progressive dysphagia, nausea, vomiting, weight loss, and anemia. Symptoms attributable to adenocarcinoma occur in advanced stages when the tumor is large enough to interfere with swallowing. Based on the pathogenesis of EAC and Barrett esophagus, chronic pyrosis, regurgitation, and chest pain due to gastroesophageal reflux are common.

Yamada's Handbook of Gastroenterology, Third Edition. Edited by Tadataka Yamada and John M. Inadomi.
© 2013 John Wiley & Sons, Ltd. Published 2013 by John Wiley & Sons, Ltd.

Diagnostic investigation

Endoscopic studies

Barrett esophagus is diagnosed using upper gastrointestinal endoscopy with biopsy, and requires the presence of circumferential or isolated islands (or tongues) of salmon-colored mucosa proximal to the esophagogastric junction in which there is histological confirmation of intestinal metaplasia. The Prague C and M criteria describe the circumferential ("C") and maximum ("M") length of columnar-appearing mucosa. Biopsy specimens should be targeted to all erosions, nodules, and strictures, as well as randomly obtained from flat-appearing columnar mucosa because dysplasia and cancer may be present in Barrett esophagus in the absence of otherwise detectable structural lesions.

Histological evaluation

The interpretation of biopsy samples from patients with Barrett esophagus requires the expertise of an experienced gastrointestinal pathologist. There is a high degree of interobserver variation in distinguishing low-grade dysplasia from no dysplasia, in addition to variability in interpreting high-grade dysplasia. It may be difficult or impossible to distinguish high-grade dysplasia from invasive carcinoma if biopsy samples fail to include the lamina propria; therefore, large-capacity or jumbo forceps should be used when sampling areas of Barrett esophagus. Flow cytometry has been used to identify aneuploid or tetraploid cell populations and shows considerable promise in predicting the development of EAC. Other markers of cell proliferation such as PCNA, Ki-67, tritiated thymidine uptake, and ornithine decarboxylase may be predictive; however, the ability of these tests to affect clinical practice positively has not been established.

Diagnostic pitfalls

Currently the US definition of Barrett esophagus requires endoscopically abnormal (columnar) mucosa in conjunction with histological confirmation of specialized intestinal metaplasia (presence of goblet cells). The British Society of Gastroenterology criteria allow the definition of Barrett esophagus to include other types of metaplastic epithelium, including gastric and junctional (cardiac) epithelium. Because the natural history of Barrett esophagus with regard to cancer risk is still poorly defined, limiting the definition of Barrett esophagus to the entity for which most data are available (intestinal metaplasia) has been accepted by US national society guidelines.

Management and prevention

See Table 19.1.

Table 19.1 Management of Barrett esophagus

Barrett's esophagus with:	Recommendation
No dysplasia	Endoscopic surveillance with biopsies every 3–5 years
Low-grade dysplasia	Endoscopic surveillance with biopsies every 12 months or endoscopic therapy
High-grade dysplasia	Endoscopic therapy (endoscopic mucosal resection, radiofrequency ablation, photodynamic therapy)
Esophageal adenocarcinoma	Esophagectomy

Screening and surveillance

Identification of the link between EAC and Barrett esophagus has led to the implementation of endoscopic screening and surveillance programs. The strategy proposed by several national societies includes screening patients with multiple risk factors for EAC (age 50 years or older, male sex, white race, chronic symptoms of gastroesophageal reflux disease, hiatal hernia, elevated Body Mass Index, intra-abdominal distribution of body fat) to detect Barrett esophagus using upper gastrointestinal endoscopy. If intestinal metaplasia is histologically confirmed in a region of the esophagus that has columnar-appearing mucosa, surveillance with high-resolution white-light endoscopy should be performed at intervals dependent on the presence and degree of dysplasia. Current guidelines suggest taking systematic four-quadrant biopsy specimens every 2 cm along the length of Barrett metaplasia. In addition, any endoscopic abnormalities such as erosions, nodules, or strictures should be biopsied.

Patients with no dysplasia are recommended to undergo surveillance at an interval between 3 and 5 years. Patients in whom low-grade dysplasia is diagnosed should have surveillance with four-quadrant biopsies every 1 cm performed every 12 months, or be considered for endoscopic ablation. High-grade dysplasia (HGD) must be confirmed on review by an experienced pathologist. Confirmation of HGD prompts a recommendation for endoscopic therapy using endoscopic mucosal resection, radiofrequency ablation or photodymic therapy. Visible lesions (ulcers, nodules, masses) associated with HGD should be removed by endoscopic mucosal resection techniques, which is both therapeutic and diagnostic by confirming the absence of invasive cancer. Invasive cancer should be staged using endoscopic ultrasound and treated by surgical resection.

Case–control studies illustrate a potential survival benefit from endoscopic surveillance of patients with Barrett esophagus; however, prospective studies to confirm the efficacy of surveillance are lacking.

Molecular markers for the presence of Barrett esophagus, dysplasia and cancer are under development; however, markers have not been validated to predict which patients with Barrett esophagus are at risk for progression. Furthermore, advanced imaging techniques such as chromoendoscopy have not been shown

---

Guidelines: Barrett's esophagus

1. American Gastroenterological Association, Spechler SJ, Sharma P, Souza RF, Inadomi JM, Shaheen NJ. American Gastroenterological Association medical position statement on the management of Barrett's esophagus. Gastroenterology 2011;140:1084–1091.

2. Wang KK, Sampliner RE. Updated guidelines 2008 for the diagnosis, surveillance and therapy of Barrett's esophagus. American Journal of Gastroenterology 2008;103:788–797.

Diagnostic pitfalls

Low-grade dysplasia has been a source of controversy regarding the risk of cancer. While some studies report increased incidence of adenocarcinoma, other studies illustrate cancer risk to be low and similar to the risk among patients with no dysplasia. One of the reasons for the difference may be the poor inter- and intraobserver correlation in the diagnosis of low-grade dysplasia. Inflammation, which is a necessary component of gastroesophageal reflux disease, can cause morphologically similar changes to dysplasia. Risk stratification based on dysplasia will be problematic; therefore, advances in molecular techniques or other tools that more accurately describe the risk of cancer will greatly improve the effectiveness and cost-effectiveness of screening and surveillance among patients with Barrett esophagus.

---

to improve the clinical outcomes of patients with Barrett esophagus and are not recommended for routine use at this time.

Squamous Cell Carcinoma

Squamous cell carcinoma (SCC) is the most common malignant tumor of the esophagus worldwide. Men have a threefold higher risk than women and in the United States, African-Americans have a fivefold increased risk for SCC relative to whites. The geographic variation in the prevalence of SCC between and within countries shows the importance of environmental factors in its pathogenesis. Alcohol and tobacco consumption increase the risk for SCC in a dose-dependent manner. This effect appears to be additive because the risk for patients who smoke and drink excessively is much higher than the risk for patients who use either substance alone. Deficiencies of vitamins A, C, E, and B_{12}, folic acid, and riboflavin are risk factors for cancer.

Achalasia is associated with a 10–30-fold increase in the rate of SCC. Synchronous or metachronous esophageal SCC develops at an annual rate of 3–7% in patients with SCC of the head and neck. Tylosis, a rare autosomal dominant condition characterized by hyperkeratosis of the palms and soles, is highly linked with esophageal SCC; 50% of patients will develop cancer by age 45 and 95% by age 65. Lye ingestion that causes an esophageal stricture has been associated with development of squamous cell tumors. Other factors associated with esophageal SCC include ionizing radiation, celiac sprue, human papillomavirus, Plummer–Vinson syndrome, and esophageal diverticula.

Clinical presentation

Patients with esophageal SCC present with progressive dysphagia. Odynophagia and weight loss may occur, as well as nausea, vomiting, hematemesis, and back pain. Involvement of adjacent mediastinal strictures may result in chronic cough caused by a tracheo-esophageal fistula, hoarseness caused by recurrent laryngeal nerve involvement, and, rarely, massive gastrointestinal hemorrhage due to invasion into the aorta.

A generalized loss of muscle mass and subcutaneous fat is often evident. In patients with early disease, the physical examination findings may be normal but patients with metastatic disease may exhibit hepatomegaly, bony pain, and supraclavicular adenopathy.

Diagnostic investigation

Radiographic studies

The diagnostic evaluation of patients with dysphagia traditionally began with esophageal radiological imaging. Barium swallow radiography is very sensitive in detecting cancers large enough to cause symptoms but its sensitivity for detecting early lesions is only 75%, which limits its usefulness as a screening test. Fluoroscopic examination can often detect motility abnormalities or proximal diverticula that may not be appreciated in endoscopic studies. However, some malignancies produce a smooth symmetrical stricture, which precludes barium radiographs from reliably distinguishing tumors from benign peptic strictures. For these reasons, endoscopy has become the first-line evaluation for patients presenting with dysphagia.

Endoscopic studies

Diagnostic confirmation of esophageal SCC requires upper gastrointestinal endoscopy. Early cancers can be detected as elevated plaques or small erythematous erosions. All mucosal abnormalities should undergo biopsy for histological examination. Because a sampling error occasionally leads to false-negative results, any lesion that highly suggests malignancy should be rebiopsied.

Staging

Esophageal cancer should be staged on the basis of the depth of invasion (T stage), the nodal status (N stage), and the presence of distant metastatic disease (M stage). Staging helps determine the therapeutic approach and assess the prognosis (Table 19.2). The tools for staging include computed tomography (CT) and endoscopic ultrasound. Although a sensitive means of documenting aortic invasion or pulmonary and hepatic metastases, CT has low accuracy in determining

Table 19.2 TNM staging system for cancer of the esophagus (American Joint Committee on Cancer criteria)

Primary tumor (T)

TX	Primary tumor cannot be assessed
T0	No evidence of primary tumor
Tis	Carcinoma *in situ*
T1	Tumor invades lamina propria or submucosa
T2	Tumor invades muscularis propria
T3	Tumor invades adventitia
T4	Tumor invades adjacent structures

Lymph node (N)

NX	Regional lymph nodes cannot be assessed
N0	No regional lymph node metastasis
N1	Regional lymph node metastasis

Distant metastasis (M)

MX	Presence of distant metastasis cannot be assessed
M0	No distant metastasis
M1	Distant metastasis
M1a	Metastasis in celiac (lower esophagus) or cervical lymph nodes (upper esophagus)
M1b	Other distant metastasis (lower or upper esophagus) or nonregional lymph nodes (midesophagus)

Stage grouping

0	Tis	N0	M0
I	T1	N0	M0
IIA	T2	N0	M0
	T3	N0	M0
IIB	T1	N1	M0
	T2	N1	M0
III	T3	N1	M0
	T4	Any N	M0
IV	Any T	Any N	M1
IVA	Any T	Any N	M1a
IVB	Any T	Any N	M1b

Reproduced with permission from the AJCC Cancer Staging Manual, 7th edition.

nodal involvement and magnetic resonance imaging does not provide an advantage over CT. Endoscopic ultrasound is superior to CT for determining the T and N stages in all types of esophageal tumors, and is therefore an important tool for predicting resectability. Endoscopic ultrasound has accuracy rates of about 90% and 85% for establishing the T and N stages of a tumor, respectively.

Treatment of cancer

Therapeutic approaches for esophageal SCC and EAC are similar. Surgical resection is the primary therapy for patients with tumors that are confined to the esophagus. However, because of the advanced stage at which most esophageal cancers are diagnosed, surgical exploration is indicated in only 60% of patients, of which only two-thirds are able to undergo resection. Overall, the 1- and 5-year survival rates are 18% and 5%, respectively. Although curative resection is unlikely for T3 or N1 lesions, palliative resection can provide 1–2 years of symptom-free survival. Locally advanced (T4) or metastatic (M1) disease is not amenable to curative resection, and the poor long-term survival of these patients makes surgical palliation an unfavorable option.

There are several accepted surgical approaches to treating esophageal cancer. The choice of procedure depends on tumor location, lymph node status, the patient's body habitus and performance status, and the preference of the surgeon and institution. Traditionally, a transthoracic esophagectomy with esophagogastric anastomosis is performed. An alternative procedure for lesions in the upper one-third of the esophagus involves a subtotal esophagectomy with a gastric pull-up into the neck and requires a combined abdominal and cervical approach. Both procedures provide the adequate exposure and tissue resection margins necessary for a cancer operation. With the increase in incidence of EAC in the distal esophagus, transhiatal resection and primary anastomosis has become the most common mode of therapy. Complications include anastomotic leak or stricture, pulmonary disease (e.g. pneumonia, pulmonary emboli), recurrent laryngeal nerve injury, and cardiac disease (e.g. myocardial infarction, arrhythmia, and congestive heart failure), leading to mortality rates of 2–13%.

The overall 5-year survival of patients who undergo resection is 12–27%. High rates of recurrence have prompted trials of perioperative chemotherapy and radiation therapy to improve systemic and regional control of the tumor. Neoadjuvant (preoperative) chemotherapy is favored and has been shown to increase resectability and improve 2-year survival rates over other modalities.

Endoscopic placement of self-expanding metal stents is the palliative therapy of choice to relieve esophageal obstruction. In addition, coated stents may be

---

Essentials of treatment

Curative

- Stage T1 and T2 lesions without nodal disease: surgical resection
- Locally advanced disease: perioperative chemotherapy and/or radiation therapy plus surgical resection

Palliation

- Local disease: external beam radiation (with or without chemotherapy), brachytherapy, endoscopic therapy (self-expanding metal stents, laser, bipolar electrocoagulation, photodynamic therapy)
- Metastatic disease: systemic chemotherapy with 5-FU and cisplatin, or paclitaxel, docetaxel, gemcitabine, irinotecan, oxaliplatin

placed across tracheo-esophageal fistulae to allow patients to swallow saliva and food without aspirating. Complications associated with stents include stent migration, chest pain, perforation, and bleeding. Endoscopic therapy using laser, argon plasma coagulation, or bipolar electrocautery may also help to relieve obstruction. Photodynamic therapy consists of administering a photosensitizer, followed by local exposure of the tumor to light of a specific wavelength (630 nm). Tumor destruction occurs as a result of singlet oxygen production that leads to ischemia and necrosis. Systemic chemotherapy with paclitaxel, docetaxel, gemcitabine, irinotecan, and oxaliplatin has shown response rates up to 60%, including increased survival and quality of life.

Other Malignant Neoplasms

Epithelial tumors

A variant of SCC characterized by a prominent spindle cell component has been variably termed carcinosarcoma, pseudosarcoma, spindle cell carcinoma, and polypoid carcinoma. These lesions are large and polypoid and may be solitary or multiple. Men are affected more often than women, and most are middle-aged or elderly at the time of presentation. Another variant of SCC is termed verrucous carcinoma because the primary lesion grows slowly and invades local tissues with only rare metastases. Adenoid cystic carcinomas are rare tumors thought to arise from submucosal glands. Adenosquamous carcinomas or adenoacantho-mas combine features of the two common forms of esophageal cancer. Mucoepidermoid carcinoma, also composed of glandular and squamous elements likely arising from submucosal glands or ducts, has a poor prognosis. Melanoma of the esophagus may be primary or metastatic, although the esophagus is a less common site of metastatic gastrointestinal disease than the stomach, small intestine, or colon.

Neuroendocrine tumors of the esophagus include small cell carcinomas, carci-noids, and choriocarcinomas. Small cell carcinoma of the esophagus may be a primary esophageal tumor or it may represent a metastatic lesion from the lung. Neoplasia may be associated with a paraneoplastic phenomenon, including inappropriate antidiuretic hormone secretion and hypercalcemia.

Nonepithelial tumors

Malignant nonepithelial tumors of the esophagus include leiomyosarcomas, metastatic cancers, and lymphomas. Leiomyosarcomas may be polypoid or infil-trative and can be located anywhere in the esophagus. Metastatic lesions are most commonly due to melanoma, followed by breast cancer; less common etiologies include gastric, renal, liver, prostate, testicular, bone, skin, lung, and head and neck cancer. Primary esophageal lymphoma may be of the Hodgkin or non-Hodgkin type and is more common among immunocompromised patients.

Benign Esophageal Tumors

Squamous cell papillomas

Squamous cell papillomas are small, sessile, polypoid lesions discovered incidentally during endoscopic examination for unrelated symptoms. Papillomas usually are solitary and are located in the distal third of the esophagus. They may be associated with chronic irritation from gastroesophageal reflux disease or may result from infection with human papillomavirus. Cancer development has not been documented in these neoplasms.

Submucosal neoplasms

Leiomyomas are the most common benign esophageal tumor. The male-to-female ratio is 2/1. Most are asymptomatic but large tumors may cause dysphagia or chest pain. They occur most commonly in the distal esophagus. The diagnosis is made by barium swallow radiography or upper gastrointestinal endoscopy. Large benign leiomyomas may be difficult to distinguish from rare malignant leiomyosarcomas. Other submucosal lesions of the esophagus are rare and include lipomas, fibromas, fibrovascular polyps, granular cell tumors, hemangiomas, and lymphangiomas. As with leiomyomas, most of these lesions are found incidentally and are not considered morbid.

CHAPTER 20
Disorders of Gastric Emptying

Disorders of gastric emptying can be classified as those with delayed or accelerated emptying. While there are variety of disorders that are associated with gastroparesis (delayed gastric emptying), accelerated emptying is clinically relevant only among patients who have undergone surgical intervention that includes vagotomy and gastric drainage.

Disorders with Delayed Gastric Emptying

Clinical presentation

Symptoms of gastroparesis include chronic or intermittent nausea, vomiting, bloating, early satiety, and postprandial abdominal pain. As the disease progresses, bloating and nausea increase slowly for several days because of incomplete gastric evacuation of multiple ingested meals, only to be relieved by voluminous vomiting of foul-smelling food ingested hours to days before. In severe cases, intractable retching may develop even if no meal has been ingested in several hours.

Evaluation of symptoms consistent with gastroparesis is outlined in Table 20.1.

Differential diagnosis

Disorders involving the stomach
Diabetic gastroparesis

Patients with long-standing diabetes (usually type 1 for >10 years with other neuropathic complications) may develop gastroparesis. Motor abnormalities that contribute to delays in gastric emptying include loss of antral contractions, increased pyloric activity (pylorospasm), increased fundus compliance, and increased intestinal motor activity, which function as a brake on gastric evacuation. The degree of hyperglycemia can exacerbate delays in gastric emptying in diabetics.

Yamada's Handbook of Gastroenterology, Third Edition. Edited by Tadataka Yamada and John M. Inadomi.
© 2013 John Wiley & Sons, Ltd. Published 2013 by John Wiley & Sons, Ltd.

Table 20.1 Management of suspected gastroparesis

History and physical
Blood tests: CBC, glucose, potassium, creatinine, total protein, albumin, calcium, amylase, pregnancy
Radiological tests: plain abdominal series
Evaluate structural disease
Upper endoscopy and/or radiological tests (UGI series, small bowel follow-through)
Evaluate motility disorder
Solid-phase gastric emptying test (4 h) or pH/pressure capsule (SmartPill)
If gastroparesis diagnosed, obtain thyroid function, antinuclear antibody, HbA1C
Treatment
Prokinetic or antiemetic agent
Refractory symptoms
Electrogastrography
Antroduodenal manometry
CT enterography

CBC, complete blood count; CT, computed tomography; UGI, upper gastrointestinal.

Essentials of diagnosis and potential pitfalls

Diabetic gastroparesis is due to a neuropathy and generally coincides with other complications of diabetes mellitus including retinopathy, nephropathy, and peripheral neuropathy. Orthostatic hypotension may be present as a manifestation of autonomic neuropathy. While generally a complication of type 1 diabetes, gastroparesis is also a complication of type 2 diabetes. Note that hyperglycemia itself decreases antral contractility, induces gastric dysrhythmias and delays gastric emptying; however, this is a reversible phenomenon and not necessarily indicative of neuropathy.

Idiopathic gastroparesis

Many patients (25–30%) with gastroparesis have no predisposing factor for their disease. In most series the majority of affected patients are young women. In a subset of these individuals, fever, myalgias, nausea, and diarrhea precede the onset of gastroparesis, which suggests an underlying viral cause.

Postoperative gastroparesis

A minority of patients (<5%) who have undergone surgery for peptic ulcer disease or malignancy experience nausea, vomiting, and early satiety secondary to postoperative stasis. Abnormalities in antral peristalsis and fundus tone have been demonstrated in this condition. Gastric stasis may also complicate gastroplasty or gastric bypass operations for morbid obesity, producing early satiety, anorexia, and weight reduction. Patients undergoing fundoplication for gastroesophageal reflux develop gastroparesis, possibly by intraoperative damage to the vagus nerve.

Table 20.2 Effects of medications on gastric emptying

Delay gastric emptying
Ethanol (high concentration)
Aluminum hydroxide antacids
Anticholinergics
β-Adrenergic receptor agonists
Calcitonin
Calcium channel antagonists
Dexfenfluramine
Diphenhydramine
Glucagon
Interferon-α
L-Dopa
Octreotide
Opiates
Progesterone
Proton pump inhibitors
Sucralfate
Tetrahydrocannabinol
Tobacco/nicotine
Tricyclic antidepressant

Accelerate gastric emptying
β-Adrenergic receptor antagonists
Clonidine
Domperidone
Erythromycin/other macrolides
Nizatidine
Metoclopramide
Naloxone
Tegaserod

Functional dyspepsia

Delayed gastric emptying is reported in 30–82% of cases of functional dyspepsia. Many affected patients also exhibit increased sensitivity to gastric balloon distension, suggesting that sensory nerve abnormalities may be involved in symptom induction.

Medication-induced delays in gastric emptying

Many prescription and over-the-counter medications delay gastric emptying (Table 20.2). Nonmedicinal compounds, including tobacco, marijuana, and intoxicating quantities of ethanol, also inhibit gastric motor function. Total parenteral nutrition has been associated with delayed gastric emptying, which may relate in part to the induction of hyperglycemia.

Disorders with diffuse gastrointestinal involvement
Rheumatological disorders

Scleroderma produces dysphagia, heartburn, nausea, vomiting, bloating, abdominal pain, and bowel disturbances as a result of diffuse dysmotility that involves the esophagus, stomach, small intestine, and colon. In most patients, gastroduodenal manometry demonstrates diffuse low-amplitude contractions that are consistent with myopathic involvement. However, a subset of patients with early disease exhibits high-amplitude, unco-ordinated contractile activity, which indicates neuropathic disease.

Chronic idiopathic intestinal pseudo-obstruction

Patients with this disorder may have associated gastric dysmotility with prominent nausea, vomiting, bloating, and early satiety. The presence of bladder dysfunction or orthostatic hypotension suggests diffuse neuromuscular disease. Pseudo-obstruction may be familial, it may occur after a viral prodrome, or it may be a paraneoplastic consequence of certain malignancies such as small cell lung carcinoma.

Nongastrointestinal disorders

Eating disorders

Delayed gastric emptying with reduced antral contractility is a common manifestation of anorexia nervosa. Causes of gastroparesis with anorexia nervosa include central nervous system inhibition and malnutrition, but no specific gastric pathology has been demonstrated. Some patients with bulimia nervosa exhibit delayed solid emptying. Rumination syndrome usually is not associated with delayed emptying, although small reductions in postprandial antral motor activity have been documented.

Cyclic vomiting syndrome

Cyclic vomiting syndrome is a disorder of unknown etiology that is characterized by intermittent symptomatic periods that begin abruptly and last for 3–5 days followed by prolonged asymptomatic intervals that last for months. Some patients with cyclic vomiting syndrome exhibit delayed gastric emptying, which suggests underlying gastric motor dysfunction although motility may also be normal. Metabolic derangements, mitochondrial disorders, atopy, and migraine headaches are associated with distinct subsets, suggesting a heterogeneous pathogenesis.

Neurological disorders

Altered gastric motility or emptying has been demonstrated after cerebrovascular accidents, with migraines, and after high cervical spinal injury. Gastric stasis may occur with disorders of autonomic function (e.g. Shy–Drager syndrome, Parkinson disease, Guillain–Barré syndrome, and multiple sclerosis).

Endocrinological and metabolic disorders

Nausea, vomiting, and anorexia are frequently reported by patients with end-stage renal disease, even after adequate dialysis, but only a minority of these patients exhibit abnormal gastric emptying. Hypothyroidism causes gastroparesis and hypothyroidism, hyperthyroidism and hypoparathyroidism are associated with intestinal pseudo-obstruction.

Diagnostic investigation

Laboratory studies

Laboratory studies may assist in determining the severity and chronicity of the patient's disorder. Hypokalemia and contraction alkalosis result from severe vomiting, whereas anemia and hypoproteinemia are consistent with long-standing malnutrition. Specific serological tests may suggest rheumatological diseases such as systemic lupus erythematosus or scleroderma, whereas antineuronal antibody tests can screen for paraneoplastic dysmotility syndromes. Blood tests also can detect diabetes, uremia, or thyroid and parathyroid disease.

Radiographic and endoscopic studies

Patients should undergo structural evaluation to exclude mechanical obstruction. Abdominal radiography screen for obstruction of the small intestine, which can be followed by barium radiography, if clinically indicated. Upper gastrointestinal endoscopy is appropriate if gastric outlet obstruction secondary to peptic ulcer disease or malignancy is suspected.

Functional testing

Gastric scintigraphic quantitation of gastric emptying is the standard for diagnosing gastroparesis. Solid-phase gastric-emptying scintigraphic images using ^{99m}Tc-sulfur colloid mixed with a solid food such as scrambled eggs exhibit a biphasic emptying profile: an initial lag phase followed by a linear emptying phase, which persists until all digestible residues have been expelled by the stomach. In normal controls, 95% of a solid meal is emptied within 4 h of ingestion. The result of a gastric emptying scan should be used in patient management in conjunction with the clinical presentation because some profoundly symptomatic patients will exhibit normal emptying, whereas other asymptomatic individuals may show pronounced gastric retention.

The SmartPill is an ingestible capsule that simultaneously measures pressure, temperature and pH, and transmits this information to a portable recording device wirelessly. With regard to gastric emptying, this technology can measure gastric emptying (and total gastrointestinal transit time) as well as pressure patterns and motility indices for the stomach (and small and large intestine). The "gastric residence time" of the SmartPill can differentiate normal from delayed gastric emptying and has a correlation with scintigraphy of approximately 85%.

Other tests of upper gut function are performed in selected cases in referral centers. Electrogastrography (EGG) noninvasively measures gastric electrical activity. EGG detects disruptions in slow-wave rhythm that are too rapid (tachygastria) or too slow (bradygastria), as well as abnormal electrical responses to meal ingestion in some patients with nausea and vomiting. Abnormal EGGs are demonstrated in approximately 70% of patients with delayed gastric emptying; thus the technique has been proposed as another means of testing gastric emptying.

Antroduodenal manometry involves the peroral or transnasal placement of a catheter that monitors pressure changes during a 6–8-h period. Specifically, fasting motility should illustrate the migrating motor complex, while the characteristic fed motor pattern should be seen 1–2 h after a meal.

Essentials of diagnosis and potential pitfalls

While gastric emptying studies are the standard for the diagnosis of gastroparesis, the accuracy of these tests is suboptimal. Even a 4-h solid-phase test can be normal in patients who are known to have emptying delays; conversely, the test can be abnormal in normal controls. While more accurate, gastroduodenal manometry and electrogastrography have limited clinical utility and should be considered research tools at this time.

Management and prevention

Dietary and nonmedicinal therapies

Nonmedicinal therapies are included in the initial recommendations for the treatment of gastroparesis. Medications that inhibit gastrointestinal motility should be discontinued if possible. Ingesting several small meals per day may produce fewer symptoms than 2–3 large meals. Solid foods with large amounts of indigestible residue should be avoided. Hyperglycemia should be treated since it delays gastric emptying of solid foods. Because lipids are the most potent nutrient inhibitors of gastric emptying, a low-fat diet may also reduce symptoms.

Prokinetic medication therapy

Medication therapy for gastroparesis focuses on agents that promote gastric emptying (Table 20.3). Metoclopramide acutely enhances gastric emptying, but a sustained prokinetic effect is not always attained and side-effects are common. Some cases of irreversible tardive dyskinesia also have been observed with this drug. Erythromycin is a potent stimulant of gastric emptying through its action on gastroduodenal receptors for motilin. Tachyphylaxis limits the beneficial effects of erythromycin with long-term use. Clonidine (α2-adrenergic agonist) can reduce symptoms and accelerate gastric emptying in diabetic gastroparesis.

Domperidone is a peripheral dopamine receptor antagonist that does not cross the blood–brain barrier, reducing the central nervous system side-effects seen with metoclopramide. The drug is not marketed in the United States but is available in most other countries. The 5-HT$_4$ receptor agonists cisapride and tegaserod accelerate gastric emptying, but substantial adverse events led to withdrawal of both from the US market.

Antiemetic medication therapy

Antiemetic drugs without prokinetic properties may serve useful adjunctive roles in managing gastroparesis. Antidopaminergic agents such as prochlorperazine,

Table 20.3 Drugs with prokinetic effects on the stomach

Medication	Mechanisms of action	Dosage
Metoclopramide	Dopamine receptor antagonism	5–20 mg qid
	5-HT$_4$ agonist facilitation of acetylcholine release from enteric nerves	
	5-HT$_3$ receptor antagonism	
Erythromycin	Motilin receptor agonism	50–250 mg qid
Domperidone	Peripheral dopamine receptor antagonism (does not cross blood-brain barrier)	10–30 mg qid

trimethobenzamide, and promethazine may provide symptom control. 5-HT$_3$ receptor antagonists such as ondansetron and granisetron, and the neurokinin-3 receptor antagonist aprepitnat do not affect gastric emptying but are commonly used for symptom control despite lack of long-term effectiveness data. Antihistamines including diphenhydramine, dimenhydranate or meclizine reduce tachygastria and reduce symptoms in motion sickness, which has been extrapolated for use in other gastric emptying disorders. Anticholinergics such as scopolamine are advocated by some clinicians, although there have been no studies proving their efficacy.

Tricyclic antidepressants reduce nausea in many patients with diabetic gastropathy and have also been used in some diabetics with delayed gastric emptying.

Endoscopic, radiographic, and surgical therapies

For patients resistant to diet and drug therapy, endoscopic and surgical treatments may be offered. Endoscopic injection of botulinum toxin into the pylorus reportedly improves gastric emptying and symptoms of gastroparesis, presumably by reducing resistance to outflow into the duodenum. Endoscopic, radiographic, or surgical placement of a gastrostomy tube can provide intermittent decompression if the stomach becomes filled with gas or fluid. Placement of a feeding jejunostomy allows the patient to continue receiving enteral nutrition when food ingestion is precluded by severe nausea and vomiting. In rare cases, home total parenteral nutrition can be given to maintain caloric and fluid sustenance.

Surgical implantation of a gastric neurostimulator using high-frequency, low-energy pulses (not to be confused with "gastric pacing" that employs low-frequency, high-energy pulses) may reduce nausea and vomiting in selected patients with diabetic or idiopathic gastroparesis. Pancreatic transplantation can stabilize the loss of neuronal function in a patient with severe diabetic complications; moreover, symptoms are improved with transplantation. Gastric resections usually are of limited benefit, although total gastrectomy reportedly reduces symptoms specifically in patients with severe gastroparesis caused by prior vagotomy and gastric drainage.

Complications and their management

Complications of gastroparesis include heartburn from delayed gastric acid clearance, hemorrhage secondary to Mallory–Weiss tears or stasis-induced mucosal irritation, and weight loss. Bezoar development may supervene and exacerbate symptoms of fullness and early satiety. In patients with gastroparesis, endoscopy may detect a bezoar. Endoscopic disruption of organized bezoars improves symptoms in some individuals.

Disorders with Rapid Gastric Emptying

Clinical presentation
Abnormally rapid gastric emptying is clinically relevant in only one subset of patients – those who have undergone vagotomy and gastric drainage for ulcer disease or malignancy. The acceleration of liquid emptying overwhelms the postprandial absorptive capabilities of the proximal intestine, leading to fluid shifts and release of vasoactive peptide hormones. The clinical manifestation of this complication is the dumping syndrome. Early dumping syndrome that occurs within 30 min after ingesting a meal is characterized by alimentary symptoms (abdominal pain, diarrhea, gas, bloating, borborygmi, and nausea) and vasomotor symptoms (flushing, palpitations, diaphoresis, light-headedness, tachycardia, and even syncope). Late dumping syndrome occurs 2–3 h after eating and presents with weakness, palpitations, diaphoresis, tremulousness, confusion, and syncope, which are believed to result from hyperinsulinemia due to the large carbohydrate load that precipitates hypoglycemia.

Differential diagnosis

Postsurgical dumping syndrome
Any surgical procedure involving vagotomy may produce the dumping syndrome. In general, the greater degrees of vagal interruption produce more severe symptoms. Characteristically, these operations produce accelerated emptying of liquids with variable effects on solid-phase gastric emptying.

Other causes of rapid emptying
Gastric emptying of fatty liquid meals is accelerated in patients with pancreatic insufficiency and marked steatorrhea. Liquid emptying may be accelerated in some individuals with duodenal ulcer disease. Patients with Zollinger–Ellison syndrome exhibit rapid liquid and solid emptying. Many newly diagnosed diabetics have accelerated rather than delayed gastric emptying. Patients with

hyperthyroidism may have accelerated emptying, as do some morbidly obese individuals. In most instances, these findings of accelerated emptying probably do not cause symptoms and are not clinically important.

Diagnostic investigation

The diagnosis of dumping syndrome is based on eliciting a characteristic constellation of symptoms in a patient who has undergone gastric surgery. Diagnostic testing usually is not necessary. A hematocrit or plasma osmolarity determination in the early postprandial period after a glucose challenge may show hemoconcentration. Measures of packed cell volume and gastric scintigraphy are occasionally obtained, but they rarely provide critical information.

Management and prevention

Dietary management
Dietary recommendations for patients with dumping syndrome include ingesting small, frequent meals of foods high in proteins and fats and low in carbohydrates with minimal fluid intake during the meal. After vagotomy, liquid emptying is more rapid while sitting; thus, some patients may benefit by assuming a supine position immediately after eating. Viscous guar and pectin have been recommended to thicken ingested liquids, but the efficacy of this practice is not proven.

Medication therapy
The somatostatin analog octreotide (50–100 µg subcutaneously 30 min before meals) reduces symptoms of early and late dumping syndrome. The effects of octreotide on gastric emptying are controversial but it clearly blunts exaggerated postprandial hormone release. Although the acute benefits of octreotide on the dumping syndrome are well documented, there is less information on its long-term efficacy. Diarrhea has been reported with long-term use of octreotide in the dumping syndrome. Oleic acid may activate the "jejunal brake" and slow intestinal transit and decrease diarrhea in patients with dumping syndrome.

Surgical therapy
Proposed surgical therapies for the dumping syndrome include Roux-en-Y gastrojejunostomy, constructing an antiperistaltic loop between the stomach and intestine, and retrograde electrical pacing of the small intestine. Efficacy of these procedures is not ensured.

Case studies

Case 1

A 54-year-old woman with type 1 diabetes presents to your office with nausea and vomiting after most meals. She has been prescribed ondansetron and metoclopramide and although initially her symptoms abated, they have returned with full severity. On physical examination, she has normal bowel sounds, no tenderness, but absent proprioception in her toes. Laboratory tests reveal a fasting glucose of 234 and a HbA1C of 10.3. A 4-h solid-phase gastric emptying test is markedly prolonged. You prescribe erythromycin 125 mg three times daily, 30 min before meals, and contact her internist to work with the patient to improve her glucose control. Her symptoms improve for several months but they remit thereafter and she returns to your office. Her HbA1C is now normal. You discontinue the erythromycin and write a prescription for domperidone 20 mg three times daily to be filled by a compounding agency.

Discussion

The diagnosis of diabetic gastroparesis is plausible only when other evidence of neuropathy is present, in this case documented by the loss of proprioception. Erythromycin in low (125–250 mg) doses has been illustrated to improve emptying and symptoms from diabetic gastroparesis. However, tachyphylaxis is common and adjunctive medical therapy is commonly necessary. If this patient were to return with more symptoms, antiemetic therapy would be reasonable for symptom relief. Difficult cases may require placement of a venting gastrostomy and feeding jejunostomy.

Case 2

A 65-year-old man who recently underwent a subtotal gastrectomy with Bilroth II anastomosis for gastric adenocarcinoma complains of increasing light-headedness, weakness and diarrhea shortly after meals. He says that these symptoms do not occur in between meals and he did not have them prior to his surgery. With the exception of a well-healed abdominal incision, his examination is normal. His laboratory tests are notable for a potassium of 3.1 and a BUN and creatinine of 19 mg/dL and 1.6 mg/dL, respectively.

Discussion

The most likely diagnosis in this patient with this constellation of symptoms shortly after gastric surgery is dumping syndrome. The "early dumping" syndrome is believed to be due to loss of gastric receptive relaxation (due to vagotomy), reduced gastric capacity, loss of controlled emptying due to loss of pyloric sphinter, and loss of duodenal feedback inhibition of gastric emptying. No specific diagnostic tests are reliable; therefore clinical recognition is necessary to pursue empirical therapy.

CHAPTER 21

Acid Peptic Disorders

Acid peptic disorders include ulcer disease and gastroesophageal reflux disease, which is discussed in Chapter 18. While the majority of ulcers are caused by nonsteroidal anti-inflammatory drugs (NSAIDs) or infection with *Helicobacter pylori*, cigarette use and stress are also established causes of ulcers.

Causes of acid peptic disease

Helicobacter pylori

Helicobacter pylori is a curved, Gram-negative rod that produces a characteristic highly active urease. Chronic *H. pylori* infection causes most cases of histological gastritis and peptic ulcer disease (PUD) and predisposes to development of gastric carcinoma. Evidence suggests that *H. pylori* is transmitted by fecal–oral routes, although contaminated water also may be a source in some populations. In the United States, the prevalence of *H. pylori* gastritis increases from 10% at age 20 to 50% at age 60; however, this finding is likely to be the result of a birth cohort phenomenon and does not indicate increased acquisition with advancing age. The age-adjusted prevalence rates are higher among Latin-Americans and African-Americans.

Helicobacter pylori colonizes the antrum, body, and fundus of the stomach and is found in 70–95% of patients with active chronic gastritis, which is characterized by histological increases in mucosal neutrophils and round cells. *H. pylori* infection affects 90% of patients with duodenal ulcers and 70–90% of those with gastric ulcers. The etiological role of this organism is supported by numerous studies showing that *H. pylori* eradication prevents ulcer recurrences. The role of *H. pylori* in complicated PUD is less defined since only 50–70% of patients with bleeding duodenal ulcers are infected with *H. pylori*.

Helicobacter pylori is a predisposing factor for developing gastric adenocarcinoma and gastric lymphoma of mucosa-associated lymphoid tissue (MALT); regression

Yamada's Handbook of Gastroenterology, Third Edition. Edited by Tadataka Yamada and John M. Inadomi.
© 2013 John Wiley & Sons, Ltd. Published 2013 by John Wiley & Sons, Ltd.

of this low-grade lymphoma may occur after *H. pylori* is eradicated. Conversely, cancers of the gastric cardia are not associated with *H. pylori* and appear to be more linked to adenocarcinoma of the esophagus.

Nonsteroidal anti-inflammatory drugs

Each year, 2–4% of persons who take NSAIDs develop serious complications, and up to 20,000 deaths per year are attributed to NSAID-related complications. Gastric erosions are diagnosed by endoscopy in 30–50% of patients on chronic NSAID therapy, although these lesions are usually superficial and are not associated with subsequent ulcer development or symptoms. The relative risk of developing gastric ulcer among NSAID users compared to non-NSAID users is 4.0 and for duodenal ulcer is 1.7–3.2. Dyspepsia in patients who take NSAIDs is more common in the first few weeks of therapy and declines with time. Only 26% of patients with dyspepsia have ulcers; conversely, 40% of patients with NSAID-induced ulcers are asymptomatic.

In addition to gastric and duodenal ulcers, complications of NSAID use include dyspepsia; ulceration and strictures of the small intestine; acute colitis; exacerbations of inflammatory bowel disease; and ulcers, strictures, or perforation of the colon.

Additional factors associated with ulcer disease

Tobacco smokers are twice as likely as nonsmokers to develop ulcers. Epidemiological studies in areas affected by natural disaster, such as the 1995 Hanshin-Awaji earthquake in Japan, report a significant rise in the diagnosis of PUD after an event, supporting stress as a factor contributing to ulcer development. In a United States study, emotional stress was associated with a relative risk of 1.4–2.9 for developing ulcers.

Diseases associated with duodenal ulcers

Specific diseases are associated with increases in PUD (Table 21.1). The prevalence of PUD is increased threefold with chronic pulmonary disease, although the role of tobacco smoking in this association is uncertain. Patients with cystic fibrosis have an increased risk of PUD because of reduced bicarbonate secretion. α_1-Antitrypsin deficiency may lead to PUD because of a lack of protease inhibitors. Cirrhosis and renal failure predispose to development of PUD by unknown mechanisms.

Seasonal variations have been reported for PUD development, as have regional and geographic differences. The effect of corticosteroid use on ulcer development, in the absence of NSAID use, is controversial. Ethanol in amounts routinely ingested has no proven ulcerogenic effect on the gastroduodenal mucosa. There are no obvious dietary components that increase the risk of PUD, although foods that induce dyspepsia should be avoided.

Table 21.1 Diseases associated with duodenal ulcers

Evidence strongly supports an association
ZollingerEllison syndrome
Systemic mastocytosis
Multiple endocrine neoplasia type I
Chronic pulmonary disease
Chronic renal failure
Cirrhosis
Kidney stones
α_1-Antitrypsin deficiency

Evidence only suggests an association
Crohn's disease
Hyperparathyroidism without multiple endocrine neoplasia type I
Coronary artery disease
Polycythemia vera
Chronic pancreatitis
Cystic fibrosis

Clinical presentation

Abdominal pain is the most common presenting symptom of PUD. The pain is usually epigastric in location without radiation, burning in quality and relieved by food or antacids. About 10% of patients with PUD, especially with NSAID-related disease, present with complications without a history of ulcer pain. Nausea, vomiting, and weight loss are also common symptoms of PUD.

Essentials of diagnosis and potential pitfalls

NSAID ulcers: among patients who develop NSAID-associated ulcer hemorrhage, 60% have no prior symptoms. Thus, the absence of dyspepsia in NSAID users does not eliminate the possibility of ulcer complications and prophylaxis should be considered in high-risk individuals. The risk of NSAID-associated hemorrhage or perforation is increased among patients with a previous history of complicated or uncomplicated PUD, use of multiple or high-dose NSAIDs, advanced age, and concurrent anticoagulant or steroid use.

H. pylori **ulcers:** the presence of *H. pylori* should be assessed using a test that detects active infection, such as a urea breath test, stool antigen test or endoscopic biopsy. Serological testing is not advised, especially to document eradication after therapy.

Differential diagnosis

The differential diagnosis of suspected peptic ulcer disease includes intra-abdominal and extra-abdominal disorders. The most common diagnosis among patients presenting with chronic epigastric pain is functional dyspepsia. Esophageal diseases such as esophagitis or esophageal dysmotility present with epigastric pain that radiates substernally and to the back, jaw, left shoulder, and arm. Small intestinal disease including inflammatory bowel disease most commonly produces periumbilical pain. Liver capsular distension produces right upper quadrant pain. Gallbladder and bile duct pain is experienced in the epigastrium and right upper quadrant. Pancreatic pain typically is felt in the epigastrium with radiation to the back. Left upper quadrant pain suggests pancreatic disease but may also result from splenic lesions, perinephric disease, and colonic splenic flexure lesions. Cholecystitis may begin in the epigastrium and migrate to the right upper quadrant. Mesenteric ischemia can present with epigastric pain, as can malignancy of the stomach or small intestine. Appendicitis generally causes right lower quadrant abdominal pain but should be considered in any differential diagnosis of abdominal pain.

Nongastrointestinal disease can present with upper abdominal pain. Renal pain from acute pyelonephritis or obstruction of the ureteropelvic junction usually is sensed in the costovertebral angle or flank but upper abdominal pain is not unusual. Pneumonia, especially basilar in location, can present with abdominal pain that is sufficiently severe to prompt exploratory laparotomy.

Diagnostic investigation

Endoscopy
Esophagogastroduodenoscopy (EGD) has emerged as the preferred test because biopsy specimens can be obtained to document the presence of *H. pylori* infection and to exclude malignancy in gastric ulcers. All suggestive gastric ulcers should be examined by repeat upper gastrointestinal endoscopy 8–12 weeks after initiating appropriate therapy. Although gastric ulcers that clearly develop in association with NSAID use do not always need biopsy, they should be observed until healed.

Helicobacter pylori testing
A variety of invasive and noninvasive methods may be used to document *H. pylori* infection. Some tests can document active infection whereas others cannot distinguish current from prior infection.

Invasive tests
Biopsy specimens obtained by endoscopy are examined using Giemsa, Warthin–Starry silver, or hematoxylin-eosin stains, which are the standard for diagnosing *H. pylori*. Biopsy specimens may also be placed in gels containing urea and an indicator (e.g. CLO test, Hpfast, PyloriTek, Pronto Dry) to detect the presence of *H. pylori*-associated urease activity. Urease tests have 90% sensitivity with specificity of 95–100%. Biopsy tests may give false-negative results in patients who are bleeding acutely or who have been given short courses of antibiotics.

Noninvasive tests

Enzyme-linked immunosorbent assays are available for detecting serum immunoglobulin G (IgG) antibodies to *H. pylori*, with sensitivities of 80–95% and specificities of 75–95%. Titers frequently remain elevated after successful eradication; therefore, serological testing is a poor means of assessing active *H. pylori* infection and is not recommended for documenting eradication after therapy. Breath tests may be performed using either ^{13}C-urea (nonradioactive isotope) or ^{14}C-urea (radioactive isotope) labels, which are orally administered. Breath tests have 90–100% sensitivities and specificities for active *H. pylori* infection; however, false-negative results can be produced by intake of proton pump inhibitors (PPIs), bismuth compounds, histamine receptor antagonists, and antibiotics. It is recommended that these drugs be held for 2–4 weeks prior to examination by breath tests. Fecal antigen tests use an enzymatic immuno-assay (HpSA) to detect *H. pylori* antigen in stool specimens with high levels of sensitivity and specificity.

Management and prevention

Most gastric and duodenal ulcers are treated medically with drugs that suppress acid secretion, neutralize gastric acid, have cytoprotective effects, and eradicate *H. pylori*. Endoscopy is indicated for control of hemorrhage and possibly gastric outlet obstruction. Surgery is required for hemorrhage not controlled by endoscopic methods and for other complications such as perforation and obstruction.

Medical therapy for ulcers

Histamine$_2$ receptor antagonists

Histamine$_2$ receptor antagonists inhibit basal, histamine-stimulated, pentagastrin-stimulated, and meal-stimulated acid secretion in a linear, dose-dependent manner with a maximal 90% inhibition of vagal-stimulated and gastrin-stimulated acid production and near-total inhibition of nocturnal and basal secretion. Plasma concentrations of H$_2$ receptor antagonists are affected by renal insufficiency; doses should be halved when creatinine clearance is less than 15–30 mL/min (cimetidine, famotidine) or less than 50 mL/min (nizatidine, ranitidine). Side-effects from these agents are rare but include cardiac rhythm disturbances with intravenous therapy, antiandrogenic effects resulting in gynecomastia and impotence (caused by cimetidine), hyperprolactinemia with galactorrhea, central neural effects (e.g. headache, lethargy, depression, memory loss), and hemato-logical effects (e.g. leukopenia, anemia, thrombocytopenia, and elevations in hepatic aminotransferases). Cimetidine (and less commonly ranitidine) binds to hepatic cytochrome P450 enzymes and strongly inhibits the metabolism of theophylline, phenytoin, lidocaine, quinidine, and warfarin.

Proton pump inhibitors

The PPIs currently available include omeprazole, esomeprazole, lansoprazole, dex-lansoprazole, rabeprazole, and pantoprazole. These substituted benzimidazoles inhibit H^+, K^+-adenosine triphosphatase activity in the gastric parietal cell canalicular membrane, leading to nearly complete inhibition of basal and stimulated acid secretion. PPIs have far greater effects on daytime (meal-stimulated) acid secretion than H_2 receptor antagonists. The optimal time for drug ingestion for most is 30 min to 1 h before meals because PPIs bind only to activated proton pumps, which are maximally stimulated by food. The exception is dexlansoprazole, which is approved for use without regard to timing of dose. PPIs are well tolerated but have been associated with side-effects, including headache, constipation, nausea, abdominal pain, and diarrhea. Various adverse events have also been associated with PPI use, including *Clostridium difficile* infection, pneumonia, bone fracture, and hypomagnesemia; however, the absolute risks of these complications are rare and should not prevent PPI use in appropriate patients. Finally, symptomatic (heartburn) rebound acid hypersecretion has been observed with discontinuation of PPI.

Cytoprotective agents

Sucralfate is a sucrose salt that binds to tissue proteins and forms a protective barrier that decreases exposure of the epithelium to acid, bile salts, and pepsin. Sucralfate may also stabilize gastric mucus and have trophic effects on the mucosa. Adverse effects of sucralfate include constipation and, in renal failure, the possibility of aluminum toxicity. The drug also binds several drugs, limiting their absorption.

Misoprostol is a prostaglandin E_1 analog that inhibits gastric acid secretion, stimulates bicarbonate and mucus secretion, enhances mucosal blood flow, and inhibits cell turnover. The major limitation on its use relates to dose-related diarrhea that occurs in 10–30% of patients. The use of misoprostol is contraindicated in women who may be pregnant.

Treatment of peptic ulcer disease induced by *Helicobacter pylori*

Most peptic ulcers are caused by *H. pylori* infection, and the presence of an *H. pylori*-related duodenal or gastric ulcer is an indication for specific therapy to eradicate the organism. Triple or quadruple therapy with antibiotics and acid suppression is advocated for treating *H. pylori*. Numerous regimens have documented efficacy but a 2-week course of bismuth subsalicylate (two tablets, four times daily), metronidazole (250 mg four times daily), and tetracycline (500 mg four times daily), plus an antisecretory drug (e.g. a PPI), is an inexpensive and effective program that has eradication rates of 80–95%. Alternative strategies include a twice-daily dose PPI with clarithromycin (500 mg twice daily) and a second antibiotic (e.g. amoxicillin 1 g twice daily or metronidazole 500 mg twice daily) for 2 weeks. Shorter courses have been proposed to enhance compliance but the eradication rates decrease significantly if treatment is less than 10 days.

Sequential therapy (amoxicillin 1 g twice daily for 5 days, followed by clarithromycin 500 mg twice daily and tinidazole 500 mg twice daily for 5 days, plus twice-daily dose PPI for the entire 10-day course) has been shown to increase eradication rates. Levofloxacin 250 mg or 500 mg twice daily may be substituted for clarithromycin in the face of clarithromycin resistance.

Essentials of treatment

Urea breath or stool antigen testing should be performed 1 month after completing therapy to document *H. pylori* eradication in patients with complicated ulcer disease, or who had gastric MALT lymphoma or early gastric cancer, or persistent or recurrent symptoms. Testing should be conducted with the patient off acid suppression therapy for at least 1 week. After successful eradication of *H. pylori*, the recurrence rate of gastric and duodenal ulcers is less than 10%. In contrast, PUD recurs within 2 years in 50–100% of patients who remain infected with *H. pylori* in the absence of acid suppression.

Treating and preventing peptic ulcer disease related to nonsteroidal anti-inflammatory drugs

Whenever possible, a patient with an NSAID-induced ulcer should discontinue NSAIDs, in which case antisecretory therapy with H_2 receptor antagonists, PPIs, or cytoprotective agents will generally induce ulcer healing within 8 weeks. If NSAIDs must be continued for their analgesic or anti-inflammatory effects, a number of regimens have demonstrated efficacy. H_2 receptor antagonists in conventional doses may heal duodenal ulcers but gastric ulcers generally are resistant to healing if NSAIDs are continued. In randomized clinical trials, PPIs have effectively healed both duodenal and gastric ulcers in the presence of continued NSAID use (95% rate of healing within 8 weeks). Misoprostol has efficacy equal to PPIs in healing ulcers associated with NSAID use.

Management of refractory ulcers

Duodenal ulcers are considered refractory if 8 weeks of therapy fail to heal the ulcer, while refractory gastric ulcers are defined by lack of response to 12 weeks of treatment. Causes of refractory ulcers include patient noncompliance, surreptitious NSAID use, tobacco use, untreated *H. pylori* infection, gastric acid hypersecretion (gastrinoma), and malignancy. Rare causes of chronic ulceration are Crohn's disease, amyloidosis, sarcoidosis, eosinophilic gastroenteritis, and infections (e.g. tuberculosis, syphilis, and cytomegalovirus). Compliance with prescribed therapy should be evaluated, and any NSAID consumption should be examined. Endoscopic follow-up is indicated with performance of multiple biopsies to exclude malignancy and nonpeptic causes of ulcer. High doses of PPIs can heal 90% of refractory ulcers after 8 weeks, reducing the need for surgical intervention. However, surgery should be considered for diagnosing and treating patients who do not respond to this aggressive regimen.

Table 21.2 Differential diagnosis of hypergastrinemia

Hypochlorhydria and achlorhydria with or without pernicious anemia
Retained gastric antrum
G-cell hyperplasia
Renal insufficiency
Massive resection of the small intestine
Gastric outlet obstruction
Rheumatoid arthritis
Vitiligo
Diabetes mellitus
Pheochromocytoma

Serum gastrin should be measured to exclude Zollinger–Ellison syndrome (ZES), a disorder of acid hypersecretion secondary to a gastrin-secreting tumor or gastrinoma; however, hypergastrinemia has many causes (Table 21.2). A serum gastrin level of more than 1000 pg/mL in a person who demonstrates gastric acid secretion is virtually diagnostic of ZES. Rarely, pernicious anemia, in the setting of achlorhydria, may produce gastrin levels that exceed 1000 pg/mL.

Complications and their management

Complications of PUD include hemorrhage, perforation, penetration, and obstruction. Hemorrhage occurs in 15% of patients with PUD and is most common after age 60, probably because of NSAID use in this age group. Acute hemorrhage is best treated initially with endoscopic hemostasis (hemoclips, thermocoagulation) after adequate resuscitation. Massive hemorrhage not responsive to endoscopic therapy should be referred for interventional radiological therapy (embolization) or surgical therapy.

Perforation occurs in 7% of patients and is increasing in incidence secondary to increased NSAID use. Duodenal ulcers perforate anteriorly and gastric ulcers perforate along the anterior wall of the lesser curvature. Radiation of ulcer pain to the back suggests a posterior penetrating duodenal ulcer. Penetration differs from perforation in that the ulcer erodes into an adjacent organ instead of the peritoneal cavity. Gastric ulcers penetrate into the left lobe of the liver or the colon, causing a gastrocolic fistula, whereas duodenal ulcers penetrate into the pancreas, producing pancreatitis. Inflammation, edema, and scarring near the gastroduodenal junction can cause outlet obstruction, which occurs in 2% of patients with PUD, producing symptoms of heartburn, early satiety, weight loss, abdominal pain, and vomiting. Surgery is generally indicated to treat ulcer perforation. If *H. pylori* is the etiology of the ulcer, eradication of *H. pylori* prevents recurrent ulcers and ulcer complications.

Key practice points

- NSAIDs and *H. pylori* infection cause the majority of gastrointestinal ulcers.

- Upper endoscopy is the preferred method for diagnosing ulcers and their etiology.

- Treatment depends on whether *H. pylori* is detected: *H. pylori*-positive patients should receive triple or quadruple eradication therapy, while patients testing negative should receive acid suppression, usually in the form of proton pump inhibitors.

- *H. pylori* detection using a test that detects active infection is recommended (stool antigen test or urea breath or tissue-based test).

CHAPTER 22
Functional Dyspepsia

Dyspepsia is a symptom characterized by persistent or recurrent upper abdominal pain or discomfort. This discomfort can be accompanied by postprandial fullness, early satiety, nausea, and bloating. Patients with dyspepsia who are evaluated and have no definable structural or biochemical abnormality are classified as having a diagnosis of functional dyspepsia, also known as nonulcer dyspepsia. Functional dyspepsia has been subclassified into different subgroups (ulcer-like, dysmotility-like, and unspecified) based on the dominant symptom (Table 22.1).

Although only a minority of individuals with dyspepsia seek medical care, it is estimated that functional dyspepsia and related functional disorders of the gut account for 2–5% of consultations with family physicians and up to half of all referrals to gastroenterology. Functional dyspepsia is at least twice as common as peptic ulcer disease. Medical attention may be sought because of symptom severity, fear of malignancy, and underlying anxiety or other psychosocial factors.

Clinical presentation

Ulcer-like functional dyspepsia is characterized by episodes of epigastric pain that is relieved by antacids or food, whereas dysmotility-like functional dyspepsia presents with discomfort that is aggravated by food or associated with early satiety, fullness, nausea, retching, vomiting, or bloating (see Table 22.1). Patients with unspecified dyspepsia report symptoms that do not fulfill criteria for ulcer-like or dysmotility-like disease.

Differential diagnosis

In evaluating a patient with unexplained dyspepsia, the clinician should consider stopping medications that may produce dyspepsia, including iron, potassium,

Yamada's Handbook of Gastroenterology, Third Edition. Edited by Tadataka Yamada and John M. Inadomi.

Table 22.1 Rome III criteria for functional dyspepsia

One or more of the following, in the previous 3 months with symptom onset at least 6 months before diagnosis:
Bothersome postprandial fullness
Early satiation
Epigastric pain
Epigastric burning
No evidence of structural disease (including at upper gastrointestinal endoscopy) that is likely to explain the symptoms; *and*
No evidence that dyspepsia is exclusively relieved by defecation or associated with the onset of a change in stool frequency or stool form (i.e. not irritable bowel syndrome)

Dyspepsia subgroups
Ulcer-like dyspepsia: pain centered in the upper abdomen is the predominant (most bothersome) symptom
Dysmotility-like dyspepsia: an unpleasant or troublesome nonpainful sensation (discomfort) centered in the upper abdomen is the predominant symptom; characterized by or associated with fullness, early satiety, bloating, or nausea
Unspecified dyspepsia: symptoms do not fulfill the criteria for ulcer-like or dysmotility-like dyspepsia

digoxin, theophylline, erythromycin, and ampicillin. Other conditions that present with dyspepsia include peptic ulcer disease, gastroesophageal reflux disease, hepatobiliary disease, chronic pancreatitis, malignancies, intestinal angina, infiltrative diseases (e.g. Crohn's disease, sarcoidosis, eosinophilic gastroenteritis, tuberculosis, and syphilis), Ménétrier disease, and abdominal wall pain from muscle strain, nerve entrapment, or myositis.

A diagnosis of functional dyspepsia can be further categorized into several disorders: altered gastric motor function, abnormal gastrointestinal sensory function, and infection or inflammation. In addition, psychological factors must be considered in order to understand the severity of symptoms and impact on quality of life.

Disturbed gastric motor function

Approximately 40% of patients with functional dyspepsia exhibit postprandial antral hypomotility or delayed gastric emptying; however, symptoms and delays in gastric emptying are weakly linked at best. Some patients with functional dyspepsia have an impaired gastric fundus accommodation reflex, which may underlie postprandial discomfort or fullness. Additional rhythm disturbances of the gastric slow wave have been reported with functional dyspepsia.

Disturbed gastric sensory function

Many patients with functional dyspepsia exhibit reduced tolerance to balloon distension of the stomach and duodenum, which is not accompanied by changes in wall compliance. This finding suggests that functional dyspepsia in these individuals stems from exaggerated responsiveness of visceral afferent nerve pathways. The pathogenesis of visceral hypersensitivity in functional dyspepsia is poorly understood. The prevalence of back pain and headache in functional dyspepsia suggests possible abnormalities in cerebral cortical processing of pain information.

Gastric acid, duodenitis, and postinfectious dyspepsia

Acid secretion is normal in most patients with functional dyspepsia. Histological duodenitis is present in 14–83% of individuals with functional dyspepsia and many of these ultimately develop duodenal ulcers. However, erosive duodenitis is more appropriately considered within the spectrum of peptic ulcer disease, rather than functional dyspepsia. *Helicobacter pylori* infection is found in 40% of patients with functional dyspepsia but similar rates are found in matched asymptomatic populations. Furthermore, eradication of *H. pylori* clearly alleviates symptoms in only a subset of patients with functional dyspepsia.

Finally, a small subgroup of patients with functional dyspepsia develops symptoms after a clearly defined acute attack of infectious gastroenteritis.

Psychological factors

Patients with functional dyspepsia are more psychologically distressed than healthy controls and have increased anxiety, depression, neuroticism, and somatization. However, some have suggested that these emotional disturbances may be consequences rather than the cause of dyspeptic symptoms. Acute stress elicits gastric motor responses similar to those observed with functional dyspepsia. As in studies of irritable bowel syndrome, the prevalence of prior physical or sexual abuse is higher in functional dyspepsia.

Diet and environmental factors

Aspirin and nonsteroidal anti-inflammatory drugs cause acute dyspepsia but their roles in chronic dyspepsia are less well established. There is no evidence that smoking tobacco or ingesting ethanol causes functional dyspepsia. Similarly, it is unlikely that food intolerance is a major contributor to the pathogenesis of functional dyspepsia. Coffee stimulates gastric acid production and may elicit dyspeptic symptoms but it is unknown if it acts via gastric irritation or induction of gastroesophageal reflux.

Diagnostic investigation

Patients younger than age 45 without weight loss, bleeding, dysphagia, or recurrent vomiting rarely harbor malignancy. In this population, peptic ulcer disease, gastroesophageal reflux disease, and functional dyspepsia are the most common etiologies of dyspepsia. Therefore, young patients presenting

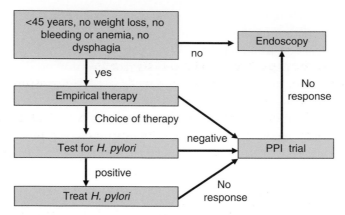

Figure 22.1 Management of uninvestigated dyspepsia. PPI, proton pump inhibitor.

uninvestigated dyspepsia without alarm findings may be initially managed using empirical therapy with an acid-suppressing drug, with consideration of endoscopy if symptoms persist (Figure 22.1). Alternatively, such patients may first undergo *H. pylori* serology, stool antigen, or ^{13}C or ^{14}C urea breath testing. If testing is positive, *H. pylori* should be eradicated. If *H. pylori* is not present, empirical acid-reducing drugs can be administered.

Initial upper gastrointestinal endoscopy is recommended for patients older than age 50, for those with long-standing or recurrent symptoms, and for those with "alarm symptoms," including weight loss, gastrointestinal bleeding, anemia or dysphagia, to assess for the presence of upper gastrointestinal malignancy. For endoscopically documented peptic ulcer disease, gastric biopsies should be obtained for urease testing and histopathology. After appropriate therapy, urea breath or stool antigen testing should be used to confirm *H. pylori* eradication.

Essentials of diagnosis and potential pitfalls

Decision analyses have been conducted to determine the most cost-effective approach to patients with dyspepsia but no one diagnostic approach is consistently favored. The decision to begin with investigation versus empiric therapy (and if the latter, which therapy to initiate first) depends largely on the prevalence of *H. pylori* in the population and the costs of diagnostic testing.

Barium radiography is less useful than endoscopy and abdominal ultrasound has a low yield and is not ordered routinely. Although other tests (ambulatory esophageal pH monitoring, gastric scintigraphic emptying scanning, biliary scanning, lactose tolerance testing) may find abnormalities in up to half of patients, the clinically relevant gain from these additional tests is small.

Management and prevention

Medication therapy for functional dyspepsia

Once a diagnosis of functional dyspepsia is made, confident reassurance by the clinician is essential to manage patients with functional dyspepsia and may obviate the need for medication therapy in many patients. Patients should avoid aggravating medications and foods if possible. Postprandial symptoms may be reduced by eating low-fat meals or more frequent but smaller meals throughout the day.

Essentials of treatment

There is no universally effective medication for treating functional dyspepsia. Many controlled trials in functional dyspepsia have yielded unimpressive results, in part due to the high placebo response rates (30–70%) in this condition.

Meta-analyses illustrate that prokinetic agents, H_2 receptor antagonists, and proton pump inhibitors (PPIs) are more effective than placebo in reducing symptoms. Conversely, there does not appear to be significant benefit with bismuth, sucralfate, or antacids. Of the functional dyspepsia subgroups, PPIs appear to be more effective in relieving symptoms among patients with ulcer-like symptoms.

Prokinetic drugs including cisapride, tegaserod, and domperidone have been shown to improve global symptoms significantly more than placebo; unfortunately, the first two have been removed from the drug market and domperidone has not been approved for use in the US. Metoclopramide is used with benefit in some patients but is associated with concerning adverse events, including extrapyramidal side-effects.

Eradicating *H. pylori* has limited benefits. Although multiple studies illustrate efficacy compared to placebo, eradication cures no more than one of every 15 patients with functional dyspepsia.

Small studies suggest potential efficacy of tricyclic antidepressant drugs such as amitriptyline and the serotonin reuptake inhibitor trazodone. Simethicone may produce improvement if gas retention or aerophagia is present. In one study, the cytoprotective drug sucralfate reduced dyspeptic symptoms. Drugs in the dopamine receptor antagonist and serotonin $5-HT_3$ receptor antagonist classes may decrease associated symptoms of nausea. Limited placebo-controlled trials have reported symptomatic improvements in functional dyspepsia with herbal medicines, such as Iberogast.

Psychological therapies

Small trials have shown the benefits of cognitive behavioral and hypnotherapy in functional dyspepsia. However, studies of psychological treatment have been suboptimal and comparisons with drug therapy have not been performed.

Key practice points

- Dyspepsia is a symptom; functional dyspepsia is a diagnosis that is made after diagnostic investigation establishes no structural etiology to explain symptoms.

- The etiology of functional dyspepsia may vary between patients, and can be attributed to gastroparesis (or other motility disturbances), sensory dysfunction (heightened visceral nociception), inflammation or infection (*H. pylori*), diet, or psychological factors.

- Initial management of dyspepsia may be empirical with either acid suppression (proton pump inhibitor) or *H. pylori* testing (with eradication treatment if positive). Investigation with upper endoscopy may be reserved for patients presenting with alarm features, patients with new symptoms over the age of 50 years of age, or those with persistent or recurrent symtoms after empirical therapy.

- No universally effective medication is available to treat functional dyspepsia.

CHAPTER 23

Tumors of the Stomach

A majority of tumors that occur in the stomach are gastric adenocarcinomas, which is the second most common cause of cancer-related mortality worldwide. Other less common gastric tumors include lymphoma, mesenchymal tumors, and endocrine tumors.

Adenocarcinoma

Clinical presentation

Patients with early gastric cancer generally are asymptomatic. Rather, most individuals present at an advanced stage, usually with nonspecific symptoms such as epigastric pain, early satiety, bloating, nausea, vomiting, and weight loss. Gastrointestinal hemorrhage and gastric outlet obstruction are rarely the initial manifestations of a gastric tumor. The results of the physical examination may be normal or evaluation may reveal occult or gross gastrointestinal blood loss, lymphadenopathy, or hepatomegaly with disease dissemination. A Virchow node indicates metastasis to the left supraclavicular lymph node, whereas a periumbilical nodule (Sister Mary Joseph node) may indicate tumor spread along peritoneal surfaces. An ovarian mass (Krukenberg tumor) or a mass in the cul-de-sac (Blumer shelf) may also be present. Paraneoplastic syndromes, such as acanthosis nigricans, membranous glomerulonephritis, microangiopathic hemolytic anemia, arterial and venous thrombi (Trousseau syndrome), seborrheic dermatitis (Leser–Trélat sign), or dermatomyositis, may also be present.

Yamada's Handbook of Gastroenterology, Third Edition. Edited by Tadataka Yamada and John M. Inadomi.
© 2013 John Wiley & Sons, Ltd. Published 2013 by John Wiley & Sons, Ltd.

Diagnostic investigation

Upper gastrointestinal endoscopy

Suggestive symptoms or findings on physical examination require further evaluation by upper gastrointestinal endoscopy or double-contrast upper gastrointestinal barium radiography. Upper gastrointestinal endoscopy may provide evidence that strongly suggests a neoplasm but endoscopic biopsy is necessary to confirm the diagnosis. The overall sensitivity and specificity of upper gastrointestinal endoscopy with biopsy are 95% and 99%, respectively. Multiple biopsies are necessary to achieve this accuracy. Further, the combined application of brush cytology and then forceps biopsy may improve sensitivity. Biopsy specimens of ulcers are best obtained from the base and the four quadrants of the edge of the ulcer. Because of sampling error, any suggestion of malignancy in the appearance of a gastric ulcer warrants re-evaluation by upper gastrointestinal endoscopy after therapy to confirm healing, and biopsy specimens should be taken of any persistent mucosal defect.

Tumors that appear as thickened gastric folds with normal overlying mucosa are caused by infiltration of the tumor into the submucosa. These cancers can be diagnosed with cautious use of a snare to obtain a biopsy specimen from the submucosa. Light-induced fluorescence endoscopy is an emerging diagnostic technique that relies on the naturally occurring fluorescence (autofluorescence) of tissue after irradiation with blue or violet light to distinguish neoplastic from normal tissue.

Radiographic studies

When performed by an experienced radiologist, upper gastrointestinal radiography detects more than 90% of gastric adenocarcinomas. Characteristic radiographic findings include an asymmetrical ulcer crater, distorted or nodular folds radiating from an ulcer, a lack of distensibility of the stomach, or a polypoid mass. However, radiography does not have the capability of obtaining histological samples and has been largely replaced by endoscopy for diagnosing gastric malignancy.

Staging evaluation

Endoscopic ultrasound (EUS) is ideally suited to the TNM classification for staging gastric cancer because it can accurately assess the depth of tumor penetration. Note, however, that EUS has limited ability to differentiate inflammatory from malignant adenopathy. And because EUS cannot detect the majority of distant metastases, computed tomographic (CT) scanning is required to evaluate the M stage. Magnetic resonance imaging (MRI) shows promise as a tool for excluding metastases but it is not yet superior to CT for staging. Positron emission tomography (PET) appears to be sensitive in detecting gastric neoplasia but poor differentiation between primary and metastatic lesions precludes its use in staging.

Histopathology

The Borrmann classification of gastric adenocarcinoma contains four distinct morphological subgroups, including polypoid, fungating, ulcerated, and diffusely infiltrating or linitis plastica. Early gastric cancer is a term that applies to tumors limited to the mucosa and submucosa. It is most commonly diagnosed during screening of asymptomatic high-risk populations and carries a favorable prognosis. The two best predictors of survival are depth of invasion (T stage) and metastases to lymph nodes (N stage) or distant sites (M stage). A TNM staging system categorizes gastric tumors into four stages that correlate with long-term survival (Table 23.1). Young patients, patients with linitis plastica, and patients with proximal tumors have poor prognoses.

Histologically, gastric cancer can be divided into an intestinal type, characterized by epithelial cells that form glandular structures, and a diffuse type, in which undifferentiated cells proliferate in sheets. The intestinal type is more common in countries where gastric cancer is endemic, whereas the diffuse type is more common in low-risk populations, such as in the United States. The intestinal type is more likely to be associated with intestinal metaplasia and atrophic gastritis and has a more favorable prognosis than the diffuse type. Gastric malignancies rarely exhibit adenomatous and squamous features. The adenosquamous variant has a poor prognosis.

Management and course

See Table 23.2.

Table 23.1 TNM staging of gastric carcinoma

Stage	T Stage	N Stage	M Stage	5-year survival (%)
IA	T1	N0	M0	91
IB	T1	N1	M0	82
	T2	N0	M0	
II	T1	N2	M0	65
	T2	N1	M0	
	T3	N0	M0	
IIIA	T2	N2	M0	49
	T3	N1	M0	
	T4	N0	M0	
IIIB	T3	N2	M0	28
	T4	N1	M0	
IV	T4	N2	M0	5
	Any T	Any N	M1	

Table 23.2 Treatment recommendations for gastric adenocarcinoma

	N0	N1	N2	N3
T1 (mucosa)	EMR or modified gastrectomy	Modified or standard gastrectomy	Standard gastrectomy	
T1 (submucosa)	Modified gastrectomy			
T2	Standard gastrectomy	Standard gastrectomy Adjuvant chemotherapy		Extended or palliative gastrectomy or chemotherapy or radiation or palliative care
T3	Standard gastrectomy Adjuvant chemotherapy			
T4	Extended gastrectomy Adjuvant chemotherapy Radiation		Extended or palliative gastrectomy Chemotherapy or radiation or palliative care	
M1 Recurrent	Extended or palliative gastrectomy Chemotherapy or radiation or palliative care			

Surgical therapy

Complete surgical resection is the only therapy that offers a potential cure for gastric adenocarcinoma but the advanced stage at which more than half of patients present precludes curative surgery. The importance of surgical resection is reflected in the 5-year survival rate of 35–45% of patients with resectable tumors, compared with the 5-year survival rate of less than 5% of patients who undergo palliative resection.

Although surgery is recognized as the best treatment option for gastric cancer, there is little consensus on the optimal curative surgical procedure for gastric adenocarcinoma, especially concerning the extent of lymph node dissection. Adenocarcinomas of the proximal fundus are treated by proximal gastric resection. Tumors of the gastroesophageal junction require *en bloc* resection of the distal esophagus and proximal stomach, often by a combined thoracic and abdominal approach. Splenectomy usually is performed if tumors are located along the greater curvature. The role of resection of isolated hepatic metastases at the time of gastrectomy has not been determined in controlled clinical trials. Palliative surgery may be indicated for obstruction, perforation, or bleeding. Bypass procedures provide significantly shorter periods of palliation compared to resection.

Endoscopic procedures

Endoscopic submucosal dissection (ESD) has been shown to cure early gastric cancer in Japanese populations. Palliative endoscopic therapy may consist of stent placement or Nd:YAG laser tumor ablation, both of which may be used to treat obstruction. Gastrointestinal hemorrhage may be controlled by Nd:YAG laser coagulation necrosis.

Medical therapy

The role of chemotherapy and radiation therapy in treating gastric adenocarcinoma is evolving. Agents shown to decrease tumor mass include 5-fluorouracil, mitomycin C, doxorubicin, cisplatin, and hydroxyurea but there is no evidence of improved survival. Postoperative radiotherapy has likewise not been shown to increase survival.

Key practice points: gastric cancer

- A Virchow node indicates metastasis to the left supraclavicular lymph node.
- A periumbilical nodule (Sister Mary Joseph node) may indicate tumor spread along peritoneal surfaces.
- Gastric cancers are associated with paraneoplastic syndromes, such as acanthosis nigricans, membranous glomerulonephritis, microangiopathic hemolytic anemia, arterial and venous thrombi (Trousseau syndrome), seborrheic dermatitis (Leser–Trélat sign), or dermatomyositis.
- Esophagogastroduodenoscopy (EGD) with biopsy is necessary to confirm the diagnosis.
- EUS provides accurate local and regional staging (T and N stages) but CT scan should be performed to assess for metastatic disease.
- The two best predictors of survival are depth of invasion (T stage) and metastases to lymph nodes (N stage) or distant sites (M stage).

Gastric Lymphoma

Clinical presentation

The presentation of gastric lymphoma is similar to that of gastric adenocarcinoma. Nonspecific symptoms include epigastric pain, weight loss, nausea, vomiting, early satiety, and anorexia. Gastrointestinal hemorrhage and perforation from extensive ulceration are less common manifestations. Physical examination may reveal an abdominal mass or peripheral adenopathy.

Diagnostic investigation

Upper gastrointestinal endoscopy and upper gastrointestinal barium radiography are the primary means for detecting gastric lymphoma; however, the ability to obtain biopsy specimens makes upper gastrointestinal endoscopy the procedure of choice. CT scans are required to determine extragastric involvement. Occasionally, lymphoma appears as a thickened fold on endoscopy and biopsy reveals a submucosal mass with normal overlying mucosa. In this setting, EUS can delineate which layers of the gastric wall are involved, and cytology or biopsy may confirm the diagnosis. Laparotomy may be necessary to define the extent of disease.

Management and course

Gastric lymphoma has a favorable prognosis compared with gastric adenocarcinoma. The 5-year survival rate is 50%. The Ann Arbor staging system for gastric lymphoma is based on the extent of disease which, once established, determines the appropriate course of management (Table 23.3). Patients with stage I tumors limited to the stomach have cure rates higher than 80% and should undergo total gastrectomy or limited gastrectomy with adequate margins. Postoperative chemotherapy and radiation therapy may improve survival of patients with this early-stage disease. Patients with stage II–IV disease are best treated with combination chemotherapy but if bulky transmural stomach tumors are present, prophylactic gastrectomy is often performed to prevent treatment-related perforation. Patients with disseminated non-Hodgkin lymphoma rarely survive for 2 years. Most mucosa-associated lymphoid tissue (MALT) lymphomas are stage I. Early mucosal tumors may respond to antibiotic therapy to eradicate *Helicobacter pylori*, whereas more advanced MALT lymphomas require systemic chemotherapy. MALT lymphomas, in particular, have relatively favorable outcomes.

Key practice points: gastric lymphoma

- EGD should be performed to obtain biopsies to establish the diagnosis of gastric lymphoma. If gastric lymphoma is suspected, a biopsy sample should be sent for flow cytometry analysis.
- CT scans are required to determine extragastric involvement.
- Gastric lymphoma has a favorable prognosis compared with gastric adenocarcinoma.
- Early MALT lymphomas may respond to antibiotic therapy to eradicate *H. pylori*.

Table 23.3 Ann Arbor staging system for gastric lymphoma

Stage	Extent of disease	Relative incidence (%)
I	Limited to stomach	26–38
II	Involvement of abdominal lymph nodes	43–49
III	Involvement of lymph nodes above the diaphragm	13–31
IV	Disseminated disease	–

Gastrointestinal Stromal Cell Tumors

Gastrointestinal stromal cell tumors (GISTs) are mesenchymal neoplasms that are thought to originate from the interstitial cells of Cajal, which is an innervated network of intestinal pacemaker cells. GISTs are composed of a heterogeneous group of neoplasms with predominantly myogenic, neural, or mixed features. Seventy percent of GIST tumors occur in the stomach. The peak incidence occurs in the fifth and sixth decades with equal gender distribution. Symptoms are similar to those of other gastric cancers, although bleeding due to ulceration is more common. Surgical resection is the treatment of choice in patients with tumors >2 cm without evidence of metastasis. High-risk features of GISTs include size >10 cm, any size tumor with >10 mitoses per 50 high-power fields (HPF), tumor >5 cm with a mitosis count >5/50 HPF, or tumor rupture into the peritoneal cavity. Chemotherapy with imatinib should be considered in patients diagnosed with GISTs with high-risk features. No effective therapy exists for advanced metastatic disease. The 5-year survival rate is 28–65% in patients with metastatic GIST.

Metastatic Tumors

Malignant neoplasms from distant sites may metastasize to the stomach. Common sources include melanoma, ovarian, colon, lung, and breast cancer. Tumors may be mucosal or submucosal with associated ulceration. Patients may experience epigastric pain, vomiting, and gastrointestinal hemorrhage.

Miscellaneous Benign and Malignant Gastric Tumors

Gastric polyps

Most gastric polyps are hyperplastic with no malignant potential. They usually are less than 1 cm in diameter and rarely produce symptoms. Some patients with Ménétrier disease (i.e. hypertrophic gastropathy) may have large numbers of fundic hyperplastic polyps. Adenomatous polyps account for 10% of gastric polyps. Their malignant potential dictates removal, followed by a program of endoscopic surveillance to detect recurrence. Patients with familial adenomatous polyposis (FAP) may have fundic gland polyposis. These polyps usually are hamartomatous, although some are adenomatous. Gastric adenomas in patients with FAP have the potential for malignant degeneration, necessitating excision and endoscopic surveillance.

Gastric carcinoids

Only 3% of all carcinoid tumors are located in the stomach. There are three types of gastric carcinoids. The most common is type 1, which is characterized by generally small multiple tumors localized to the fundus and body. Type 1 gastric carcinoids have the lowest metastatic rate of the three types (9–23%). Associated findings include chronic atrophic gastritis, achlorhydria, and pernicious anemia. Type 2 is associated with multiple endocrine neoplasia type I (MEN I) and has an intermediate risk of metastasis. Type 3 is the least common but the most aggressive and most prone to metastasis. Type 3 gastric carcinoids are not associated with a hypergastrinemic state. The tumors are sporadic and generally solitary and large.

Gastric carcinoids are endocrine tumors that produce multiple bioactive substances, including serotonin, histamines, somatostatin, and kinins, but they rarely produce the carcinoid syndrome, which is characterized by flushing, diarrhea, and cardiopulmonary symptoms. Carcinoids usually are submucosal lesions, although they can cause ulceration of the overlying mucosa. Metastatic tumors may require systemic chemotherapy to control tumor bulk. The somatostatin analog octreotide improves symptoms in many patients with the carcinoid syndrome.

Leiomyoma and leiomyosarcoma

Leiomyomas are benign gastric subepithelial masses. They usually cause no symptoms and are often detected incidentally during upper gastrointestinal endoscopy. Leiomyomas rarely undergo malignant transformation to leiomyosarcomas, which account for less than 1% of gastric malignancies. A leiomyosarcoma is a highly vascular tumor that often manifests with massive gastrointestinal hemorrhage. The differentiation of a leiomyoma from a leiomyosarcoma is often problematic and is based on the number of mitotic figures and invasiveness seen on histological examination. The 5-year survival rate of patients is about 50% after resection of a leiomyosarcoma.

Key practice points: miscellaneous gastric tumors

- GISTs are neoplasms with variable malignant potential. High-risk features of GISTs include size >10 cm, any size tumor with >10 mitoses per 50 HPF, tumor >5 cm with a mitosis count >5/50 HPF, or tumor rupture into the peritoneal cavity.

- Malignant neoplasms from distant sites may metastasize to the stomach, including melanoma, ovarian, colon, lung, and breast cancer.

- Gastric adenomas in patients with FAP have the potential for malignant degeneration, necessitating excision and endoscopic surveillance.

Case studies

Case 1

A 67-year-old man presents to his gastroenterologist with complaints of early satiety and 15 lb unintentional weight loss over the past 3 months. Physical exam demonstrates an enlarged left supraclavicular lymph node and mild epigastric tenderness to palpation. Labs are notable for a hematocrit of 32%. Endoscopy demonstrates diffusely abnormal gastric mucosa and the lumen does not expand to air insufflation. When taking biopsies, the mucosa is noted to be friable and firm. Stacked biopsies are obtained due to the suspicion of linitis plastica, as these tumors are known to infiltrate the submucosa and mucosal biopsies can be falsely negative. Histology confirms the diagnosis of gastric carcinoma with poorly differentiated, diffuse type histology. A CT scan is performed that shows evidence of metastatic disease to multiple lymph nodes and to the liver. The patient is diagnosed with stage IV gastric cancer and is referred to an oncologist for consideration of palliative chemotherapy.

Case 2

A 55-year-old man is referred for EGD to evaluate new-onset symptoms of epigastric pain. The patient reports a 2-month history of epigastric pain that has increased in severity over the last 2 weeks. He denies any unintentional weight loss, fevers, night sweats, nausea, or vomiting. Physical examination is unremarkable. EGD is performed demonstrating a 3 cm diameter area of mucosal nodularity in the gastric body. Biopsies is obtained for histology and flow cytometry. Histology is consistent with a lymphoma of MALT type. *Helicobacter pylori* organisms are also identified in the gastric mucosal biopsy specimens. Flow cytometry demonstrates a clonal B-cell population consistent with extranodal marginal zone B-cell lymphoma MALT type. EUS demonstrates the mucosal nodularity to be limited to the mucosal layer without evidence of extension into the submucosa. There are no abnormal perigastric lymph nodes identified. It is determined that the patient has early-stage MALT type lymphoma and he is treated for *H. pylori* eradication. Urea breath test is performed 4 weeks following therapy, which confirms eradication. Repeat EGD is performed at 2 months following eradication therapy demonstrating a decrease in the mucosal nodularity. Repeat biopsies demonstrate residual MALT lymphoma. EGD is repeated at 2-month intervals and eventually demonstrates no evidence of lymphoma at 8 months following eradication therapy.

CHAPTER 24
Celiac Disease

Celiac disease, also known as celiac sprue and gluten-sensitive enteropathy, is characterized by intestinal mucosal damage and malabsorption from dietary intake of wheat, rye, or barley. Symptoms may appear with the introduction of cereal into the diet in the first 3 years of life. A second peak in symptomatic disease occurs in adults during the third or fourth decade, although disease onset as late as the eighth decade has been reported. Serological testing of blood donors indicates that the prevalence of celiac disease is approximately 1 in 250 adults. In Ireland, the prevalence may be as high as 1 in 120. The disorder occurs in Arabs, Hispanics, and Israeli Jews but is rare in individuals with a pure Afro-Caribbean or Chinese background.

Celiac disease results from an interplay of environmental factors, genetic predisposition, and immunological interactions (Table 24.1). The alcohol-soluble gliadin fraction of wheat gluten and similar alcohol-soluble proteins (prolamins) in rye and barley contain the disease-promoting moieties in these grains. The α, β, γ, and ω subfractions of gliadin are toxic to celiac small intestinal mucosa and exacerbate clinical disease.

Jejunal biopsies from celiac disease patients show dense lamina propria lymphocyte and plasma cell infiltrates as well as increased intraepithelial lymphocytes. Patients with untreated celiac disease have high circulating antibody titers to gliadin, reticulin, and endomysium. The antigen for antiendomysial antibody is tissue transglutaminase (tTG). Symptomatic or asymptomatic celiac disease can occur in 10% of first-degree relatives of patients with defined celiac sprue. Three-quarters of identical twins are concordant for the disorder. Celiac sprue is strongly associated with HLA class II D region genes, which may be important determinants of disease susceptibility.

Yamada's Handbook of Gastroenterology, Third Edition. Edited by Tadataka Yamada and John M. Inadomi.
© 2013 John Wiley & Sons, Ltd. Published 2013 by John Wiley & Sons, Ltd.

Table 24.1 Factors and diseases associated with celiac disease

Factor/disease	Incidence
First-degree relative of celiac patient	10%
HLA-DQ2 or HLA-DQ8	99%
IgA deficiency	2.5%
Hyposplenism	100%
Arthritis	26%
Aphthous ulceration	5%
Thyroid disease	6%
Diabetes mellitus	6%
Small intestinal T-cell lymphoma	10%
Dermatitis herpetiformis	Unknown
Other immune diseases	Unknown
Down syndrome	Unknown
Neurological disorders (peripheral neuropathy, ataxia)	Unknown

Clinical presentation

Adult patients with celiac disease often, but not always, have gastrointestinal symptoms, fatigue, weight loss, or pallor when diagnosed. Typically, affected individuals pass 3–4 loose stools daily, which are frothy or difficult to flush, in association with flatulence, loud borborygmi, as well as rare nausea, vomiting, or abdominal pain. Some patients report anorexia, whereas others experience voracious appetites. The magnitude of weight loss depends on the extent (lesions begin proximally in the duodenum), the severity of the intestinal lesion, and the degree to which the patient increases dietary intake. Rare cases of celiac disease present with intestinal pseudo-obstruction. Conversely, some patients are asymptomatic and the diagnosis is considered after detecting unexplained iron deficiency anemia. In children, celiac disease produces failure to thrive, pallor, developmental delay, and short stature, in addition to variable abdominal symptoms. Children with celiac sprue typically present in the first to third years of life. Symptoms often disappear during adolescence but may recur during early adulthood.

Other regions of the gastrointestinal tract may exhibit inflammatory changes in patients with celiac disease. Ten percent of patients also have lymphocytic gastritis. Microscopic colitis represents a cause of unexplained watery diarrhea and is diagnosed on colonic biopsy. When this is diagnosed, coexistent celiac disease should be entertained. Depending on whether a thickened subepithelial collagen band is demonstrated, microscopic colitis may be subclassified as collagenous or lymphocytic colitis.

Patients with celiac disease can present with extraintestinal manifestations (see Table 24.1). Anemia may be secondary to iron or folate malabsorption or, in the case of severe ileal disease, vitamin B_{12} deficiency. Osteopenic bone disease results from calcium and vitamin D malabsorption. Hypocalcemia (and hypomagnesemia) may be associated with tetany and may lead to secondary hyperparathyroidism. Cutaneous bleeding, epistaxis, hematuria, and gastrointestinal hemorrhage may result from vitamin K malabsorption. Neurological manifestations include peripheral sensory neuropathy, patchy demyelination of the spinal cord, and cerebellar atrophy with ataxia. Psychiatric findings include mood changes, irritability, and depression. The cause of the neurological and psychiatric manifestations is unknown; furthermore, these symptoms may not resolve by excluding gluten from the diet. Muscle weakness may result from a proximal myopathy. Vitamin A deficiency may lead to night blindness. Women may experience amenorrhea, delayed menarche, and disturbed fertility. Men may report impotence and infertility. Some patients exhibit hyposplenism, which may increase the risk of bacterial infection. These persons should be given prophylactic antibiotics before invasive procedures or dental work.

A number of immunological conditions are associated with celiac disease (see Table 24.1). The main cutaneous complication is dermatitis herpetiformis, a skin disease with intensely pruritic papulovesicular lesions on the elbows, knees, buttocks, sacrum, face, scalp, neck, and trunk. Approximately 5% of patients with celiac disease report symptomatic dermatitis herpetiformis. Most patients who present initially with dermatitis herpetiformis exhibit celiac sprue-like findings on intestinal biopsy specimens and may respond slowly to a gluten-free diet, although this is not universal. In most patients, a granular or speckled pattern of IgA deposits is noted at the epidermal-dermal junction of uninvolved skin; a linear pattern is less common. Celiac disease exhibits clinical associations with other immune-mediated diseases such as insulin-dependent diabetes mellitus, thyroid disease, IgA deficiency, Sjögren syndrome, systemic lupus erythematosus, mixed cryoglobulinemia, vasculitis, pulmonary disease, pericarditis, mesenteric lymph node cavitation, inflammatory bowel disease, neurological disorders, ocular abnormalities, IgA mesangial nephropathy, primary sclerosing cholangitis, and primary biliary cirrhosis. Other skin diseases found in patients with celiac sprue include psoriasis, eczema, pustular dermatitis, cutaneous amyloid, cutaneous vasculitis, nodular prurigo, and mycosis fungoides.

Physical findings depend on disease severity. Patients with mild disease exhibit no abnormal physical symptoms. In more severe disease, emaciation, clubbed nails, dependent edema, ascites, ecchymoses, pallor, cheilosis, glossitis, decreased peripheral sensation, and a positive Chvostek or Trousseau sign may be detected. Hyperkeratosis follicularis may result from vitamin A deficiency. The abdomen may be distended and tympanitic and have a doughy consistency.

Diagnostic investigation

Screening blood tests for celiac disease may detect anemia (microcytic resulting from iron deficiency or macrocytic resulting from folate or vitamin B_{12} deficiency), hypocalcemia, hypophosphatemia, hypomagnesemia, metabolic acidosis, hypo-albuminemia, hypoglobulinemia, low serum vitamin A levels, prolonged prothrombin time, and an elevated serum alkaline phosphatase level. Fecal fat levels may be increased on qualitative (i.e. Sudan stain) or quantitative assessment. Patients with celiac disease may have flat glucose tolerance test results.

Antibody testing

If celiac disease is a diagnostic consideration in a patient with unexplained gastrointestinal symptoms, serological antibody tests are informative but do not replace the need for small intestinal biopsy. The sensitivity and specificity of IgA antigliadin antibodies are 83% and 82%, respectively, calling into question their role in the diagnosis of celiac disease. More recently developed antibody tests provide more reliable screens for celiac disease. Antiendomysial antibodies have a sensitivity and specificity for disease detection of 90% and 99%, whereas tTG serological testing is 93% sensitive and 95% specific. Of patients with celiac disease, 2–3% have selective IgA deficiency, which may produce false-negative tests in antigliadin, antiendomysial, and anti-tTG antibody testing. Some clinicians obtain IgG titers of the same antibodies or measure serum IgA levels to exclude this possibility. A suggested algorithm for the evaluation of suspected celiac disease is shown in Figure 24.1.

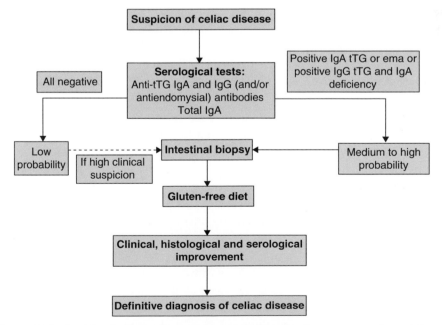

Figure 24.1 Algorithm for the evaluation of a patient for celiac disease. ema, endomysial antibody; tTG, tissue transglutaminase. (Source: Yamada T et al. (eds) *Textbook of Gastroenterology*, 5th edn. Oxford: Blackwell Publishing Ltd, 2009.)

Clinical indications for serological testing

- Chronic diarrhea with and without malabsorption
- Irritable bowel syndrome
- Unexplained weight loss
- Iron deficiency anemia
- Folate deficiency
- Vitamin E or K deficiency
- Osteoporosis
- Hypocalcemia or vitamin D deficiency, secondary hyperparathyroidism, persistently low urinary calcium excretion
- Unexplained elevation of transaminases
- First-degree relatives of patients with celiac disease
- Associated autoimmune diseases: type 1 diabetes, Sjögren syndrome, primary biliary cirrhosis
- Down and Turner syndromes
- Neurological disorders: unexplained peripheral neuropathy, epilepsy, and ataxia

---

Histology of the small intestine

To confirm the diagnosis of celiac disease, biopsy of the small intestinal mucosa is mandatory. With active disease, the endoscopic appearance of the duodenal mucosa is a loss of normal folds with scalloping. Different grades of enteropathy can be graded on microscopic examination.

Grade 0, or preinfiltrative, histology appears normal but can produce antibody to gluten and endomysium, is found in some cases of dermatitis herpetiformis, and characterizes latent disease. Grade 1 is an infiltrative lesion with increased epithelial lymphocytes but no villous atrophy; it usually does not produce gastrointestinal symptoms. Grade 2 is similar to grade 1 but the crypts are hypertrophic. The destructive grade 3 lesion is characterized by the typical flat mucosa of untreated celiac disease. With this finding, the total thickness of the mucosa is increased by crypt hyperplasia and lamina propria infiltration by plasma cells and lymphocytes. Epithelial cells lose their columnar appearance and become pseudostratified. Subtotal villous atrophy may be observed in milder disease or in disease that has been treated with a gluten-restricted diet. The grade 4 lesion is a hypoplastic histology that is not responsive to a gluten-free diet and is associated with nonneoplastic and neoplastic complications of celiac disease.

Other infectious or inflammatory diseases produce histological findings similar to celiac disease, including giardiasis, tropical sprue, collagenous sprue, HIV enteropathy, tuberculosis, radiation enteritis, Whipple disease, lymphoma and Crohn's disease. Thus, a presumptive diagnosis of celiac disease should be supported by the response to a gluten-free diet.

Findings of imaging studies

In 85% of celiac disease patients, barium radiography of the small intestine exhibits the loss of the fine, feathery mucosal pattern with thin mucosal folds. Additional findings in some individuals include straightening of the valvulae conniventes, thickened mucosal folds, lumenal dilation, and flocculation of contrast. Such radiographic exams are most important in excluding ulcerative and neoplastic complications of celiac disease. Abdominal computed tomography and magnetic resonance imaging may detect hyposplenism and abdominal lymphadenopathy in some patients. The bone density of patients with celiac disease is measured to exclude osteopenia.

Essentials of diagnosis of celiac disease

- Maintain a high index of suspicion for celiac disease.
- Serological testing for tissue transglutaminase and/or endomysial antibiodies.
- Biopsy of the small intestine is the gold standard for the diagnosis of celiac disease.
- Because other conditions can have a similar histological appearance to celiac disease, documenting normal villous histology on a gluten-free diet is recommended.

Potential pitfalls in the diagnosis of celiac disease

- Early histological changes (i.e. Marsh I: normal villous architecture with intraepithelial lymphocytosis) are not specific for celiac disease. Other causes include giardiasis, tropical sprue, eosinophilic gastroenterology, HIV enteropathy, radiation enteritis, Crohn's disease and many others.
- Selective IgA deficiency occurs more commonly in patients with celiac disease. Since the most sensitive serological tests for celiac disease are based upon the use of IgA isotypes, total IgA levels should also be assessed.
- Though the the sensitivity of the IgA anti-tTG assay is greater than 90%, it is not as specific as the IgA endomysial antibody.
- Over- and underinterpretation of villous atrophy on small bowel biopsies can result from poorly oriented biopsy specimens.
- Histological findings may be milder than expected due to gluten restriction in the diet and use of immunosuppressant medications.

Management

The mainstay for treating celiac sprue is the initiation of a gluten-free diet. Commitment to this diet is lifelong. It requires completely eliminating wheat (including triticale, spelt, and semolina), rye, and barley products from the diet. Corn, rice, sorghum, buckwheat, and millet do not activate the disease. While oats have traditionally been excluded from a gluten-free diet, multiple studies have demonstrated that most patients with celiac disease tolerate oats. Gluten is not present in distilled liquor so whisky and other spirits are well tolerated. However, barley-containing beer and ale should be avoided. Because of the loss of brush border lactase activity, dairy products should initially be avoided but these substances can be reintroduced after symptoms improve on a gluten-restricted diet. Symptomatic improvement with these dietary recommendations may be reported as soon as 48h after they are initiated. Recovery of normal intestinal histological features often takes much longer (i.e. months), and abnormalities persist in 50% of patients despite strict adherence to the diet. The distal intestinal mucosa heals more rapidly than the proximal mucosa.

Supplemental iron or folate (and rarely vitamin B_{12}) may be needed to treat anemia early in therapy. Vitamin K may be required to treat a coagulation deficit. Osteopenic bone disease is treated with calcium and vitamin D replacement or bisphosphonate therapy. Corticosteroid therapy should be reserved for patients unresponsive to dietary gluten restriction or for patients with complications. Azathioprine or 6-mercaptopurine can be used as steroid-sparing agents, if needed. Cyclosporine and infliximab are used as second-line therapies for refractory sprue.

Complications and their management

Enteropathy-associated T-cell lymphoma of the small intestine may complicate long-standing celiac disease and is often multifocal and diffuse. Diagnosing lymphoma may be difficult because of the insidious onset of symptoms in many patients. Carcinoma of the small intestine as well as of the mouth, pharynx, and esophagus is more common in patients with celiac disease than in the normal population. Evidence strongly suggests that adherence to a gluten-free diet reduces the subsequent incidence of malignancy. Chronic ulcerative jejunoileitis is characterized by multiple ulcers and strictures of the small intestine and presents with anemia, hemorrhage, perforation, or stricture. Patients with celiac disease who have this complication often are refractory to gluten restriction and are further predisposed to developing lymphoma. Other causes of refractoriness to dietary therapy include refractory sprue and collagenous sprue in which a thick band of collagen-like material is deposited under the intestinal epithelial cells. Some patients with refractory sprue have circulating antienterocyte antibodies. Although many refractory patients respond to corticosteroids or other immunosuppressive drugs, some individuals require permanent parenteral hyperalimentation to maintain adequate nutrition and hydration.

CHAPTER 25

Short Bowel Syndrome

Short bowel syndrome refers to the symptoms and pathological disorders associated with a malabsorptive state resulting from surgical resection, congenital defect or disease-associated loss of absorption from a substantial portion of small or large intestine. Parenteral nutrition is usually required if less than 40 cm of small intestine in children or less than 150 cm in adults is conserved. The consequences of small bowel resection are variable but in general relate to the extent of resection, the site of resection, and subsequent adaptive processes.

Clinical presentation

The clinical presentation of short bowel syndrome is divided into three phases: early (1–2 weeks after surgery), intermediate, and late. Watery diarrhea characterizes the the *early* (postoperative) phase, resulting in dehydration and electrolyte deficiencies (hyponatremia, hypokalemia, hypocalcemia, and hypomagnesemia). An *intermediate* phase of up to 1 year follows during which intestinal adaptation occurs. Although oral feedings may be initiated, enteral or parenteral supplements may still be needed to treat malabsorption, weight loss, and malnutrition. During the *late* phase after maximal intestinal adaptation has been achieved, weight often stabilizes and normal oral intake may be possible. However, some patients never reach a stage where they can supply all needs orally, and home parenteral nutrition may be needed.

Diarrhea results from a reduction in the absorptive surface area, decreased transit time, increased osmolality of the lumenal contents (as a result of carbohydrate malabsorption), bacterial overgrowth, and fluid hypersecretion from the stomach, small and large intestine.

After surgery, fluid losses may exceed 5 L per day, especially with concomitant colectomy. Gastric hypersecretion evokes intestinal mucosal damage, impaired micelle formation, and inhibition of pancreatic enzyme function. Nutritional

Yamada's Handbook of Gastroenterology, Third Edition. Edited by Tadataka Yamada and John M. Inadomi.

deficiencies produce weight loss, weakness, fatigue, and growth retardation (in children). Consequences of fatty acid malabsorption include tetany, osteomalacia, and osteoporosis secondary to hypocalcemia and hypomagnesemia. Depletion of the bile salt pool with ileal resection contributes to steatorrhea. Undigested and unabsorbed carbohydrates may be metabolized by colonic bacteria to short-chain fatty acids that cause diarrhea by osmotic and secretory effects. Proteins also are metabolized by colonic flora and contribute to osmotic diarrhea to a lesser degree. Zinc deficiency, which may impair intestinal adaptation, is common, as is fat-soluble vitamin deficiency and vitamin B_{12} deficiency. However, other water-soluble vitamins and trace metals are generally well absorbed even if the resection is extensive.

Potential pitfalls

Short bowel syndrome presents with a variety of symptoms that may require individualized therapy. Diarrhea is universal and multifactorial. Fat malabsorption (steatorrhea) and carbohydrate malabsorption induce an osmotic diarrhea, while hypersecretion of gastric fluid secondary to hypergastrinemia contributes to a secretory diarrhea. Mineral deficiencies often complicate short bowel syndrome, and vitamin B_{12} is especially common after ileal resection; however, other water-soluble vitamins are absorbed throughout the small intestine and deficiencies are not typical. Similarly, protein absorption is generally preserved.

Differential diagnosis

Causes of short bowel syndrome

The most common disorders in adults that lead to massive resection of the small intestine are vascular insults and Crohn's disease (Table 25.1). Risk factors for vascular disease include advanced age, congestive heart failure, atherosclerotic and valvular heart disease, chronic diuretic use, hypercoagulable states, and oral contraceptive use. Less common adult causes include jejunoileal bypass, abdominal trauma, neoplasm, radiation enteropathy, and gastrocolic fistulae. Pediatric causes of short bowel syndrome are intestinal atresia, midgut or segmental volvulus, abdominal wall defects, necrotizing enterocolitis, Hirschsprung disease, hypercoagulable states, cardiac valvular vegetations, Crohn's disease, and abdominal trauma.

Factors that influence absorption after intestinal resection

The amount of small intestine that remains after resection determines the transit time as well as the surface area available for nutrient, fluid, and electrolyte absorption. Approximately 50% of the small intestine can be resected without significant nutritional sequelae but resections of 75% or more almost invariably produce severe malabsorption that requires enteral or parenteral replacement therapy. Long-term survival has been reported with only 15–48 cm of residual jejunum in addition to the duodenum.

Table 25.1 Causes of short bowel syndrome

Adult causes	Pediatric causes
Intestinal vascular insults	Prenatal causes
Superior mesenteric artery embolus or thrombosis	Vascular accidents
Superior mesenteric vein thrombosis	Intestinal atresia
Volvulus of the small intestine	Midgut or segmental volvulus
Strangulated hernia	Abdominal wall defect
Postsurgical causes	Postnatal causes
Jejunoileal bypass	Necrotizing enterocolitis
Abdominal trauma with resultant resection	Trauma
Inadvertent gastroileal anastomosis for peptic ulcer disease	Inflammatory bowel disease
Miscellaneous	Midgut segmental volvulus
Crohn's disease	Hirschsprung disease
Radiation enteritis	Radiation enteritis
Neoplasms	Venous thrombosis
	Arterial embolus or thrombosis

Resection of different small intestinal regions produces distinct consequences. Removal of the jejunum causes only limited defects in macronutrient, electrolyte, and water absorption. Jejunal resection reduces secretion of mucosal hormones that leads to gastric hypersecretion and pancreatic insufficiency. Removal of more than 100 cm of ileum usually precludes bile acid absorption and leads to bile salt-induced secretory diarrhea. The body compensates for this loss by increasing bile acid synthesis up to eightfold. Steatorrhea also results from loss of long ileal segments. The ileum is the primary site for vitamin B_{12} absorption. Malabsorption of vitamin B_{12} occurs with resection of as little as 60 cm. Because ileal nutrients regulate gastric emptying and small bowel transit, ileal resection may shorten intestinal transit times, magnifying the absorptive defect. A combined resection of the small intestine and colon usually increases dehydration and sodium and potassium depletion compared with a resection of the small intestine alone. Preservation of at least 50% of the colon reduces morbidity and mortality after massive small intestinal resection. Removal of the ileocecal junction accelerates small intestinal transit and increases bacterial colonization of the residual intestine, producing bile salt deconjugation, fat and fat-soluble vitamin malabsorption, vitamin B_{12} malabsorption, and bile salt diarrhea.

In human biopsy specimens, mucosal hyperplasia has been demonstrated after small bowel resection. Increased ileal absorption of glucose, maltose, sucrose, bile acids, vitamin B_{12}, and calcium after proximal resection has been documented in animals, as has increased activity of the enzymes involved in DNA and pyrimidine synthesis. In humans, there is a gradual improvement in the absorption of fat, nitrogen, and carbohydrate after extensive resection of the small intestine. The colon also undergoes adaptive dilation, lengthening, and mucosal proliferation and acquires the ability to absorb glucose and amino acids to a limited degree. Enteral nutrients elicit intestinal adaptation by direct effects on epithelial cells and by stimulating trophic gastrointestinal and pancreatico-biliary hormone secretion. Disaccharides are more potent stimulants of adaptation than monosaccharides, whereas highly saturated fats are more effective than those that are less saturated. Hormones that may have relevant trophic effects include gastrin, cholecystokinin, enteroglucagon, and neurotensin. Growth factors such as epithelial growth factor and insulin-like growth factor 1, prostaglandins, glutamine, arginine, short-chain fatty acids, and polyamines such as putrescine, spermidine, and spermine also may participate in the adaptation process. Conversely, intestinal hypoplasia may result from complete reliance on parenteral nutrition.

Diagnostic investigation

Laboratory testing

Laboratory abnormalities relate to the severity of nutrient, vitamin, and mineral deficiencies. Electrolyte determinations may reveal hyponatremia, hypokalemia, hypocalcemia, and hypomagnesemia, whereas a complete blood count may show anemia caused by vitamin B_{12} deficiency or, less commonly, folate and iron deficiencies. Fat-soluble vitamin deficiencies (i.e. A, D, E, and rarely K) may be evident. Urine oxalate levels may be elevated in patients predisposed to oxalate calculi. Fecal analysis reveals elevated fat levels. Bacterial overgrowth is diagnosed by quantitative culture of intestinal fluid obtained endoscopically or from a fluoroscopically placed aspiration catheter. Hydrogen breath testing is less reliable because of rapid transit of the substrate into the colon.

Radiographic studies

Small intestinal barium radiography can be performed if the length of residual bowel is uncertain. Bone radiography and bone densitometry can be used to assess for osteomalacia and osteoporosis in a patient with calcium and vitamin D malabsorption. Ultrasound may be of value in detecting gallstones. Computed tomography, intravenous pyelography, or renal ultrasound may detect renal calculi.

Management and prevention

Medical therapy

Controlling diarrhea and malnutrition is a major goal of treating a patient with short bowel syndrome. Opiate agents, the most effective antidiarrheal agents for this condition, act by delaying transit in the small intestine and increasing intestinal capacity. Loperamide may be effective in some cases but many patients require more potent opiates such as codeine or tincture of opium to control symptoms. In patients with limited ileal resection, cholestyramine may be effective for treating bile salt diarrhea. Subcutaneous octreotide reduces fluid and electrolyte losses in some patients with short bowel syndrome as a result of retarded propulsion, decreased digestive juice secretion, and altered mucosal fluid and electrolyte transport. Proton pump inhibitors may reduce gastric hypersecretion, minimizing ulcer complications and inhibiting the gastric secretory contribution to diarrhea. Oral broad-spectrum antibiotics are warranted if intestinal bacterial overgrowth is suspected. Pancreatic enzyme supplements are given to patients with proximal intestinal resections because of the loss of cholecystokinin and secretin release and to those with severe protein-calorie malnutrition.

Nutritional therapy

During the initial postoperative phase, total parenteral nutrition is required to prevent diarrhea, dehydration, and fluid and electrolyte losses. Over time, many patients can be slowly weaned from intravenous feedings. If more than 25% of the intestine remains, it should be possible to stop parenteral nutrition eventually. The length of remaining small intestine, preservation of the colon, and ileocolonic anastomosis predict the ability to wean from intravenous hyperalimentation. Patients who receive long-term parenteral nutrition at home require a permanent intravenous catheter that must be placed surgically.

Limited oral intake to stimulate intestinal adaptation should be resumed when stool output is less than 2 L per day. A liquid solution that contains an isotonic sodium and glucose mixture takes advantage of the small intestinal sodium/glucose cotransport carrier to enhance fluid absorption. For patients with more than 60–80 cm of remaining small intestine, consumption of dry solids can be started slowly. Foods low in lactose content may be needed to limit diarrhea. If oxalate stones are a concern, administering oral calcium or cholestyramine may reduce dietary oxalate absorption. Fat content may need to be limited in a patient with an intact colon because colonic bacterial fat metabolites such as hydroxyl fatty acids promote secretory diarrhea. Medium-chain triglycerides can be used as nutritional supplements because they are absorbed directly from the proximal intestine into the portal circulation in the absence of bile salts. However, medium-chain triglycerides are unpalatable, may induce diarrhea, and do not provide essential fatty acids. The role of fiber supplements is controversial. In some patients, oral conjugated bile acids may improve fat absorption.

Patients who cannot tolerate oral feedings and those with less than 60–80 cm of remaining small intestine may benefit from enteral feedings. Elemental or semi-elemental formulas are recommended initially because they require minimal absorptive surface area. These formulas contain sucrose or glucose polymers, easily digested proteins, or free amino acids or short peptides, vitamins and minerals, and minimal amounts of fat. Because of their poor taste and their propensity to induce osmotic diarrhea, these formulas are often administered by slow infusion through a nasogastric or nasoenteric tube. Polymeric formulations provide 30% of calories as fat and contain intact protein sources. These solutions are more palatable and can be introduced when adaptation has progressed.

In general, vitamin and mineral supplements are included in oral feedings and enteral and parenteral solutions. Liquid solutions should be given because the hard matrix of solid pills may not dissolve during rapid transit through the shortened small intestine. Multivitamin preparations that contain 2–5 times the recommended dietary allowances are advocated. Patients with ileal resections of more than 90 cm should receive intramuscular vitamin B_{12}. Serum retinol, calcium, 25-hydroxyvitamin D, and urinary calcium are monitored to assess the adequacy of vitamin A and D supplementation. Calcium intake of 1000–1500 mg per day is encouraged. Symptomatic hypomagnesemia may mandate intravenous magnesium replacement because oral magnesium supplements worsen diarrhea. Iron and zinc deficiency can develop, requiring specific supplementation. Deficiencies of other minerals usually are averted by multivitamins.

Key practice points

Nutrional management of short bowel syndrome evolves over the course of the disease state. One of four long-term outcomes will emerge, depending on the length of intestinal resection and the degree of postsurgical adapation:

- maintenance of a balanced nutritional status using an oral diet (normal or modified)
- requirement for defined enteral formula diet
- requirement for parenteral electrolyte and fluid supplementation
- necessity of total or partial parenteral nutritional intake supplemented by variable amounts of enteral intake.

Surgical therapy

A variety of surgical procedures may benefit selected patients with short bowel syndrome. Antiperistaltic segments that retard intestinal transit can increase water, fat, and nitrogen absorption in 70% of patients. Interposition of colonic segments into the shortened small intestine also has been tried to slow propulsion. Tapering enteroplasty may improve intestinal function in patients with short bowel syndrome who have had a dilated small intestine.

Small intestinal transplantation has become a life-saving treatment for patients with irreversible intestinal failure who cannot be maintained on parenteral nutrition because of liver disease, recurrent sepsis, or loss of venous access. Contraindications to intestinal transplant include profound neurological difficulty, life-threatening illness, and multiple system immune disease. Transplantation should be considered prior to development of parenteral nutrition-associated cirrhosis because combined liver-intestine transplants have higher mortality rates than intestinal transplantation alone. One-year survival rates after intestinal transplantation range from 66% to 75%, depending on the need for other grafts or transplanted organs. Causes of death after intestinal transplant include sepsis, lymphoproliferative disease, nontransplant organ failure, thrombosis, ischemia, bleeding, and graft rejection.

Complications and their management

Short bowel syndrome has significant systemic sequelae. Calcium oxalate renal calculi develop because of increased colonic absorption of dietary oxalate, decreased urinary concentrations of phosphate and citrate, and reduced urinary volume. The incidence of gallstones is increased twofold to threefold by ileal resection. This phenomenon has been attributed to bile salt malabsorption, which secondarily causes cholesterol supersaturation of gallbladder bile. However, calcium-containing cholesterol stones and pigment stones are also prevalent after small bowel resection, indicating that other mechanisms are involved.

Intrahepatic steatosis and hepatic dysfunction occur secondary to parenteral nutrition and sepsis, and may lead to liver failure, especially in children.

CHAPTER 26

Tumors and Other Neoplastic Diseases of the Small Intestine

Tumors of the small intestine account for less than 2% of all gastrointestinal malignancies. Primary cancers of the small intestine include adenocarcinomas, carcinoids, lymphomas, sarcomas, and leiomyosarcomas; however, benign neoplasms such as adenomas, leiomyomas, lipomas, and hamartomas are more common (Table 26.1).

Adenocarcinoma

Clinical presentation

Eighty-five percent of patients with small intestinal adenocarcinomas present after age 50. Symptoms may include abdominal pain, nausea, vomiting, and weight loss. Occult blood loss with anemia may be present. Ileal tumors may cause intussusception, and periampullary tumors (i.e. tumors of the ampulla of Vater) may cause gastric outlet obstruction, biliary obstruction with jaundice, or pancreatitis. Patients with celiac sprue may present with new-onset weight loss and abdominal pain after years of quiescent disease. Similarly, patients with Crohn's disease exhibit symptoms of obstruction that may mistakenly be attributed to a flare of their underlying disease.

The physical examination of patients with adenomas and adenocarcinomas of the small intestine is often normal. A minority of patients have abdominal distension, abdominal masses, gastric outlet obstructions, or evidence of fecal occult blood loss.

Diagnostic investigation

Upper gastrointestinal endoscopy using both forward-viewing and side-viewing endoscopes may be necessary to diagnose small intestinal adenocarcinoma. Most

Yamada's Handbook of Gastroenterology, Third Edition. Edited by Tadataka Yamada and John M. Inadomi.

Table 26.1 Classification of tumors of the small intestine

Benign epithelial tumors
Adenoma
Hamartomas (Peutz–Jeghers syndrome, Cronkite–Canada syndrome, juvenile polyposis, Cowden disease, Bannayan–Riley–Ruvalcaba syndrome)

Malignant epithelial tumors
Primary adenocarcinoma
Metastatic carcinoma
Carcinoid tumors

Lymphoproliferative disorders
B-cell
  Diffuse large cell lymphoma
  Small, noncleaved cell lymphoma
  Mucosa-associated lymphoid tissue (MALT) lymphoma
  Mantle cell lymphoma (multiple lymphomatous polyposis)
  Immunoproliferative small intestinal disease (IPSID)
T-cell
  Enteropathy-associated T-cell lymphoma

Mesenchymal tumors
Gastrointestinal stromal cell tumors (GISTs)
Fatty tumors (lipoma, liposarcoma)
Neural tumors (schwannomas, neurofibromas, ganglioneuromas)
Paragangliomas
Smooth muscle tumors (leiomyoma, leiomyosarcoma)
Vascular tumors (hemangioma, angiosarcoma, lymphangioma, Kaposi sarcoma)

Table 26.2 Distribution of malignant tumors of the small intestine

Tumor	Duodenum (%)	Jejunum (%)	Ileum (%)
Primary adenocarcinoma	40	38	22
Malignant carcinoid	18	4	78
Primary lymphoma	6	36	58
Leiomyosarcoma	3	53	44

adenomas in patients with familial adenomatous polyposis (FAP) are located in the proximal duodenum and periampullary region, whereas up to half of sporadic carcinomas occur in the jejunum and ileum (Table 26.2). Lesions in the proximal or middle jejunum can be identified and biopsy specimens obtained with enteroscopy. Wireless capsule endoscopy of the small intestine may be useful for visualizing tumors that are too small to detect by radiographic techniques if clinical suspicion remains elevated despite normal radiographic studies.

Computed tomographic (CT) scans are helpful in staging tumors of the small intestine by identifying lymph node and hepatic metastases.

Management and course

Surgical resection is the treatment of choice for adenocarcinoma of the small intestine. Tumors in the jejunum and proximal ileum are treated with segmental resection. A right hemicolectomy is required to treat adenocarcinoma of the distal ileum. Lesions that involve the ampulla of Vater require pancreaticoduodenectomy (i.e. the Whipple procedure). The long-term survival for primary small bowel adenocarcinoma is 47.6% (local disease), 33% (regional disease), and 3.9% (distal disease). Neither chemotherapy nor radiation therapy is effective for small bowel adenocarcinoma.

Key practice point: small bowel adenocarcinoma

Most adenomas in patients with FAP are located in the proximal duodenum and periampullary region, whereas up to half of sporadic carcinomas occur in the jejunum and ileum.

Carcinoids

Clinical presentation

The most common clinical presentation of a symptomatic carcinoid tumor of the small intestine is intermittent abdominal pain. Additional complications include intestinal ischemia, intussusception, and gastrointestinal hemorrhage.

The carcinoid syndrome affects 10–18% of patients with small bowel carcinoids. Although localized foregut carcinoids may produce the carcinoid syndrome, carcinoids of the small intestine cause this syndrome only after hepatic metastasis. The characteristic symptoms of the carcinoid syndrome are flushing of the face and neck and intermittent watery diarrhea. Less common symptoms include bronchospasm and right-sided heart failure. Patients with carcinoid syndrome may experience a hypotensive crisis during the induction of general anesthesia.

Diagnostic investigation

Laboratory testing

Measuring the urinary excretion of 5-hydroxyindoleacetic acid (5-HIAA), the major metabolite of serotonin, is a sensitive and specific test for the carcinoid syndrome, but it is less accurate for detecting localized carcinoids. Excretion of more than 30 mg of 5-HIAA in a 24-h urine sample after provocative testing is diagnostic of the carcinoid syndrome. False-positive tests may be caused by celiac disease, Whipple disease, tropical sprue, and ingesting food rich in serotonin (e.g. walnuts, bananas, and avocados). Elevation of chromogranin A can also be used for diagnosing carcinoid tumors, as well as for monitoring treatment response or recurrence. The measurement of neuron-specific enolase levels has also been used, but it is a less accurate diagnostic test for carcinoid tumors than the measurement of chromogranin A.

Imaging studies

Because most carcinoids occur in the ileum, upper gastrointestinal endoscopy and colonoscopy have limited roles in identifying these tumors. Most symptomatic lesions are visible in barium radiographs of the small intestine. The desmoplastic distortion of the mesentery may be evident as kinking and tethering of the intestine. A CT scan is also helpful in demonstrating these mesenteric changes; it is the procedure of choice for documenting hepatic metastases. Scintigraphy with iodine-123 (^{123}I) or ^{131}I-labeled metaiodobenzylguanidine (I-MIBG), indium-labeled pentetreotide, or octreotide may identify primary and metastatic carcinoids not detected by conventional imaging techniques. Positron emission tomography (PET) can also be used to identify metastatic carcinoids.

Management and course

Localized carcinoids of the small intestine should be completely resected, either endoscopically or surgically. Asymptomatic lesions smaller than 1 cm in diameter may be treated with local excision, but lesions larger than 1 cm require a wide surgical excision. Duodenal lesions require a Whipple procedure, whereas distal ileal lesions require ileocecectomy and lesions in the jejunum and proximal ileum require segmental resection with 10 cm margins. When localized disease is resected, the overall 5-year survival is 75%, compared with 20–40% for metastatic disease.

Tumors with regional spread require wide surgical resection. Five-year survival after resection and nodal dissection for regional disease is 65–71%, compared to 38% for patients who do not have surgery.

Patients with metastatic disease and the carcinoid syndrome may benefit from debulking surgery. The somatostatin analog octreotide inhibits serotonin release and reduces flushing in more than 70% and reduces diarrhea in more than 60% of patients with carcinoid syndrome. Initial doses range from 50 to 250 μg subcutaneously 2–3 times daily but as the disease progresses, larger doses may be necessary.

Treatment with interferon is associated with substantially longer survival (median 80 months) compared to combination chemotherapy with streptozocin and 5-fluorouracil (8 months); the addition of hepatic chemoembolization to interferon may be associated with even longer survival.

Key practice points: small bowel carcinoid tumors

- The carcinoid syndrome affects 10–18% of patients with small bowel carcinoids.
- Measuring the urinary excretion of 5-HIAA, the major metabolite of serotonin, is a sensitive and specific test for the carcinoid syndrome, but it is less accurate for detecting localized carcinoids.
- Most carcinoids occur in the ileum.
- Most symptomatic small bowel lesions are visible in barium radiographs of the small intestine.
- Localized carcinoids of the small intestine should be completely resected, either endoscopically or surgically. When localized disease is resected, the overall 5-year survival is 75%, compared with 20–40% for metastatic disease.

Mesenchymal Tumors

Clinical presentation and diagnosis

Most small gastrointestinal stromal tumors (GISTs) are discovered incidentally and are asymptomatic. Larger tumors may be associated with symptoms of abdominal pain, nausea, vomiting, weight loss, or gastrointestinal hemorrhage. In some series, up to 40% of patients with ileal GISTs present with intussusception.

Small bowel radiography, CT scan, and angiography are useful in diagnosing GISTs. Because the lesions are submucosal, endoscopic diagnosis is often difficult unless ulceration is present. Biopsy specimens or resected tissue should be stained for CD117 to confirm the diagnosis of a GIST.

Management

The treatment of choice for small bowel GISTs is segmental intestinal resection. Despite complete resection with negative margins, recurrence rates approach 50–80% for GISTs with high-risk features (see Chapter 23). Patients found to have GISTs with high-risk features should be evaluated by an oncologist for consideration of chemotherapy with imatinib.

Key practice points: small bowel gists

- Small bowel GISTs should be surgically resected as long as there is no evidence of metastatic disease or if the lesion is causing a bowel obstruction.
- Patients found to have GISTs with high-risk features should be evaluated by an oncologist for consideration of imatinib therapy.

Lymphoma

Clinical presentation

A discrete mass lesion characterizes primary small bowel lymphoma (PSBL). Intermittent abdominal pain caused by obstruction is the most common complaint. Weight loss is often marked, and a small percentage of patients presents with perforations. Lymphoma should be suspected in patients with celiac sprue who complain of abdominal pain and weight loss after years or decades of quiescent disease. Misinterpreting these symptoms as a flare of celiac sprue may delay diagnosis.

Patients with immunoproliferative small intestinal disease (IPSID) present earlier than those with PSBL. Patients report profuse diarrhea and weight loss in addition to symptoms of obstruction. Many patients have associated clubbing of the digits. Unlike PSBL, a palpable abdominal mass is uncommon.

Diagnostic investigation

Barium radiography of the small intestine is the primary means of detecting small bowel lymphomas. Because most PSBLs occur in the ileum, upper gastrointestinal endoscopy may not visualize the lesion. Tumors within the distal 5–10 cm of the terminal ileum are accessible to colonoscopic biopsy. Double balloon enteroscopy may also identify the lesion. CT scans may be able to stage the tumor based on detecting malignant intra-abdominal and intrathoracic lymph nodes. Because of the diffuse nature of IPSID, a laparotomy may be required to establish the diagnosis. There are no specific laboratory features of PSBL but serum protein electrophoresis demonstrates an α-heavy chain paraprotein in 20–70% of patients with IPSID.

Management and course

Staging lymphomas of the small intestine is similar to that of gastric lymphomas. Patients with PSBL should be treated with surgical resection with lymph node sampling. Even if curative resection is not possible, palliative resection will prevent perforation resulting from chemotherapy-induced tumor necrosis. Combination chemotherapy is indicated for disease that is incompletely resected or unresectable but the role of adjuvant therapy after curative resection is undefined. Patients with IPSID may respond to antibiotic therapy in the prelymphomatous stage (tetracycline or metronidazole for 6–12 months). Nonresponders or patients in the lymphomatous stage have responded to anthracycline-based chemotherapy. The 5-year survival rate after curative resection for PSBL is 44–65%, whereas the corresponding survival rate for unresectable disease is only 20%. A poor prognosis is associated with IPSID, enteropathy-associated T-cell lymphoma, and mantle cell lymphoma.

Key practice points: small bowel lymphomas

- Most PSBLs occur in the ileum.
- Because of the diffuse nature of IPSID, a laparotomy may be required to establish the diagnosis.
- Patients with PSBL should be treated with surgical resection with lymph node sampling.
- Patients with IPSID may respond to antibiotic therapy in the prelymphomatous stage (tetracycline or metronidazole for 6–12 months).

Case studies

Case 1

A 45-year-old woman with Peutz–Jeghers syndrome (PJS) presents to the gastrointestinal clinic for an annual clinic visit. She states that she feels well overall; however, she reports occasional episodes of severe crampy midabdominal pain associated with abdominal fullness, nausea, and vomiting. The episodes typically last for only a few hours and always resolve spontaneously. She denies any weight loss. The patient has already had a colectomy due to multiple adenomatous polyps. She undergoes annual surveillance of her upper GI tract due to extensive polyposis in her stomach and multiple adenomas that have been resected and/or ablated in her duodenum. Physical exam is notable for mucocutaneous pigmentation involving the lips and buccal mucosa. Otherwise, her abdomen is benign with no palpable masses. A barium radiograph of the small bowel demonstrates a 3 cm polyp in the midjejunum. A double balloon enteroscopy is then performed and the polyp is endoscopically removed. Histology demonstrates the polyp to be hamartomatous.

Discussion

Peutz–Jeghers syndrome is an autosomal dominant disorder. Gastrointestinal polyps in patients with PJS are common. Polyps are typically hamartomatous and can occur in the stomach, small bowel, and colon. Obstruction of the small bowel is a common presenting symptom and is due to intussusceptions or obstruction of the lumen by the polyp.

Diagnosis of PJS should be suspected in a patient found to have a hamartomatous polyp. The diagnosis is established clinically if two of the three following criteria are present:

- family history of PJS
- mucocutaneous hyperpigmentation
- small bowel polyps.

In addition, genetic testing should be considered. Patients with PJS are at increased risk for GI (colorectal, stomach, small bowel, and pancreas) and non-GI (lung, breast, uterus, and ovary) cancers.

Case 2

A 64-year-old woman presents to her primary care provider with complaints of intermittent crampy right lower quadrant abdominal pain. She denies any blood in her stool and does not report any change in her bowel habits. The patient had a normal screening colonoscopy 1 year prior. Physical exam is unremarkable. A CT scan is performed and a 3 cm tumor in the ileum is identified. No other lesions are identified. The patient has the tumor surgically resected and histology demonstrates the tumor to be a carcinoid with extension through the muscularis propria without penetration of the overlying serosa. There is also evidence of nodal metastasis. The patient is staged as stage IIIB (T3N1M0). Six months following resection the patient is found to have a normal urinary 5-HIAA and no evidence of recurrence on CT scan.

Discussion

Small bowel carcinoids are typically found in the ileum. They often are found incidentally or present with nonspecific symptoms of vague abdominal pain. Small bowel carcinoids can metastasize irrespective of size. They often present with multiple lesions. Carcinoid syndrome is usually present only with hepatic metastasis. Following surgical resection of nonmetastatic carcinoid tumors, the patient should be followed clinically to monitor for evidence of recurrence, typically with urinary 5-HIAA measurements and CT scans.

National Comprehensive Cancer Network (NCCN) guidelines for neuroendocrine tumors are available at www.nccn.org.

CHAPTER 27
Diverticular Disease of the Colon

A diverticulum (plural: diverticula) is a sac-like protrusion of the wall of the colon. Diverticular disease encompasses a spectrum from diverticulosis to diverticulitis and diverticular hemorrhage.

Uncomplicated Diverticulosis

Diverticulosis is an acquired condition characterized by the presence of diverticula. Typical colonic diverticula herniate through defects in the muscle layer where arteries pass (vasa recta), on either side of the mesenteric taenia and on the mesenteric aspect of the antimesenteric teniae (Figure 27.1). Because they do not possess muscular layers, they are false or pulsion diverticula. In industrialized nations, 33–50% of the population older than age 50 has colonic diverticula, which may relate to low levels of dietary fiber. Ninety-five percent of patients with diverticulosis have diverticula in the sigmoid colon. Twenty-four percent of patients have diverticula in other regions in addition to the sigmoid colon; 7% have pancolic involvement. Sigmoid diverticulosis is accompanied by thickening of the circular muscle, shortening of the taenia coli, and narrowing of the lumen. Most diverticula are 0.1–1.0 cm in diameter, whereas larger diverticula may be the consequence of prior diverticulitis. Rectal diverticula are rare because of the presence of the circumferential longitudinal muscle layer.

Development of diverticulosis depends on the strength of the colon wall and the pressure difference between the lumen of the colon and the peritoneal cavity. Muscle thickening in the sigmoid colon is likely to represent a prediverticular condition resulting from high intralumenal pressures in an area of small diameter, with no corresponding increase in wall strength. The elasticity and tensile strength of the colon decrease with age, an effect that is most marked in the sigmoid colon. Deterioration in colonic structural proteins in Ehlers–Danlos

Yamada's Handbook of Gastroenterology, Third Edition. Edited by Tadataka Yamada and John M. Inadomi.
© 2013 John Wiley & Sons, Ltd. Published 2013 by John Wiley & Sons, Ltd.

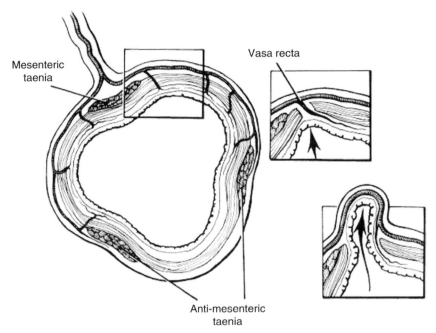

Figure 27.1 Cross-section of the sigmoid colon. The main illustration indicates the points of penetration of the vasa recti around the bowel circumference. *Inset*: The development of a diverticulum at one such point of weakness. (By permission of Mayo Foundation for Medical Education and Research. All rights reserved.)

and Marfan syndromes may explain the premature development of diverticula in these conditions. The role of primary colonic motor disorders in the pathogenesis of diverticulosis is undefined, and the relationship of diverticulosis and irritable bowel syndrome is controversial.

Clinical presentation

Seventy percent of persons with diverticulosis never develop significant symptoms. Some patients have mild, intermittent abdominal pain, bloating, flatulence, and altered defecation, although coexistence of irritable bowel syndrome is possible. Three-quarters of the remaining patients develop diverticulitis and one-quarter report hemorrhage.

Diagnostic investigation

On barium enema radiography, diverticula appear as contrast-filled colonic protrusions that may persist after evacuation. The presence of diverticula reduces the accuracy of barium enema radiography in detecting coexisting colonic neoplasia. Colonoscopy may reveal diverticular orifices, sigmoid tortuosity, and thickened folds consistent with prior diverticulitis.

Management and prevention

Therapy for symptomatic but uncomplicated diverticular disease relies on increased intake of dietary fiber or the use of fiber supplements. The role of low dietary fiber in the pathogenesis of diverticular disease is controversial. However, lack of vigorous physical activity is associated with diverticulosis, and obesity is associated with an increased risk of complications. Therefore, exercise and weight loss for overweight individuals are recommended.

Diverticulitis

Diverticulitis is symptomatic inflammation of a diverticulum and begins as peridiverticulitis caused by a microperforation of the colon. Diverticulitis can be classified as simple or complicated in presentation. The incidence of diverticulitis increases with age. Most cases of diverticulitis in westernized countries are left-sided but inflammation of diverticula at other sites, including the rectum and appendix, may occur.

Clinical presentation

Early manifestations of diverticulitis include pain and tenderness over the site of inflammation (usually in the lower abdomen or pelvis), nausea and vomiting, ileus, fever, a possible palpable mass, and tenderness or a mass effect on rectal examination. Complications of progressive inflammation include abscess, perforation, fistulization, and obstruction.

Differential diagnosis

The differential diagnosis of acute diverticulitis is broad and needs to be considered prior to embarking on therapy specific to diverticulitis. Acute appendicitis, Crohn's disease, ischemic colitis, peptic ulcer disease, and pseudomembranous colitis can all present with symptoms similar to acute diverticulitis. Ectopic pregnancy and ovarian cysts, torsion or abscess should be suspected in female patients. Neoplasia, especially colorectal carcinoma, should also be considered, particularly in patients with weight loss or bleeding.

Diagnostic investigation

Computed tomography (CT) scanning is indicated if the diagnosis is uncertain, complications are suspected, medical therapy has failed, or the patient is immunocompromised. CT scans may reveal thickening of the colon wall, pericolic inflammation, fistulae, sinuses, abscess cavities, and obstruction. Ultrasound is occasionally useful for detecting and draining pericolonic fluid collections. Barium enema radiography is not recommended during the acute attack, although water-soluble contrast enemas may be used to detect diverticula. Careful flexible sigmoidoscopy is used during an episode of suspected diverticulitis to differentiate a neoplasm from an inflammatory diverticular mass, but colonoscopy is contraindicated in cases of acute diverticulitis because of the risk of complications, including perforation.

Management and prevention

The initial management of diverticulitis includes fluid replacement, nasogastric suction for ileus or obstruction, and broad-spectrum antibiotics to treat possible infection with anaerobes, Gram-negative bacilli, and Gram-positive coliform organisms, such as ceftriaxone with metronidazole. Oral quinolones, amoxicillin/clavulanate, or a cephalosporin may be given to outpatients who have no peritoneal signs. Indications for surgery include perforation, abscess, fistula, obstruction, recurrent diverticulitis, or the inability to exclude carcinoma. In the case of urgent surgery, primary anastomosis is not attempted because anastomotic breakdown is possible. However, a one-stage operation with anastomosis can be performed in the absence of advanced age, sepsis, hemodynamic instability, an unprepared colon, local contamination, friable tissues, malnutrition, steroid use, or poor blood supply. Percutaneous CT-guided abscess drainage may benefit patients who are stable and without signs of sepsis. Fistulae usually can be resected in a one-stage procedure, whereas obstruction usually mandates a two-stage operative approach. Surgical resection can reduce the likelihood of recurrent diverticulitis from 30% to between 5% and 10%. In most cases, distal sigmoid resection must be complete to minimize recurrent diverticular inflammation. An algorithm for the treatment of acute diverticulitis is shown in Figure 27.2.

Historically, patients with diverticular disease were advised to avoid seeds, corn and nuts out of concern that these could obstruct the diverticula and cause complications. Data to support these recommendations are lacking. In fact, a prospective cohort study found an inverse association between the consumption of nut and popcorn consumption and the risk of diverticulitis.

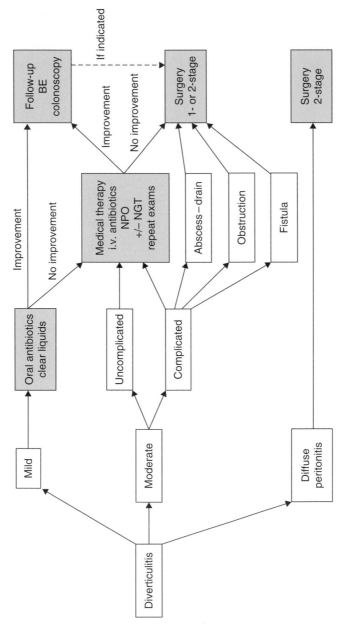

Figure 27.2 Algorithm for treatment of acute diverticulitis. (Source: Yamada T et al. (eds) *Textbook of Gastroenterology,* 5th edn. Oxford: Blackwell Publishing Ltd, 2009.)

Diverticular Hemorrhage

Diverticular hemorrhage is the most common cause of acute massive colonic blood loss. Massive bleeding from colonic diverticula occurs in 5% of patients; minor bleeding occurs in up to 47%. The close proximity of diverticula and arteries accounts for the propensity of these lesions to bleed. Paradoxically, although most diverticula are sigmoid in location, half of diverticular hemorrhages emanate from a right colonic source.

Clinical presentation

Diverticular hemorrhage is characterized by the sudden, painless passage of large amounts of bright-red blood from the rectum and may be associated with hypotension, tachycardia, or syncope. Bleeding stops spontaneously in 80% of patients. Complications of diverticular hemorrhage are related to hypovolemia and involve the heart, brain, kidneys, and lungs.

Differential diagnosis

It is important to bear in mind that hematochezia may result from a variety of lower gastrointestinal sources, as well as from massive upper gastrointestinal hemorrhage. This topic is discussed in more detail in Chapter 3.

Management and prevention

The initial management of diverticular hemorrhage, as for other types of gastrointestinal hemorrhage, requires aggressive fluid resuscitation and replacement of colloid including blood products. The patient's cardiovascular system must be stabilized, the airway protected, and ventilation support established, as needed. Because massive hemorrhage is statistically more likely to be from an upper rather than lower gastrointestinal source, upper gastrointestinal lavage or upper gastrointestinal endoscopy should be performed to exclude definitively a source proximal to the ligament of Treitz. Combinations of radionuclide imaging, mesenteric angiography, and colonoscopy may be required to determine the type and location of the bleeding lesion. Diverticular bleeding can be treated with cautery or endoscopic clip placement. Even though endoscopic therapy to stop diverticular hemorrhage may fail, localization of the bleeding site may allow limited resection of the appropriate colonic segment. Scintigraphy with technetium-99 m (^{99m}Tc) sulfur colloid or ^{99m}Tc-tagged erythrocytes in conjunction with angiography may confirm the presence of active bleeding and assists in localizing the approximate site of hemorrhage. The rate of bleeding must be 0.1 mL/min or more for this modality to reveal the source. Selective mesenteric angiography may show extravasation of the contrast agent if the bleeding rate is higher than 0.5 mL/min. In such cases, the angiocatheter may also be used to deliver intra-arterial vasopressin or synthetic emboli to stop bleeding in patients who are not surgical candidates.

Minor hemorrhage (<2 units transfused) with spontaneous cessation is managed conservatively. Persistent hemorrhage (2–4 units transfused) typically indicates the need for further evaluation to localize the site of bleeding and attempt to achieve hemostasis, or to identify the involved segment so that it may be surgically resected on a semi-elective basis. More urgent surgery is necessary for major hemorrhage (>4 units transfused) that does not stop. If the site of bleeding cannot be determined, total abdominal colectomy may be needed.

CHAPTER 28
Irritable Bowel Syndrome

Irritable bowel syndrome (IBS) is a disorder characterized by abdominal pain or discomfort with altered bowel habits in the absence of organic disease. The most widely accepted definition is provided by the Rome criteria: recurrent abdominal pain or discomfort at least 3 days/month in the last 3 months associated with two or more of the following criteria: (1) improvement of discomfort by defecation, (2) onset associated with a change in the frequency of stool, and (3) association of discomfort with altered stool form (Table 28.1). Using symptom-based criteria, approximately 14% of the United States population reports symptoms consistent with a diagnosis of IBS. Only one-quarter of this number seeks medical attention because of symptom severity and other factors, including psychosocial dysfunction. Most affected individuals report disease onset before age 45, although the condition is recognized in both adolescents and the elderly. IBS is 2–4 times more common in women.

Clinical presentation

The intensity, location, and timing of abdominal discomfort or pain in patients with IBS are highly variable. The pain may be so intense as to interfere with daily activities. Abdominal discomfort is most often described as crampy or achy but sharp, dull, and gas-like pains are also reported. Abdominal pain in IBS commonly is exacerbated by ingesting a meal or by stress and may be relieved by defecation or passage of flatus. Despite this, the pain rarely leads to significant weight loss or malnutrition and infrequently interrupts sleep. Abdominal discomfort may be associated with significant complaints of bloating, which may or may not produce visible distension.

Different bowel habit disturbances characterize distinct IBS subsets. Constipation-predominant IBS patients report stools that are hard or pellet-like,

Yamada's Handbook of Gastroenterology, Third Edition. Edited by Tadataka Yamada and John M. Inadomi.
© 2013 John Wiley & Sons, Ltd. Published 2013 by John Wiley & Sons, Ltd.

Table 28.1 Rome III diagnostic criteria* for irritable bowel syndrome

Recurrent abdominal pain or discomfort at least 3 days/month in the last 3 months, associated with two or more of the following three features related to bowel habit:
1. improvement of discomfort by defecation
2. onset associated with a change in the frequency of stool
3. onset associated with a change in the form (appearance) of stool

*Criteria should be fulfilled for the last 3 months with symptom onset at least 6 months prior to diagnosis.

are difficult to pass, and are associated with a sensation of incomplete fecal evacuation. Diarrhea-predominant patients pass soft or loose stools of normal daily volume, which may occur after eating or during stress. Many individuals exhibit a pattern of diarrhea alternating with constipation and report characteristics of each subtype. Passage of fecal mucus is reported by 50% of patients. Rectal bleeding, nocturnal diarrhea, malabsorption, or weight loss warrants an aggressive search for organic disease.

Irritable bowel syndrome patients frequently report symptoms referable to other organs. Large subsets have associated heartburn, early satiety, nausea, vomiting, and dyspepsia. High incidences of genitourinary dysfunction (dysmenorrhea, dyspareunia, impotence, urinary frequency, and incomplete urinary evacuation), fibromyalgia, low back pain, headaches, fatigue, insomnia, and impaired concentration have been observed in individuals with IBS.

Physical examination of the person with IBS usually is unimpressive. The patient may appear anxious and have cold, clammy hands. Diffuse tenderness or a palpable bowel loop may be evident on abdominal examination. Organomegaly, adenopathy, or occult fecal blood is not consistent with a diagnosis of IBS and warrants a search for organic disease.

Differential diagnosis

While the diagnosis of IBS is based upon identifying symptoms that are consistent with the condition (see Table 28.1), many other conditions may present in a similar manner and need to be excluded in a cost-effective manner. Patients with inflammatory bowel disease, microscopic colitis, celiac disease, thyroid dysfunction, colorectal neoplasia, and infectious diarrhea can have symptoms that mimic IBS. The presence of "alarm features" such as weight loss or gastrointestinal bleeding, refractory diarrhea or a family history of colorectal cancer should be used to help direct the evaluation. In the absence of "alarm features" the Rome criteria for diagnosing IBS are very specific.

Diagnostic investigation

Diagnosing IBS confidently involves a directed evaluation to confirm that organic disease is not present. The extent of the diagnostic investigation depends on patient age and the predominant symptoms.

Laboratory studies

Normal values of selected laboratory tests help to confirm a diagnosis of IBS. In contrast, anemia, leukocytosis, leukopenia, or elevations of the sedimentation rate suggest organic disease. Thyroid chemistries are performed in some cases of diarrhea-predominant or constipation-predominant disease to exclude hyperthyroidism or hypothyroidism, respectively. Celiac disease serologies, including endomysial and tissue transglutaminase antibodies, are obtained in individuals with possible celiac disease. Stool samples may be obtained to exclude giardiasis in some patients with diarrhea-predominant disease.

Structural studies

Structural testing is recommended for many patients with suspected IBS. In patients older than age 45–50, colonoscopy is recommended to screen for colorectal cancer. Sigmoidoscopy or colonoscopy may be performed in younger individuals, especially if the diagnosis is uncertain. Biopsy of the colon during lower endoscopy is indicated in some patients with prominent diarrhea to rule out microscopic colitis as a cause of symptoms. Upper endoscopy may be performed for reflux or dyspeptic symptoms. Endoscopic small intestinal biopsy is indicated if serological testing suggests celiac disease.

Other testing

Other tests occasionally are indicated to evaluate for other diagnostic possibilities in patients with IBS symptoms. Hydrogen breath testing often is used to exclude lactase deficiency or small intestinal bacterial overgrowth. Patients with constipation refractory to medical management may undergo colonic transit testing using radio-opaque markers, anorectal manometry, and defecography to test for slow transit constipation, pelvic floor abnormalities, and anal sphincter dysfunction. Individuals with severe diarrhea may be evaluated for secretory or malabsorptive processes. Screening for laxatives should be considered because laxative abuse is common in patients with unexplained diarrhea. Liver chemistry studies and ultrasound are performed for suspected biliary tract disease. Computed tomography is obtained if malignancy is a concern in a patient with prominent pain, whereas gastric scintigraphy or gastroduodenal manometry may be indicated for a patient with prominent nausea, vomiting, or early satiety. In very rare instances, screening for porphyria or heavy metal intoxication is performed.

Management

After a confident diagnosis of IBS, the clinician should provide reassurance and education to the patient and impart awareness that IBS is a functional disorder without long-term health risks. In some individuals, education and dietary advice will be sufficient. However, most patients receive medications to reduce their symptoms. Some affected persons will be refractory to drug treatment and are considered for psychological therapies. IBS usually persists in a waxing and waning fashion for many years. Despite this, the quality of life for patients with IBS can be improved by appropriate physician involvement; patients can cope with their symptoms and experience an improved sense of well-being. Patients likely to report good outcomes include those who are male, have a brief history of symptoms, have acute symptom onset, exhibit predominant constipation, and have a good initial response to therapy.

Dietary recommendations

Changes in diet can be recommended for selected patients with IBS. Reducing fat content may decrease abdominal discomfort evoked by lipid-stimulated motor activity. Increasing fiber content in the diet or consuming a fiber supplement (psyllium, polycarbophil, or methylcellulose) may improve bowel function in constipated IBS patients. Fiber supplements may take several weeks to produce satisfactory results and can produce gaseous symptoms if large quantities are ingested rapidly. Low-gas diets have been devised to reduce bloating and excess flatulence in patients with IBS. Some patients with diarrhea and excess gas may respond to exclusion of dairy products or fruits and soft drinks that contain the poorly absorbed sugars fructose and sorbitol.

Medication therapy

Medication regimens for patients with IBS should be customized to treat the predominant symptoms of each individual. Individuals with constipation who do not respond to fiber supplements may experience relief with osmotic laxatives such as milk of magnesia or a poorly absorbed sugar (e.g. lactulose, sorbitol). Isotonic solutions that contain polyethylene glycol are useful for constipation and may produce fewer side-effects than hypertonic osmotic laxatives. Lubiprostone, a chloride channel activator, has been shown to be effective at treating constipation-predominant IBS. Opiate agents (e.g. loperamide, diphenoxylate with atropine) are the most useful initial agents for treating diarrhea-predominant IBS. Other medications used for some individuals with diarrhea include the bile acid binder cholestyramine and disodium cromoglycate for rare cases of food hypersensitivity.

The 5-HT$_3$ receptor antagonist alosetron is a potent treatment for refractory diarrhea-predominant IBS. Because this agent increases the risks of severe constipation and ischemic colitis, it is prescribed only through a restricted program. Because it has not been adequately studied in men, it is only approved for women with severe diarrhea-predominant IBS.

Antispasmodic anticholinergic agents are the initial therapy of choice to reduce pain in IBS. These drugs also blunt the gastrocolonic response and may also be useful in preventing postprandial diarrhea. Oral antibiotics provide benefit to some individuals with IBS and associated bacterial overgrowth. Rifaximin, a minimally absorbed antibiotic, has demonstrated efficacy for improving global IBS symptoms and bloating. Tricyclic antidepressants exhibit significant potency in patients with significant pain. Tricyclics may also reduce symptoms in those with prominent diarrhea. Conversely, this class of drugs can exacerbate constipation. The gonadotropin-releasing hormone analog leuprolide has been evaluated for patients with severe pain. However, this agent induces amenorrhea and osteoporosis and should be used with care.

Over-the-counter and alternative therapies are sometimes used for treating IBS. Antigas products, such as simethicone, activated charcoal, and bacterial α-galactosidase, have been proposed for patients with bloating but controlled trials of these agents have not been performed. Selected herbal remedies reportedly provide benefits to some patients. Probiotic compounds reduce gaseous symptoms in some IBS trials.

Psychological therapies

Recent research has demonstrated that mindfulness-based stress reduction training, typically in a group setting, can result in improvements in bowel symptom severity and quality of life, while reducing distress among IBS patients. Biofeedback and relaxation training may also reduce symptoms. Hypnosis has been effective in selected patients with medically refractory symptoms. Some studies of psychotherapy report reductions in abdominal pain, diarrhea, and somatic symptoms as well as anxiety. Consistent problems with most of these investigations include poor definitions of symptom response or lack of appropriate control populations.

Complications and their management

Long-term studies show that more than 75% of patients have symptoms persisting beyond 5 years, despite appropriate therapy. IBS has a significant impact upon the quality of life of affected individuals and some have considerable disability. Studies have shown that counseling, reassurance and education, along with judicious use of medication and continued interest in the patients' well-being, can promote successful outcomes in many patients with IBS.

Society guidelines

AGA Technical Review and Medical Position Statement on Irritable Bowel Syndrome (*Gastroenterology* 2002;123:2105–2107 and *Gastroenterology* 2002;123:22108–2131). Available at: www.gastro.org/practice/medical-position-statements.

Key practice points

- Irritable bowel syndrome may be diagnosed without extensive testing. In addition to symptom criteria, limited structural examination to rule out inflammatory bowel disease, celiac disease and chronic infection should be sufficient.

- Management of irritable bowel syndrome focuses on reassurance and providing insight to the patient to understand the waxing and waning nature of this disorder. Depending on the subtype, additional treatment may include loperamide, tricyclic antidepressants or rifaximin (diarrhea predominant), lubiprostone or selective serotonin reuptake inhibitors (constipation predominant).

- Alternatives to medication for management of IBS include mindfulness-based stress reduction therapy or behavioral modification therapy.

CHAPTER 29

Inflammatory Bowel Disease

Chronic inflammatory bowel diseases (IBD) include ulcerative colitis, a disorder in which inflammation affects the mucosa and submucosa of the colon, and Crohn's disease, in which inflammation is transmural and may involve any or all segments of the gastrointestinal tract.

Clinical presentation

Ulcerative colitis

The dominant symptom in ulcerative colitis is diarrhea, which is often bloody. Bowel movements may be frequent but of low volume as a result of rectal inflammation. Abdominal pain (usually lower quadrant or rectal), fever, malaise, and weight loss may also be reported. Localized rectal involvement may be characterized only by bloody diarrhea, with or without urgency, tenesmus, pain, or incontinence. Elderly patients rarely report constipation as a result of rectal spasm.

Patients with ulcerative colitis can be classified according to disease severity, which helps to direct disease management (Table 29.1). Diarrhea and rectal bleeding are the only complaints of mild disease, which is often associated with a normal physical examination. Most patients with ulcerative proctitis have mild disease. Moderate disease, which occurs in 27% of patients, is characterized by five or six bloody stools per day, abdominal pain, abdominal tenderness, low-grade fever, and fatigue. Nineteen percent of patients exhibit severe ulcerative colitis, which is characterized by frequent episodes of bloody diarrhea (>6 stools per day), profound weakness, weight loss, fever, tachycardia, postural hypotension, significant abdominal tenderness, hypoactive bowel sounds, and anemia and hypoalbuminemia on laboratory investigation. Abdominal distension with severe disease raises the possibility of toxic megacolon.

Yamada's Handbook of Gastroenterology, Third Edition. Edited by Tadataka Yamada and John M. Inadomi.
© 2013 John Wiley & Sons, Ltd. Published 2013 by John Wiley & Sons, Ltd.

Table 29.1 Classification of ulcerative colitis

Severe
Diarrhea: six or more bowel movements per day, with blood
Fever: mean evening temperature >37.5°C or >37.5°C on at least 2 of 4 days at any time of day
Tachycardia: mean pulse rate higher than 90 beats/min
Anemia: hemoglobin of <7.5 g/dL, allowing for recent transfusions
Sedimentation rate: >30 mm/h

Mild
Mild diarrhea: fewer than four bowel movements per day, with only small amounts of blood
No fever
No tachycardia
Mild anemia
Sedimentation rate: <30 mm/h

Moderately severe
Intermediate between mild and severe

Severe ulcerative colitis can cause life-threatening complications. If the inflammatory process extends beyond the submucosa into the muscularis, the colon dilates, producing toxic megacolon. Clinical criteria suggestive of toxic megacolon include a temperature higher than 38.6°C, a heart rate higher than 120 beats per minute, a neutrophil count of more than 10,500 cells/µL, dehydration, mental status changes, electrolyte disturbances, hypotension, abdominal distension, tenderness (with or without rebound), and hypoactive or absent bowel sounds. Toxic megacolon usually occurs in patients with pancolitis, often early in the course of their disease. Medications that impair colonic motor function may initiate or exacerbate megacolon. Perforation of the colon may complicate toxic megacolon or may occur in cases of severe ulcerative colitis without megacolon. Strictures are uncommon but lumenal narrowing is observed in 12% of patients after 5–25 years of disease, usually in the sigmoid colon and rectum. Strictures present as increases in diarrhea or new fecal incontinence and may mimic malignancy on endoscopic or radiographic evaluation.

Crohn's disease

There are three main patterns of disease distribution in Crohn's disease: (1) involvement of the small and large intestine (40% of patients); (2) disease confined to the small intestine (30%); and (3) disease of only the colon (25%), which is pancolonic in two-thirds and segmental in one-third. Less commonly, the disease affects the proximal gastrointestinal tract (5%). Predominant symptoms in Crohn's disease include diarrhea, abdominal pain, and weight loss. They may exist for months to years before a diagnosis is made (Table 29.2). With

Table 29.2 Frequency of clinical features in Crohn's disease

Feature	Ileitis (%)	Ileocolitis (%)	Colitis (%)
Diarrhea	~100	~100	~100
Abdominal pain	65	62	55
Bleeding	22	10	46
Weight loss	12	19	22
Perianal disease	14	38	36
Internal fistulae	17	34	16
Intestinal obstruction	35	44	17
Megacolon	0	2	11
Arthritis	4	4	16
Spondylitis	1	2	5

colonic disease, diarrhea may be of small volume with urgency and tenesmus whereas, if disease is extensive, small intestinal involvement produces larger stool volumes with steatorrhea. Diarrhea from small intestinal disease occurs from loss of mucosal absorptive surface area (producing bile salt-induced or osmotic diarrhea), bacterial overgrowth from strictures, and enteroenteric or enterocolonic fistulae. Pain results from intermittent partial obstruction or serosal inflammation. Commonly, pain and distension from terminal ileal disease are reported in the right lower quadrant. Weight loss occurs in most patients because of malabsorption and reduced oral intake; 10–20% of patients lose more than 20% of their body weight. Gastroduodenal involvement in Crohn's disease produces epigastric pain, nausea, and vomiting secondary to stricture or obstruction. Fatigue, malaise, fever, and chills are constitutional symptoms that contribute to the morbidity of Crohn's disease. The Crohn's Disease Activity Index assigns numerical scores to stool frequency, abdominal pain, sense of well-being, systemic manifestations, the use of antidiarrheal agents, abdominal mass, hematocrit, and body weight, and has been used as a quantitative measure of disease activity in clinical studies.

Crohn's disease often is associated with gastrointestinal complications. Abscesses and fistulae result from extension of a mucosal breach through the intestinal wall into the extraintestinal tissue. Abscesses occur in 15–20% of patients and most commonly arise from the terminal ileum but they may occur in iliopsoas, retroperitoneal, hepatic, and splenic regions, and at anastomotic sites. Abscesses present with fever, localized tenderness, and a palpable mass. Infection usually is polymicrobial (e.g. *Escherichia coli*, *Bacteroides fragilis*, *Enterococcus*, and α-hemolytic *Streptococcus* species). Twenty percent to 40% of patients with Crohn's disease have fistulous disease. Fistulae may be enteroenteric, enterocutaneous, enterovesical, or enterovaginal or perianal. They develop when disease is active and may persist after remission. Large enteroenteric fistulae produce diarrhea, malabsorption, and weight loss. Enterocutaneous fistulae produce persistent drainage that usually is refractory to medical therapy. Rectovaginal fistulae lead to foul-smelling vaginal discharge, and enterovesical fistulae produce pneumaturia and recurrent urinary infection. Obstruction, especially of the small intestine, is a common complication caused by mucosal thickening, muscular hyperplasia and scarring from prior inflammation, or adhesions. Perianal disease, including anal ulcers, abscesses, and fistulae, can also affect the groin, vulva, or scrotum and is a complication that often is difficult to treat. Fistulae drain serous or mucous material, whereas perianal abscesses cause fever, redness, induration, and pain that is exacerbated by defecation, sitting, and walking.

Extraintestinal features

Extraintestinal manifestations of IBD are divided into two groups: those in which clinical activity follows activity of bowel disease and those in which clinical activity is unrelated to bowel activity. Extraintestinal disease is more common with ulcerative colitis and Crohn's colitis than with ileal Crohn's disease. Colitic arthritis is a migratory arthritis of the knees, hips, ankles, wrists, and elbows that usually lasts a few weeks, rarely produces joint deformity, and usually responds to treatment of bowel inflammation. In contrast, the activities of sacroiliitis and ankylosing spondylitis do not follow the course of the bowel disease and may not respond to therapy for intestinal inflammation. Sacroiliitis often is asymptomatic and is found incidentally by radiography. The prevalence of ankylosing spondylitis, which is characterized by morning stiffness, low back pain, and stooped posture, increases 30-fold with ulcerative colitis and is associated with the HLA-B27 phenotype. Unlike colitic arthritis, ankylosing spondylitis can be relentlessly progressive and unresponsive to medications.

Hepatobiliary manifestations of IBD include steatosis, pericholangitis, chronic active hepatitis, cirrhosis, sclerosing cholangitis, and gallstones. Sclerosing cholangitis is a chronic cholestatic disease marked by fibrosing inflammation of the intrahepatic and extrahepatic bile ducts; it occurs in 1–4% of patients with ulcerative colitis and in lesser numbers of patients with Crohn's disease. Conversely, the prevalence of IBD is so high in patients with sclerosing cholangitis that colonoscopy should be performed even on those without intestinal symptoms. Cholangiocarcinoma develops in 10–15% of patients with IBD who have long-standing sclerosing cholangitis. Cholesterol gallstones develop in patients with Crohn's disease because of the bile salt depletion that occurs with ileal disease or resection.

Diagnostic investigation

Laboratory studies

Laboratory studies that reflect disease activity in ulcerative colitis are hemoglobin level, leukocyte count, electrolytes, serum albumin, erythrocyte sedimentation rate, and C-reactive protein. Neutrophil-derived fecal markers, including calprotectin and lactoferrin, represent a novel tool for monitoring intestinal mucosal inflammation. Anemia, hypoalbuminemia, hypokalemia, and metabolic alkalosis may be prominent in severe disease. Stool should be inspected for leukocytes and cultures should be obtained to rule out infectious etiologies of diarrhea, including *Campylobacter*, *Shigella*, *Salmonella*, *Yersinia*, and *Giardia lamblia*. Even if antibiotics have not been taken recently, stool should be tested for *Clostridium difficile* toxin.

Laboratory findings in Crohn's disease are nonspecific. Anemia results from chronic disease, blood loss, and iron, folate, and vitamin B_{12} deficiency, and bone marrow suppression from medication. Active Crohn's disease elevates leukocyte counts and sedimentation rate but marked increases suggest abscess formation. Hypoalbuminemia may indicate severe disease, malnutrition, or protein-losing enteropathy. For patients with diarrhea, testing of stools for infection is indicated as for ulcerative colitis. Measurement of fecal fat, either qualitatively (Sudan stain) or quantitatively, can provide evidence of ileal disease.

Complications and extraintestinal manifestations of IBD can be suggested by selected laboratory studies. Profound leukocytosis with a neutrophil predominance in ulcerative colitis is worrisome for perforation or toxic megacolon or *C. difficile* infection. Pericholangitis and sclerosing cholangitis produce elevations of alkaline phosphatase. Pyuria in a patient with Crohn's disease suggests a possible enterovesical fistula, whereas hematuria raises concern for renal stones.

Diagnostic pitfalls

Serological markers have been promoted to diagnose and differentiate ulcerative colitis from Crohn's disease. Perinuclear antineutrophil cytoplasmic antibodies (pANCA) are found in 60% of ulcerative colitis patients and 10% of individuals with Crohn's disease. Anti-*Saccharomyces cerevisiae* antibodies (ASCA) are found in 60% of Crohn's disease patients and 10% of individuals with ulcerative colitis. However, these tests have not reliably differentiated between ulcerative colitis and Crohn's in patients with indeterminant colitis, which represents the group that could have benefited most from this test.

Endoscopy

Colonoscopy at the initial presentation of a patient with suspected IBD can establish the diagnosis and define the extent of disease. With severe disease, sigmoidoscopy may provide enough information to initiate therapy without the risks of perforation associated with colonoscopy in this setting.

In ulcerative colitis, the inflammation begins in the rectum and extends proximally to the point where visible disease ends without skipping any areas (Table 29.3). Mild disease is characterized by superficial erosions, loss of vascularity, granularity, and exudation. In severe disease, large ulcers and denuded mucosa may dominate. With chronic disease, the mucosa flattens and inflammatory

Table 29.3 Colonoscopic findings in inflammatory bowel disease

Feature	Ulcerative colitis	Crohn's disease
Inflammation		
Distribution		
Colon		
Contiguous	+ + +	+
Symmetrical	+ + +	+
Rectum	+ + +	+
Friability	+ + +	+
Topography		
Granularity	+ + +	+
Cobblestoned	+	+ + +
Ulceration		
Location		
Colitis	+ + +	+
Ileum	0	+ + + +
Discrete lesion	+	+ + +
Features		
Size >1 cm	+	+ + +
Deep	+	+ +
Linear	+	+ + +
Aphthoid	0	+ + + +
Bridging	+	+ +

Specificity index range: 0 (not seen) to + + + + (diagnostic).

polyps (pseudopolyps) develop. Pseudopolyps are not premalignant and do not need to be resected.

Crohn's colitis exhibits a different appearance in many but not all cases. Aphthous ulcers predominate in early or mild disease, whereas severe disease is characterized by cobblestoning and large, deep, linear or serpiginous ulcers. With gastroduodenal Crohn's disease, antral aphthous and linear ulcers may be seen on upper endoscopy. Unlike ulcerative colitis, mucosal involvement in Crohn's disease is not always contiguous; patches of colon are often relatively disease free (areas skipped), and the rectum may or may not be involved. Ileal disease is common in Crohn's disease. The ileum is normal in most ulcerative colitis patients, although backwash ileitis is seen in 10–20% of cases of pancolitis.

Strictures are more common with Crohn's disease, as is perianal involvement. Strictures and mass lesions in patients with long-standing IBD (>10 years) strongly suggest malignancy. In addition to its diagnostic capability, colonoscopy has therapeutic potential (e.g. pneumatic dilation) in patients with colonic strictures.

Capsule endoscopy has been used in some cases to exclude subtle small intestinal Crohn's disease in patients without obstruction.

Specialized endoscopy can help assess the extraintestinal manifestations of IBD. Endoscopic retrograde cholangiopancreatography (ERCP) can diagnose sclerosing cholangitis and cholangiocarcinoma and can be used to dilate or stent biliary strictures in sclerosing cholangitis, possibly reducing pruritus and other manifestations of obstructive jaundice.

Radiography

Findings of radiographic evaluation complement those of endoscopy in patients with IBD. Plain abdominal radiography may be normal or show colonic dilation in toxic megacolon, air–fluid levels from intestinal obstruction in Crohn's disease, or pneumoperitoneum with perforation. Computed tomography (CT) may also characterize malignant and benign obstruction in Crohn's disease and is superior to endoscopy for detecting fistulae and strictures. CT detects abscesses and may assist in their percutaneous drainage. Magnetic resonance imaging has an increasing role in characterizing small intestinal Crohn's disease. Scintigraphic scans have been used to localize and characterize areas of intestinal inflammation or abscess.

Imaging studies are useful in characterizing complications and extraintestinal manifestations of IBD. Spine radiography shows squaring of the vertebrae, straightening of the spine, and lateral and anterior syndesmophytes in ankylosing spondylitis, whereas pelvic radiographs of the pelvis in sacroiliitis reveal blurring of the margins of the sacroiliac joints, with patchy sclerosis. Ultrasound is performed on patients with suspected biliary colic or cholecystitis secondary to gallstones in Crohn's disease. Magnetic resonance cholangiopancreatography and percutaneous transhepatic cholangiography are used in some cases to screen for sclerosing cholangitis or cholangiocarcinoma. Intravenous pyelography or CT may demonstrate enterovesical fistulae or renal stones.

Pathology

Histological evaluation of colonic biopsy specimens is usually able to distinguish ulcerative colitis from Crohn's disease, and both forms of IBD from acute colitis. Distortion of the crypt architectural structure and acute and chronic inflammation of the lamina propria are more common with ulcerative colitis than with acute, self-limited colitis. The presence of granulomas is the best histological distinction of Crohn's disease. In one series, granulomas were found in 60% of Crohn's disease patients versus 6% of patients with ulcerative colitis. Crypt atrophy, neutrophilic infiltration, and surface erosions are more common in ulcerative colitis than in Crohn's disease. Despite these variations, histological discrimination between the two forms of chronic IBD cannot be made in 15–25% of cases.

Ulcerative colitis and Crohn's disease exhibit characteristic findings on gross surgical specimens. Findings in ulcerative colitis are generally limited to the mucosa and submucosa; the muscularis propria is involved only in fulminant disease. Conversely, in Crohn's disease the bowel wall is thickened and stiff and the mesentery is thickened, edematous, and contracted because of transmural involvement. Adipose tissue creeps over the serosal surface, and intestinal loops may be matted together. Lymphoid aggregates may be observed involving the submucosa and occasionally the muscularis propria. Granulomas are found in many surgically resected intestinal, lymph node, mesentery, peritoneal, and liver specimens in Crohn's disease. Axonal necrosis of autonomic nerves is considered characteristic of Crohn's disease.

Management and prevention

Nutritional management

In most cases, the only nutritional therapy required is a well-balanced diet. Some patients with small intestinal Crohn's disease have secondary lactase deficiency and should restrict lactose intake or use supplemental lactase. Patients with strictures should avoid high-residue foods. Oral or parenteral iron supplements may be indicated for significant blood loss. Specific calcium, magnesium, zinc, vitamin B_{12}, vitamin D, or vitamin K supplements may be required to counter clinical or biochemical evidence of deficiency caused by Crohn's enteritis. Extensive terminal ileal resections (>100 cm) promote vitamin B_{12}, fat, and bile salt malabsorption. Steatorrhea may be reduced by consuming a low-fat diet. Medium-chain triglycerides, which are absorbed in the proximal intestine and do not require bile salts, are substituted for conventional long-chain triglycerides in some cases. The bile salt-binding resin cholestyramine can reduce bile salt diarrhea but may worsen fat malabsorption.

When oral intake is inadequate, enteral feedings may be provided through nasogastric, gastrostomy, or jejunostomy tubes. The use of elemental feedings that consist of amino acids, monosaccharides, vitamins, minerals, and essential fatty acids is controversial due to mixed outcomes from controlled trials. Severe IBD exacerbations or extensive small intestinal resections with Crohn's disease may warrant initiating total parenteral nutrition. Parenteral nutrition also is helpful in improving the nutritional status of patients with ulcerative colitis before colectomy.

Medication therapy
5-Aminosalicylate preparations

Drugs that contain 5-aminosalicylate (5-ASA) have been shown to effectively treat mild-to-moderate ulcerative colitis but their efficacy is less certain in Crohn's disease. Sulfasalazine is started at low doses and is gradually increased to 4g per day, as tolerated, in mild-to-moderate ulcerative colitis. After remission is achieved, doses can be tapered to 2g per day for long-term maintenance therapy, which reduces relapses from 75–20% at 1 year. Dose-related side-effects of sulfasalazine stem from the sulfapyridine component and include nausea, vomiting, headache, dyspepsia, abdominal discomfort, and hemolysis. Hypersensitive dose-independent reactions include rash, fever, aplastic anemia, agranulocytosis, and autoimmune hemolysis. Other side-effects of sulfasalazine include reduced sperm counts (which recover 3 months after stopping the drug), folate deficiency (caused by inhibition of intestinal folate conjugase), and, rarely, bloody diarrhea (caused by the 5-ASA component).

Other 5-ASA preparations are commonly prescribed in selected IBD subsets. Enemas that contain 5-ASA are effective for treating distal ulcerative colitis and induce remission in 93% of patients. 5-ASA suppositories are useful in ulcerative proctitis. Several oral 5-ASA (mesalamine) preparations are available and used because of their efficacy and favorable side-effect profiles. They differ in the vehicle, which allows some differentiation in the primary site of action. Other 5-ASA drugs include olsalazine and balsalazide. All 5-ASA products exhibit potential nephrotoxicity; thus caution should be exercised when using these drugs in patients with renal dysfunction, and routine monitoring of renal function should be performed in all patients on aminosalicylate therapy.

Corticosteroids

Corticosteroids are effective in inducing remission in ulcerative colitis and Crohn's disease but are not advocated for maintaining remission. Oral prednisone is effective in moderate ulcerative colitis and produces improvement within 3 weeks. Intravenous methylprednisolone is useful for inpatients with more severe ulcerative colitis. Corticosteroids also produce remission in 60–92% of cases of Crohn's disease within 7–17 weeks; however, the presence of an abscess should be excluded to minimize the risk of sepsis on therapy. Maintenance steroid therapy is ineffective in preventing recurrences in ulcerative colitis and Crohn's disease. Steroid enemas are effective in treating left-sided ulcerative colitis reliably up to the level of the mid-descending colon. Systemic absorption of steroid enemas is significant and increases the risks of long-term use.

The side-effects of corticosteroids may limit their use in IBD. Prednisone at a dose of 10mg or more taken for longer than 3 weeks may suppress the hypothalamic-pituitary-adrenal axis for 1 year after therapy is discontinued. Individuals thus treated should receive supplemental steroids for surgery or severe illness. Common side-effects of steroid therapy include increased appetite, centripetal obesity, moon facies, acne, insomnia, depression, psychosis, growth retardation (in children), increased infections, hypertension, glucose intolerance, cataracts, irreversible glaucoma, and (in rare cases) blindness. Avascular necrosis of the femoral head can produce permanent disability. Osteoporosis is a devastating side-effect that can occur with prednisone doses as low as 8–10mg per day.

Patients on long-term steroid therapy should receive supplemental calcium and vitamin D and should undergo periodic bone densitometry studies. More aggressive therapies including bisphosphonates, calcitonin, and hormonal treatments may be indicated in some cases.

Budesonide is a steroid whose systemic toxicity is diminished by rapid first-pass metabolism in the liver. Although observed less frequently than with prednisone, budesonide does suppress plasma cortisol levels. The drug is useful for inducing remission of Crohn's disease but has an undefined role in maintaining remission.

Immunomodulators

Azathioprine and 6-mercaptopurine (6-MP) are useful as steroid-sparing agents, and may be beneficial in healing fistulae in Crohn's disease. In contrast, these agents are less effective for acute IBD exacerbations because clinical responses may not be observed for 3–4 months after initiating therapy. Blood counts are monitored frequently because of the bone marrow-suppressive effects of these agents (especially leukopenia). Liver chemistry levels also are monitored to detect possible hepatotoxicity. Other side-effects of azathioprine and 6-MP include pancreatitis, infections, and allergic reactions. The therapeutic efficacy and toxicity of these drugs relate to their metabolites. These drugs are metabolized by thiopurine methyltransferase (TPMT) to the inactive metabolite, 6-methylmercaptopurine (6-MMP). Low TPMT activity increases 6-thioguanine (6-TG) production due to less drug inactivation. The therapeutic efficacy and hematological toxicity of 6-MP and azathioprine relate to serum 6-TG levels, whereas elevated 6-MMP levels correlate with hepatotoxicity. TPMT genotyping can identify individuals predisposed to drug toxicity. There is a risk of lymphoma associated with thiopurines.

Methotrexate is considered an effective alternative to 6-MP and azathioprine for induction and maintenance of remission in Crohn's disease. Prominent side-effects of methotrexate include nausea, bone marrow suppression, elevated liver chemistry levels, and a long-term risk for development of cirrhosis.

Intravenous cyclosporine is effective for severe ulcerative colitis refractory to intravenous steroid therapy. It is unclear if this approach prevents the ultimate need for colectomy in many patients; however, it may defer surgery to a time when the procedure can be elective. Oral cyclosporine has not shown convincing efficacy in Crohn's disease. In addition to an increase in serious and opportunistic infections, side-effects of cyclosporine include renal insufficiency, hypertension, paresthesias, tremor, and headache.

Antibiotics

Broad-spectrum antibiotics are important in treating suppurative complications of Crohn's disease, including abscesses and perianal disease, as well as small intestinal bacterial overgrowth from stasis proximal to a stricture. Metronidazole has efficacy for perianal Crohn's disease and may reduce disease activity in Crohn's colitis. Side-effects include peripheral neuropathy, dysgeusia, and disulfiram-like reactions. Ciprofloxacin has also shown efficacy in some patients with mild-to-moderate Crohn's disease, especially of the colon. Rifaximin has mixed outcomes in clinical trials.

Biological therapy

Infliximab is an intravenously administered mouse-human chimeric monoclonal IgG1 antibody directed against tumor necrosis factor α (TNF-α). The drug has demonstrated efficacy in treating refractory flares of Crohn's disease and ulcerative colitis. Infliximab also is useful for closing fistulae secondary to Crohn's disease and is increasingly used as maintenance therapy for patients with IBD who do not respond to or who have unacceptable toxicity from other immunosuppressive agents. Responses may also diminish with time in some patients secondary to development of anti-drug antibodies.

Other biological drugs include adalimumab and certolizumab, which are also anti-TNF therapies. Adalimumab differs from infliximab in that it is a fully humanized IgG antibody administered subcutaneously. Certolizumab pegol is a pegylated Fab' fragment targeted against TNF. Both adalimumab and certolizumab pegol have proven efficacy in patients with Crohn's disease who previously responded to infliximab but discontinued therapy due to loss of response or intolerance. Adverse events associated with biologicals include hypersensitivity reactions (rash, fever, myalgias, and arthralgias) and infectious complications (varicella zoster virus, *Candida* esophagitis, tuberculosis). It should be noted that the combination of biological agents in conjunction with 6-MP or azathioprine has been associated with γ-δ hepatosplenic T-cell lymphoma, a very rare and aggressive lymphoma seen primarily in young male patients.

Natalizumab is a humanized monoclonal antibody that binds to α-4 integrin, thereby inhibiting leukocyte migration. Prospective studies illustrate efficacy for Crohn's disease. Unfortunately, natalizumab has been associated with fatal progressive multifocal leukoencephalopathy and currently this drug is limited to patients with Crohn's disease who have failed anti-TNF therapies.

Medical management of ulcerative colitis

The medical management of ulcerative colitis depends on the extent and severity of disease. 5-ASA suppositories or corticosteroid foam may be used for proctitis. 5-ASA or steroid enemas can be given nightly for mild disease extending to 60 cm of the distal colon. Oral 5-ASA preparations also can be used for mild or moderate distal ulcerative colitis but responses are slower with these agents than with rectal therapy. Patients with refractory disease or severe distal colitis may respond to oral corticosteroids (40–60 mg daily), whereas those with very mild disease may need only antidiarrheal agents.

Mild-to-moderate cases of pancolitis are usually treated with an oral 5-ASA compound. Patients who do not respond within 6–8 weeks should receive alternative therapy. Patients with severe diarrhea, bleeding, or systemic symptoms are initially given 40 mg per day. If symptoms are controlled, the dose can be reduced by 5 mg every 1–2 weeks. If steroids cannot be withdrawn and the patient continues to take more than 15 mg prednisone per day for 6 months, steroid-sparing therapy should be initiated with 6-MP or azathioprine or a TNF antagonist.

The mainstays for treating severe ulcerative colitis are intravenous steroids (methylprednisolone 40–60 mg; hydrocortisone 200–300 mg), hydration, and parenteral antibiotics for signs of infection. Prophylaxis against venous thrombosis should be given (heparin 5000 IU three times daily or enoxaprin 40 mg subcutaneously daily). Total parenteral nutrition is provided if oral nutrition is to be withheld for a prolonged period. If there is no response within 7–10 days, infliximab or intravenous cyclosporine should be considered, in addition to surgical consultation.

The agent used to induce remission is usually the one that is required for maintenance of remission, with the exception of corticosteroids. Steroid weaning may be achieved with the addition of immunomodulators such as azathioprine, 6-MP or methotrexate. For severe or refractory disease, maintenance biological therapy has been shown to be effective.

Medical management of Crohn's disease

It is difficult to provide generally applicable guidelines for managing Crohn's disease because of the varied clinical presentations. Moreover, there is considerable debate over whether to initiate therapy with traditional drugs and treat failures with biological agents, or to start with biological agents to achieve remission as rapidly as possible. It is likely that the management of Crohn's disease will evolve during the lifecycle of this handbook; however, the algorithm proposed here is reasonable at the time of printing.

For mild ileocolonic or colonic disease, an oral 5-ASA preparation is reasonable initial therapy. Because of their relatively greater release in the small intestine, Pentasa (2 g/day increased to 4 g/day) or Asacol (2.4 g/day increased to 4.8 g/day) may be better choices for ileitis or ileocolitis. Sulfasalazine (2–4 g/day) is a reasonable first choice for colonic disease.

Oral prednisone (40–60 mg daily) may be used for moderate-to-severe Crohn's disease, and for patients who have failed to respond to 5-ASA compounds. Oral budesonide is an alternative, and has fewer systemic side-effects due to its high first-pass hepatic metabolism. Patients who have persistent symptoms despite steroids, who relapse after having achieved remission with steroids, or who relapse after steroids are reduced are candidates for biological therapy. Immunological therapy with azathioprine (2.5 mg/kg daily), 6-MP (1.5 mg/kg daily) or methotrexate (25 mg intramuscularly weekly) may also be used to induce remission, although these agents are best used for maintenance due to the prolonged time to effect. Fistulae and perianal disease are treated with immunosuppressants or biological therapy.

Severe flares of Crohn's disease should be treated with intravenous steroids or anti-TNF therapy. CT scans can identify abscesses that require radio-lographically guided or surgical drainage, and obstruction or fistulae can be evaluated using CT or magnetic resonance enterography. Fistulae are treated with antibiotics, immunomodulators, or biologicals; refractory disease should be managed surgically.

Maintenance therapy with immunosuppressive agents (azathioprine, 6-MP, or methotrexate) is indicated for patients who required steroids to achieve remission. Maintenance biological therapy is offered for steroid-resistant individuals who do not tolerate other immunosuppressives. Maintenance therapy with antibiotics, immunomodulators or biologicals are necessary for patients who have undergone multiple surgical resections.

Surgical management of inflammatory bowel disease

Urgent indications for colectomy in ulcerative colitis include perforation, toxic megacolon, refractory fulminant colitis in the absence of dilation, and severe hemorrhage. Nonurgent indications include failure of medical therapy, dysplasia, carcinoma, and severe drug side-effects that prevent adequate medication regimens. For ulcerative colitis, colectomy cures the colonic disease and many but not all of the extraintestinal manifestations. Uveitis, pyoderma gangrenosum, and colitic arthritis usually respond to colectomy, whereas ankylosing spondylitis and sclerosing cholangitis do not.

A colectomy, mucosal proctectomy, with ileal pouch–anal canal anastomosis is the procedure of choice for most patients with uncomplicated ulcerative colitis who undergo colectomy, because it preserves normal continence. In this operation, the colon is completely removed, and the mucosa and submucosa are dissected and removed from the rectum. A pouch is constructed from the distal 30 cm of ileum and sewn to the dentate line. Complications include incontinence, intractable diarrhea, infection, or anastomotic breakdown. In severely ill patients an ileostomy may be performed with proctocolectomy in a one-stage or two-stage (colectomy and ileostomy followed by proctectomy) procedure. Complications of an ileostomy include stomal prolapse, retraction, herniation, and stenosis.

In contrast to ulcerative colitis, surgery does not cure Crohn's disease. Thus, the extent and frequency of resections should be minimized. Indications for surgery in Crohn's disease include failure of medical therapy, obstruction, fistulae, and abscess formation. Stricturoplasty represents an alternative to resection for Crohn's strictures. For extensive colitis with rectal involvement, total proctocolectomy with an ileostomy is the procedure of choice. Subtotal colectomy with ileoproctostomy is only for patients with absolutely normal rectums.

Complications and their treatment

Toxic megacolon refers to the condition in which signs of systemic compromise (fever, tachycardia, leukocytosis and anemia) accompany colonic dilation and colitis. Medical therapy consists of nasogastric suction, intravenous steroids and broad-spectrum antibiotics. Fluid and electrolyte replacement should be aggressive because electrolyte disturbances may contribute to impaired colonic motor function. A successful medical response is defined by improvement within 24–48 h in signs of toxicity and reduction in colonic diameter on abdominal radiography. If there is no improvement within 48 h, colectomy should be performed because of the high risk of perforation.

Broad-spectrum antibiotics with percutaneous or surgical drainage are indicated for abscesses in Crohn's disease. After the abscess has been drained and the inflammation subsides, resection of the affected bowel usually is required. Strictures are a common complication of Crohn's disease, which can be managed by endoscopic dilation or surgery. Surgical excision also is required for fistulae that are proximal to strictures.

Specific therapies are indicated for selected extraintestinal manifestations of IBD. Colitic arthritis usually responds to corticosteroid therapy. Pruritus secondary to sclerosing cholangitis may respond to cholestyramine. Ursodeoxycholic acid decreases liver chemistry abnormalities in sclerosing cholangitis but does not alter the the natural history, which may require liver transplantation.

Complications of IBD may involve other organ systems. Osteoporosis or osteopenia occurs in up to half of IBD patients from malabsorption, malnutrition, smoking, persistent inflammation, and steroid use. Oxalate renal stones form with ileal Crohn's disease because of intralumenal calcium binding by malabsorbed fatty acids. Other urological complications include urinary tract infection resulting from fistulae, ureteral obstruction caused by localized inflammation, and renal amyloidosis. Pyoderma gangrenosum, a discrete ulcer with a necrotic base usually found on the lower extremities, occurs in 1–5% of patients with ulcerative colitis and less frequently in Crohn's disease. Lesions almost always develop during a bout of acute colitis. Erythema nodosum appears as raised, tender nodules found usually over the anterior surface of the tibia, and is particularly common in children with Crohn's disease. The lesions respond well to treatment of the intestinal disease. Sweet syndrome (acute febrile neutrophilic dermatosis) also is associated with IBD. Uveitis is an inflammation of the anterior eye chamber resulting in blurred vision, headache, eye pain, photophobia, and conjunctival irritation. Episcleritis is characterized by scleral injection and burning eyes. Uveitis may respond to local steroids and atropine. Topical steroids also are beneficial for episcleritis. Deep vein thrombosis, pulmonary emboli, and intracranial and intraocular thromboembolic events may result from clotting factor activation and thrombocytosis.

Surveillance for colonic neoplasia (see also
Chapter 30)

Patients with ulcerative colitis have an increased likelihood of developing colon carcinoma. Risk factors for colon cancer in ulcerative colitis include younger age at diagnosis, increased duration and extent of disease, sclerosing cholangitis, backwash ileitis, and a family history of colon cancer. In contrast to the normal population, development of colon cancer in ulcerative colitis does not follow the standard progression of adenoma to carcinoma. Thus, surveillance programs are designed to detect premalignant dysplasia in mucosal areas that appear no different from surrounding regions. Areas of special concern are dysplasia-associated lesions or masses, which are nodular, or raised colonic regions that are malignant in 40% of cases. The usual approach to surveillance of pancolitis is colonoscopy every 1–3 years beginning 8–10 years after diagnosis and taking four biopsy specimens every 10 cm of colon. If high-grade dysplasia is found and confirmed by an experienced pathologist, colectomy should be performed. The approach to low-grade dysplasia is more controversial, and an informed discussion should be undertaken with the patient about the risks and benefits of continued surveillance versus colectomy. For left-sided colitis, some have recommended deferring surveillance until 15–20 years after diagnosis.

The incidence of colon cancer in patients with Crohn's colitis is clearly higher than that in the general population. The risk for extensive Crohn's colitis appears to be similar to that of ulcerative pancolitis; thus a surveillance strategy similar to that for ulcerative colitis has been advocated for extensive Crohn's colitis.

Key practice points

- Treatment of IBD depends on the location, extent, and severity of disease.
- Mild disease may be treated with 5-ASA compounds; however, Crohn's disease does not respond as well as ulcerative colitis to these agents.
- Topical and systemic steroids are the mainstay of treatment in moderate-to-severe disease, transitioning to immunomodulators or biologicals for maintenance therapy.
- Biological therapy is generally reserved for refractory disease; however, consideration of "top-down" therapy, initiating treatment with biologicals, is an emerging concept for patients with Crohn's disease.

CHAPTER 30
Colonic Neoplasia

Colorectal cancer is the second leading cause of cancer death in the United States. Screening with fecal occult blood testing or flexible sigmoidoscopy has been proven to reduce colorectal cancer incidence and mortality. Most colorectal cancers arise from neoplastic polyps and the colonoscopic removal of these polyps has also been shown to reduce colorectal cancer incidence and mortality. Although several histopathological types of colonic polyps exist, over 90% are adenomatous or hyperplastic (Table 30.1).

Adenomatous Polyps

Clinical presentation

Three-quarters of the polyps detected by colonoscopy are adenomas. The prevalence of adenomas is higher in men than in women and increases with age. The overall prevalence of adenomas in the United States has been estimated to be about 40%, though recent studies utilizing high-definition videocolonoscopy suggest the lifetime prevalence may exceed 50%.

Adenomatous polyps generally do not cause symptoms unless they are larger than 1 cm; consequently most polyps are detected during screening examinations or during evaluation for symptoms unrelated to the polyps. When symptomatic, the most common manifestations include rectal bleeding (overt and occult), change in bowel habits, abdominal pain, and rectal prolapse. Large villous adenomas may be associated with a syndrome of profuse watery diarrhea and volume depletion. Polyps will occasionally autoamputate, which causes rectal bleeding. The physical examination of a patient with colonic adenomas is often unrevealing. Digital rectal examination may detect polyps in the distal 7–10 cm of the rectum.

Yamada's Handbook of Gastroenterology, Third Edition. Edited by Tadataka Yamada and John M. Inadomi.
© 2013 John Wiley & Sons, Ltd. Published 2013 by John Wiley & Sons, Ltd.

Table 30.1 Classification of colorectal polyps according to tissue plane and pathology

Epithelial		
Neoplastic	Nonneoplastic	Submucosal
Premalignant (adenomas)	**Inflammatory**	Lymphoid collection
Tubular	Hyperplastic	Pneumatosis cystoides intestinalis
Tubulovillous		Colitis cystica profunda
Villous		Lipoma
Low-grade dysplasia		Carcinoid
High-grade dysplasia (intraepithelial		Metastatic lesions
carcinoma)		Hemangioma
Serrated		Fibroma
		Endometriosis
		Leiomyoma
Malignant (carcinomas)	**Hamartoma**	
Carcinomatous or malignant	Juvenile	
polyp	Peutz–Jeghers	

Source: Yamada T et al. (eds) *Textbook of Gastroenterology*, 5th edn. Oxford: Blackwell Publishing Ltd, 2009.

Although colonic adenomas are premalignant lesions, the proportion that progresses to adenocarcinoma is unknown. Older literature reporting the long-term follow-up of patients with polyps that had been identified but not removed suggested that the risk of developing adenocarcinoma from a 1 cm polyp was 3% at 5 years, 8% at 10 years, and 24% at 20 years after diagnosis. Both the rate of growth and the malignant potential of individual polyps vary substantially. Serial examinations over several years illustrate that many polyps remain stable or even regress. The difference between the mean age at diagnosis of colonic adenoma and at diagnosis of adenocarcinoma leads to an estimate of the mean time of progression from adenoma to colorectal cancer of about 7 years. Since the lifetime cumulative incidence of colorectal cancer is about 4–6% in western countries, it is estimated that only about 1 in 20 adenomas progresses to malignancy.

Diagnostic investigation

Laboratory studies

The results of laboratory studies usually are normal in patients with colonic adenomas. Intermittent bleeding from large polyps may produce a positive result on a fecal occult blood test or may lead to iron deficiency anemia. Large secreting villous adenomas may cause electrolyte abnormalities.

Radiographic studies

Research shows that double-contrast barium enema radiography detects only 50% of colonic polyps over 1 cm in size, with a specificity of 85%. Air insufflation enhances mucosal detail and exposes polyps, which appear as intralumenal protrusions coated with barium or as discrete rings with barium collected at their bases or along the stalks of pedunculated polyps. The rectosigmoid region is often difficult to visualize, even by experienced radiologists. Therefore, flexible or rigid sigmoidoscopy is necessary for complete evaluation of the colon. Barium enema radiography does not afford the capability to obtain histological specimens; thus colonoscopy is required when a barium study suggests the presence of a colonic polyp. Computed tomography colonography (CTC) technology has been progressing rapidly, and can now be performed with contrast tagging of stool to allow for digital subtraction of intraluminal contents. CTC has been shown to have a 90% sensitivity for polyps 1 cm in size or larger with a specificity of 86%. However, to optimize performance, experienced radiologists and state-of-the-art software and hardware are needed.

Endoscopic studies

Colonoscopy is the procedure of choice if the clinical presentation suggests that a patient has a colonic polyp. Colonoscopy possesses the highest sensitivity and specificity of any diagnostic modality for detecting adenomatous polyps, and it also allows for biopsy and removal of polyps, thereby fulfilling a therapeutic role. However, colonoscopy is not infallible. Studies of patients undergoing two colonoscopies within a short time demonstrate that 22% of polyps are missed. Although methods to distinguish polyp histology during colonoscopy are being studied, it is not yet possible to reliably distinguish polyp subtypes by endoscopic appearance alone. Therefore, histopathological analysis is the definitive diagnostic test. It also informs assessment of future risk of colorectal cancer.

Diagnostic pitfalls

Colonoscopy has long been considered the "gold standard" for the evaluation of neoplasia in the colon. However, several studies have demonstrated that colonoscopy often misses small polyps and even large polyps and cancer can be missed. While colonoscopy reduces the risk of cancer for up to 10 years, the protection is not absolute, particularly for right-sided colorectal cancer. This may results from a variety of factors, including technical issues (e.g. failure to reach the cecum or to identify polyps, incomplete polypectomy or poor bowel preparation) or biological factors (e.g. fast-growing polyps).

Histological evaluation

Adenomas are classified by their dominant histology. Tubular adenomas are the most common (85%); tubulovillous adenomas (10%), villous adenomas (5%), and serrated adenomas (hyperplastic intermingled with adenomatous features,

1%) account for the remainder. In general, the risk of high-grade dysplasia or invasive adenocarcinoma correlates with the size of the polyp and the degree of villous architecture.

Management and prevention

Endoscopy and surgery

Most adenomatous polyps can be removed by endoscopic polypectomy using either a snare (with or without electrocautery) or biopsy forceps. Most polyps can be completely removed in a single resection, and the intact polyp can be examined histologically to confirm the absence of adenomatous tissue at the resection margin. Large, broad-based, sessile polyps may require saline injection to lift the polyp, followed by piecemeal snare resection. In general, polypectomy is safe; the major complication rate is less than 2%. If endoscopic removal of large or multiple polyps is not possible, laser ablation, argon plasma coagulation, or surgical resection may be necessary. The safe removal of large, sessile polyps sometimes requires surgery.

Because synchronous polyps are common (50%) in patients with adenomatous polyps, a patient with a documented colonic adenoma should undergo a colonoscopic examination of the entire colon. Similarly, the prevalence of recurrent (metachronous) polyps warrants a surveillance program of follow-up colonoscopies to detect the development of new polyps before they progress to adenocarcinoma. The data from the National Polyp Study suggest that the recurrence rate for metachronous polyps is about 10% per year. Polyps with high-grade atypia and multiple polyps have a higher recurrence rate. Current recommendations advise surveillance colonoscopy every 3 years if three or more adenomas are removed or if any polyp is over 1 cm in size or contains villous histology or high-grade dysplasia. A 5–10-year interval is appropriate if 1–2 small (<1 cm diameter) adenomas are found. More frequent surveillance is advised when there is doubt about the adequacy of the polyp resection or if the patient has multiple (e.g. >10) neoplasms.

Malignant polyps

Colonic adenomas with severe atypia or noninvasive carcinoma do not metastasize because there are no lymphatic channels above the muscularis mucosae. These lesions are cured by colonoscopic polypectomy. When malignant cells penetrate the muscularis mucosae, the polyp is considered an invasive carcinoma. In this case, the decision to perform colonoscopic resection only or surgical resection is based on the characteristics of the malignant polyp. Poor prognostic features include the presence of incomplete endoscopic resection, a poorly differentiated carcinoma, a carcinoma within 2 mm of the polypectomy margin, venous or lymphatic invasion, sessile (not pedunculated) morphology, or extension beyond the base of the polyp stalk. Surgical resection of the under-lying bowel is recommended if one or more of these features is present. Pedunculated polyps that can be completely resected and that lack all high-risk features may be treated with polypectomy alone. All patients with malignant polyps who are treated with polypectomy alone should have surveillance colo-noscopy within 1–3 months and at 1 year.

Chemoprevention

Nonsteroidal anti-inflammatory drugs (NSAIDs) including aspirin have been associated with reduced incidence and mortality from colorectal cancer. Several NSAIDs including sulindac and celecoxib have been shown to effectively decrease the incidence of recurrent adenomas in patients with familial adeno-matous polyposis. However, the US Preventive Services Task Force recommends against the use of aspirin or NSAIDs for the primary prevention of colorectal cancer due to concerns about potential harms.

Familial Adenomatous Polyposis

Familial adenomatous polyposis (FAP), also known as adenomatous polyposis coli (APC) or familial polyposis coli, is an autosomal dominant disease character-ized by the early onset of hundreds or thousands of intestinal polyps with an inevitable progression to colon cancer. FAP is one of many known polyposis syn-dromes (Table 30.2). Three adenomatous polyposis syndromes are variants of FAP: Gardner syndrome, attenuated adenomatous polyposis coli (attenuated FAP), and Turcot syndrome.

Clinical presentation

Gastrointestinal polyposis

Patients with FAP usually develop adenomatous polyps in adolescence or young adulthood, but colonic adenomas have been reported as early as age 4 and as late as age 40. Polyps often carpet the colon and number in the hundreds to thousands, but they rarely produce symptoms until late in the course of disease. Patients not previously identified as having FAP may present with rectal bleeding, diarrhea, and abdominal pain in the third and fourth decades, at which time they likely harbor colon cancer. Cancer is diagnosed at the mean age of 39, and more than 90% of patients develop cancer by age 50. Patients with attenuated FAP often have fewer polyps, and the onset of adenomas and progression to adenocarcinoma is delayed by 10 years. Differentiating these patients from patients with hereditary nonpolyposis colorectal cancer (HNPCC) may be difficult, but the presence of duodenal polyps or extraintestinal features of FAP may be helpful clues.

Table 30.2 Polyposis syndromes

Syndrome	Gene mutation	Risk for colorectal cancer	Histology	Distribution	Extraintestinal features
Familial adenomatous polyposis	*APC* (regulator of Wnt signaling)	100%	Adenomatous	Stomach, small intestine, colon	Desmoid tumors, epidermoid cysts, fibromas, osteomas, CHRPE, dental abnormalities
Peutz–Jeghers syndrome	*STK11* (*LKB1*) (regulator of apoptosis through p53)	39%	Hamartomatous	Stomach, small intestine, colon	Orocutaneous melanin pigment, other malignancies (pancreatic, breast, ovarian, uterine, lung)
Juvenile polyposis	*SMAD4* (*DPC4*), *BMPR1A* (regulators of TGF-β signaling)	9–68%	Hamartomatous	Stomach, small intestine, colon	Macrocephaly, hypertelorism
Cowden syndrome	*PTEN* (regulator of cell cycling, translation, and apoptosis)	Minimal	Juvenile, lipoma, inflammatory, ganglioneuroma, lymphoid hyperplasia	Esophagus, stomach, small intestine, colon	Facial trichilemmomas, oral papillomas, multinodular goiter, fibrocystic breast, other malignancies (thyroid, breast, uterine)
Hereditary mixed polyposis syndrome	Chromosome 6	Unknown	Atypical juvenile, adenomatous, hyperplastic	Colon	None
Gorlin syndrome	*PTCH* (regulator of TGF-β and Wnt signaling)	Unknown	Hamartoma	Gastric	Mandibular bone cysts, pits of palms and soles, macrocephaly, basal cell carcinoma

CHRPE, congenital hypertrophy of the retinal pigment epithelium; TGF, transforming growth factor.

Gastric polyps are present in 23–100% of patients with FAP. If present, they usually are numerous, asymptomatic, located in the proximal fundus or body, and have a hamartomatous (nonneoplastic, fundic gland) histology. Adenomatous polyps of the stomach occur in 10% of patients with FAP, usually in the antrum but occasionally in the body or fundus.

Duodenal polyps occur in 50–90% of patients with FAP, and in contrast to gastric polyps, they usually are adenomatous. These polyps tend to be multiple, developing in the periampullary region, where they may rarely cause biliary obstruction or pancreatitis. The lifetime risk of developing cancer from duodenal adenomas is 3–5%. Cancer develops most commonly in the periampullary region and is one of the most common causes of death in patients with FAP who have undergone prophylactic colectomy. Adenomas may also develop in the jejunum (50%) and ileum (20%), but malignant transformation is rare.

Extraintestinal manifestations

Gardner syndrome is a subtype of FAP with characteristic extraintestinal manifestations. Desmoid tumors are benign mesenchymal neoplasms that occur throughout the body but frequently in the mesentery and other intra-abdominal regions. These masses may infiltrate adjacent structures or compress adjacent visceral organs or blood vessels, producing abdominal pain. Abdominal examination may demonstrate a mass lesion. Osteomas are benign bony growths that occur throughout the skeletal system but most commonly involve the skull and mandible. They have no malignant potential and generally do not cause symptoms. Dental abnormalities include dental cysts, unerupted teeth, supernumerary teeth, and odontomas. These lesions are benign and generally cause no symptoms.

Cutaneous lesions associated with FAP include epidermoid cysts, sebaceous cysts, fibromas, and lipomas. Epidermoid cysts are located on the extremities, face, and scalp. Fibromas most commonly occur on the scalp, shoulders, arms, and back. Infected cysts may cause symptoms.

Congenital hypertrophy of the retinal pigment epithelium (CHRPE), or pigmented ocular fundus lesion, affects 60–85% of patients with FAP. This retinal abnormality is characterized by hamartomas of the retinal epithelium, which appear as multiple, discrete, round or oval areas of hyperpigmentation. Although the pathogenesis of CHRPE remains unknown, the presence of multiple lesions in both eyes is essentially pathognomonic for FAP.

Turcot syndrome is characterized by adenomatous polyposis in association with central nervous system malignancies, such as medulloblastomas, astrocytomas, and ependymomas, which usually manifest within the first two decades of life. Neurological surveillance may be indicated for persons at risk of developing FAP, especially in families with Turcot syndrome. Two-thirds of those with Turcot syndrome have *APC* mutations, but the remaining one-third appears to have a variant of HNPCC. Cerebellar medulloblastoma develops in those with the HNPCC-like form at a rate 90 times higher than that in the general population.

Diagnostic investigation

Screening and surveillance

Genetic testing for FAP is performed to confirm a suspected diagnosis of FAP, to identify the mutation in a patient with known FAP, and to screen relatives of a proband with established FAP. Children who carry mutated genes should be screened by endoscopy. Because polyps are distributed throughout the colon in FAP, flexible sigmoidoscopy is considered an adequate screening procedure. Screening should begin at age 10–12 and continue every 1–2 years until age 35. After that, the examination interval can be increased to 3 years. If genetic testing is unsuccessful or unavailable, all relatives should be screened by endoscopy. If the diagnosis of FAP is established, patients should be screened every 1–3 years for synchronous duodenal adenomatous polyps, supplementing a forward-viewing endoscope with a side-viewing duodenoscope to assess the periampullary region.

Relatives of a proband with attenuated FAP require screening by colonoscopy because this syndrome produces fewer polyps that may spare the colon examined by sigmoidoscopy. Screening for these persons should be initiated at an age 10 years younger than the earliest age at which colon cancer is diagnosed within the family.

Radiographic studies

Radiological tests are not recommended for imaging the colon of patients with suspected FAP. However, bone radiography may be required to document the sclerotic lesions characteristic of osteomas to establish a diagnosis of Gardner syndrome. Patients with Gardner syndrome who complain of abdominal pain or in whom a palpable mass is detected are best examined by computed tomographic (CT) scanning to evaluate for intra-abdominal desmoid tumors. CT or magnetic resonance imaging scans of the brain can identify malignancies in the central nervous system of patients with Turcot syndrome.

Management and prevention

Therapy for colonic polyposis

Patients with FAP may initially have only a few polyps but the number and size of adenomas gradually increase over several years. Left untreated, patients with FAP invariably develop colon adenocarcinoma at a mean age of 39, and more than 90% develop cancer by age 50. After the diagnosis of FAP is established, elective surgery to remove the colon is recommended. Sulindac, which promotes polyp regression in a subset of patients, may be useful if surgery is delayed. Before surgery, all patients should undergo colonoscopy to survey the colon for gross evidence of malignancy. In addition, upper gastrointestinal endoscopy with a side-viewing duodenoscope and barium radiography of the small intestine should be performed to exclude concurrent malignancy in the small intestine and to remove accessible small polyps.

The surgical options for FAP include total proctocolectomy with ileostomy, total colectomy with ileal pouch–anal canal anastomosis, and subtotal colectomy with ileorectal anastomosis. In the last procedure, the rectal stump remains at risk of developing adenomatous polyps and cancer, and surveillance sigmoidoscopy is required every 3–6 months. Sulindac may slow the progression of adenomatous polyps in the retained rectal mucosal segment but does not obviate the need for surveillance and endoscopic ablation of incident rectal adenomas. Up to 30% of patients who undergo subtotal colectomy eventually require completion of the rectal resection because of the inability to control polyps or to prevent progression to cancer. This has prompted many clinicians to consider a continence-sparing colectomy with ileal pouch–anal canal anastomosis as the procedure of choice.

Therapy for duodenal neoplasms

Progression of duodenal adenoma to adenocarcinoma, particularly periampullary cancer, occurs in 3–5% of patients with FAP, usually at an age later than colonic malignancy (mean age at diagnosis is between 45 and 52). The optimal treatment for adenomatous duodenal polyps is undefined, though endoscopic approaches are appropriate for selected individuals. It is not known if sulindac alters the natural course of duodenal adenomas.

Therapy for extraintestinal manifestations

Occasionally, extraintestinal tumors are a source of symptoms in patients with FAP. Desmoid tumors in Gardner syndrome invade or compress blood vessels, nerves, and hollow viscera, and account for 10% of deaths in FAP. Patients with small asymptomatic lesions should be observed but patients with enlarging or symptomatic desmoids should be given tamoxifen or sulindac. Failure of this conservative treatment may necessitate chemotherapy, radiation therapy, or surgery.

Colorectal Adenocarcinoma

Clinical presentation

Colorectal cancer is the second leading cause of death from cancer in the United States. More than 143,000 cases of colorectal cancer are diagnosed annually in the US, resulting in nearly 52,000 deaths per year. Most colorectal cancers are diagnosed in patients older than age 50. Colorectal cancer generally grows slowly, and symptoms or signs are due to complications of obstruction, hemorrhage, local invasion, or cancer cachexia. Approximately 15% of patients present with acute complications of colorectal cancer, including severe pain, obstruction, perforation, and bleeding. Colonic obstruction develops most commonly in the transverse, descending, and sigmoid colons where lumenal diameters are smaller than the proximal colon. Incomplete colonic obstruction may present initially with intermittent abdominal pain. However, as obstruction becomes complete, nausea, vomiting, distension, and obstipation may occur.

Colorectal adenocarcinomas bleed as a result of tumor friability and ulceration. Although most bleeding is occult, hematochezia occurs in a minority of patients. Patients with tumors in the distal colon are more likely to have hematochezia or a positive result on a fecal occult blood test (FOBT) as the presenting feature, whereas patients with right-sided colonic lesions are more likely to present with iron deficiency anemia.

Local invasion of tumor into adjacent structures may produce tenesmus (rectum), or pneumaturia, recurrent urinary tract infections, and ureteral obstruction (bladder). A patient may present with an acute abdomen if the tumor causes colonic perforation. Fistulae may develop between the colon and stomach or small intestine. Malignant ascites results from local tumor extension through the serosa, with peritoneal seeding. Advanced metastatic disease to the liver may be characterized by abdominal pain, jaundice, and portal hypertension.

A wasting syndrome consisting of anorexia with muscle and weight loss may occur that appears to be out of proportion to tumor burden. The cause of this metabolic disorder may stem from the systemic effects of mediators such as tumor necrosis factor.

Diagnostic investigation

Diagnostic testing for colorectal cancer should be separated into the evaluation of patients with symptoms or signs consistent with colorectal cancer, including patients with positive results on FOBTs, and the screening of asymptomatic populations to decrease mortality from colorectal cancer.

Evaluation of symptomatic patients
Laboratory studies
Results of laboratory tests may be normal or may indicate an iron deficiency anemia. Liver chemistry abnormalities raise the possibility of hepatic metastases. The serum level of carcinoembryonic antigen (CEA) is elevated in most but not all cases of colorectal adenocarcinomas. A baseline CEA level should be obtained in a patient diagnosed with colorectal cancer as a reference for comparison with levels obtained after treatment to assess for incomplete tumor resection or recurrence. However, because many conditions cause nonspecific elevations of CEA, measuring the CEA level is not reliable as a primary screening test.

Endoscopic studies

Patients with symptoms suggestive of colonic obstruction, bleeding, or invasion should undergo diagnostic evaluation to exclude colorectal cancer. Colonoscopy is the procedure of choice because of its superior accuracy in detecting colonic neoplasms and because biopsies and endoscopic polypectomy can also be performed. The sensitivity of colonoscopy for detecting small malignancies is superior to barium enema radiography, and exceeds 90% for neoplasms larger than 1 cm. If colorectal cancer is diagnosed in the distal colon, it is imperative to visualize the entire colon because there is a 5% incidence of synchronous malignancies. The major complication rate (e.g. perforation and hemorrhage) of colonoscopy is approximately 1 in 200 cases.

Radiographic studies

Double-contrast barium enema radiography can detect most colon cancers if performed by experienced personnel. Technical limitations may preclude adequate imaging of the rectosigmoid region; therefore, if barium enema radiography is chosen to evaluate a patient with suspected colonic adenocarcinoma, flexible sigmoidoscopy should be performed to exclude a neoplasm in this region. The sensitivity of barium enema radiography is highly dependent on the skill of the radiologist; diagnostic misinterpretation is common in inexperienced hands. In addition, many patients cannot comply with the changes in body position necessary for an adequate examination. When colorectal malignancy is diagnosed, an abdominal CT scan is recommended to exclude hepatic metastases. Similarly, chest radiography may be required to exclude pulmonary dissemination.

Management and prevention

The prognosis in colorectal cancer can be estimated by the tumor stage. The 5-year survival rates for colorectal adenocarcinoma by stage are stage I 93%, stage II 74–85%, stage III 44–83%, stage IV 8%. Other features correlate with the natural history of patients with colonic adenocarcinoma. Poorly differentiated and mucinous tumors are associated with a poor 5-year survival rate, and each comprises about 20% of all colonic adenocarcinomas. Despite the predictive value of tumor stage, there is no evidence that the size of the tumor mass is an independent predictor of survival.

Except for colonoscopic removal of malignant polyps with favorable prognostic features, the only reliable method for curing colorectal adenocarcinoma is surgical resection. A right hemicolectomy is indicated for tumors in the cecum, ascending colon, and transverse colon; lesions in the splenic flexure and descending colon are treated with a left hemicolectomy. Sigmoid and proximal rectal malignancies can be removed with a low anterior resection. Localization and staging of rectal tumors are critical because lesions that invade the muscularis propria require an extensive abdominoperineal resection with colostomy, whereas lesions confined to the submucosa may be amenable to a sphincter-sparing transanal resection. Transrectal ultrasound can be used to determine the depth of invasion. Solitary hepatic metastases or a small number of lesions localized to one hepatic lobe may also be surgically removed. Aggressive surgical resection of hepatic metastases can result in a 25–35% 5-year disease-free survival rate. Those hepatitis metastases that are not amenable to surgical resection may be treated with ablative therapy, such as intra-arterial chemoembolization or radiofrequency ablation. It is not known if resecting a solitary pulmonary metastasis improves survival.

One-third of patients who undergo surgical resections with curative intent will develop recurrent disease. Adjuvant chemotherapy is used in an attempt to reduce the postoperative recurrence of colorectal cancers. Based on its location beneath the peritoneal reflection, rectal cancer is considered separately with regard to the need for adjuvant therapy. Several studies have reported decreased pelvic recurrences and improved survival with adjuvant therapy for rectal carcinoma. Preoperative (neoadjuvant) chemotherapy and radiation therapy for patients with unresectable rectal tumors may sufficiently decrease the tumor size to make resection possible.

Management of unresectable disease

Despite the presence of distant metastatic disease, palliative resection should be considered for patients with colonic lesions because untreated colonic adenocarcinoma is associated with a high incidence of obstruction. If resection is deferred until symptoms of obstruction develop, operative morbidity and mortality can be excessive. Endoscopic placement of self-expanding metal stents or fulguration of the tumor with laser ablation may palliate rectal cancer in patients who are not operative candidates.

Therapy for patients with extensive metastatic disease in the liver and other sites is rapidly evolving, necessitating that healthcare providers continually review the primary medical literature for the latest treatment strategies. Biological agents that interrupt cellular pathways (e.g. bevacizumab) have been available since 2004. These agents are used in combination with traditional adjuvant chemotherapy agents (e.g. irinotecan, 5-fluorouracil and leucovorin) and have been demonstrated to prolong survival.

Prevention through colorectal cancer screening

Given the prevalence of colorectal cancer, the presence of an identifiable precursor lesion (adenomatous polyp) that, when treated, alters the natural history of the disease, and screening tests that have been proven to improve patient outcomes, colorectal cancer screening is strongly recommended. Screening strategies include the FOBT, flexible sigmoidoscopy, combinations of FOBT with sigmoidoscopy colonoscopy, and CTC (also known as "virtual colonoscopy"). The most accessible screening test is the FOBT. The two most commonly used approaches to detect occult blood in the stool are the guaiac-based FOBT (e.g. Hemoccult II) and the fecal immunochemical test (FIT). In the guaiac-based FOBT (gFOBT), colorless guaiac is converted to a pigmented quinone in the presence of peroxidase activity and hydrogen peroxide. Because hemoglobin contains peroxidase activity, the addition of hydrogen peroxide to the guaiac reagent transforms the slide to a blue color. The sensitivity of Hemoccult II for detecting colorectal malignancy ranges from 50% for a single test to 70% for six tests performed over 3 days. Although the false-positive rate is less than 1%, the low prevalence of colonic adenocarcinoma in healthy populations reduces the positive predictive value to less than 10%.

These performance characteristics can be modified by dietary factors. Ingestion of red meats or peroxidase-containing legumes may increase the false-positive rate, particularly with rehydrated slides. Although iron supplements do not result in activating the color indicator, the dark color of the stool may be misinterpreted as a positive test by an inexperienced processor. High doses of antioxidants (e.g. vitamin C) may interfere with guaiac oxidation to quinone and result in false-negative results. For these reasons, patients should be counseled to avoid ingesting red meats, peroxidase-containing legumes, and vitamin C several days before testing. Newer gFOBT (e.g. Hemoccult SENSA) have been developed to increase the sensitivity though the specificity of the test is lower, resulting in more false-positive results.

The FIT test uses a specific antibody to detect human globin, thereby avoiding the need for any dietary modification prior to screening. Since globin is rapidly degraded by digestive enzymes, the FIT is selective for occult bleeding of colorectal origin and many available FIT tests require only a single fecal sample each year (compared to three for the gFOBT). Studies comparing FIT to gFOBT have demonstrated improved adherence and overall improved sensitivity and specificity.

Prospective controlled studies have confirmed the efficacy of an annual FOBT in reducing the mortality from and incidence of colorectal adenocarcinoma. A 33% reduction in colon cancer mortality among subjects screened annually with a FOBT was seen in a large trial. Unfortunately, patient adherence to screening programs using FOBTs is less than 40%. Two prospective studies have shown that screening flexible sigmoidoscopy reduces colorectal cancer mortality by 26–31% and colorectal cancer incidence by 21–23%. Large-scale, randomized, controlled studies of colonoscopy are now under way. Small randomized studies, prospective cohort studies, and retrospective case–control studies estimate that screening colonoscopy reduces the incidence of colorectal cancer by 50–90% and decreases mortality from colorectal cancer by about 60%. These studies estimate that the protective effect of endoscopic procedures lasts up to 10 years. Recent studies have demonstrated that colonoscopy offers greater protection against colorectal cancer in the distal colon than the proximal colon, likely related to a combination of biological (e.g. microsatellite unstable tumors in the proximal colon) and technological factors (e.g. more difficult to see sessile polyps in the proximal colon).

The sensitivity of CTC for detecting colonic lesions varied widely when compared to conventional colonoscopy in several large prospective studies. It is likely that variation in the methods of performing virtual colonoscopy, including the colonic preparation, use of contrast agents, and interpretation based on primary two-dimensional or three-dimensional reconstruction, form the basis of the discrepancy. CTC has not been recommended by the US Preventive Services Task Force due to lack of information about the relative risks and benefits. Fecal DNA testing is available, though results from large-scale studies have been disappointing. Further developments in this test are ongoing.

Recommendations for screening average-risk asymptomatic populations

The US Preventive Services Task Force has recommended routine screening for colorectal neoplasia in adults with average risk between the ages of 50 and 75. Screening between ages 76 and 85 is not routinely recommended and screening is not recommended over age 85. Specific screening recommendations are shown in Table 30.3. Patients with positive screening results obtained through noncolonoscopic strategies should be further evaluated by colonoscopy to diagnose

Table 30.3 US Preventive Services Task Force recommendations for colorectal cancer screening

Population	Adults age 50–75 years	Adults age 76–85 years	Adults >85 years
Recommendation	Screen with high-sensitivity FOBT, sigmoidoscopy or colonoscopy	Do not screen routinely	Do not screen
	For all populations, evidence is insufficient to assess the benefits and harms of screening with CT colonography and fecal DNA testing		
Screening test intervals	**Intervals for recommended screening strategies** • Annual screening with high-sensitivity FOBT • Sigmoidoscopy every 5 years, with high-sensitivity FOBT every 3 years • Screening colonoscopy every 10 years		
Implementation	Focus on strategies that maximize the number of individuals who get screened Practice shared decision making; discussions with patients should incorporate information on test quality and availability Individuals with a personal history of cancer or adenomatous polyps are followed by a surveillance regimen, and screening guidelines are not applicable		

CT, computed tomography; FOBT, fecal occult blood test.
Source: www.uspreventiveservicestaskforce.org/uspstf/uspscolo.htm.

neoplasia and perform polypectomy. A diagnosis of adenomatous polyps typically necessitates surveillance.

Priniciples of prevention through surveillance

As opposed to screening, which is defined as the use of tests to detect prevalent disease in an average-risk population, patients at high risk of developing adeno-carcinoma of the colon undergo surveillance, which is defined as the use of repeated tests to detect incident disease in a high-risk population. The guidelines for surveillance of patients with adenomatous polyps and persons at risk of polyposis syndromes are discussed above.

Patients with a family history of colorectal cancer in a single first-degree relative have a 75–80% increase in the risk of cancer, compared to patients who have no history of colorectal cancer. Persons with multiple first-degree relatives or with one first-degree relative younger than age 60 with colon cancer are at higher risk and should be considered for surveillance colonoscopy 10 years earlier than the earliest age at onset of colon cancer in the family or at age 40, whichever comes first. The subsequent surveillance procedures and intervals are then tailored according to the extent of the family history, though every 5 years is recommended by the US Multi-Society Task Force. Patients with a family history that suggests HNPCC or attenuated familial adenomatous polyposis may require annual or biennial colonoscopy.

Surveillance should be considered for first-degree relatives of a patient diagnosed with HNPCC, also known as Lynch syndrome (Table 30.4). The cause of HNPCC is a mutation in one of the DNA mismatch repair genes. Individuals with germline MMR gene mutations develop microsatellite instability in the DNA of colorectal neoplasia. Patients may be diagnosed with HNPCC by detecting mutations of the mismatch repair genes in circulating lymphocytes or in tumor cells. Even if the Amsterdam II criteria are not fulfilled, detection of the familial clustering of colon cancers or other Lynch syndrome malignancies should prompt consideration of molecular genetic testing of the affected patient to identify relatives who should undergo surveillance colonoscopy. The clinical guidelines for microsatellite instability testing of colorectal tumors (revised Bethesda criteria) are shown in Table 30.5. The initial colonoscopy in such relatives should be performed every 1–2 years, starting at age 20–30, and annually after 40 years of age.

Table 30.4 Amsterdam II criteria for the diagnosis of hereditary nonpolyposis colorectal cancer (HNPCC)

1. Three or more relatives with histologically verified HNPCC-associated cancer (colorectal, endometrial, small bowel, ureter, or renal pelvis), one of whom is a first-degree relative of the other two: familial adenomatous polyposis should be excluded.
2. HNPCC-associated cancer involving at least two successive generations.
3. One or more cancer cases diagnosed before the age of 50.

Table 30.5 Revised Bethesda guidelines for microsatellite instability testing of colorectal tumors

1. Colorectal cancer diagnosed in a patient less than 50 years of age.
2. Presence of synchronous or metachronous colorectal, or other HNPCC-associated tumors, regardless of age.*
3. Colorectal cancer with the MSI-H[†] histology[‡] diagnosed in a patient less than 60 years of age.
4. Colorectal cancer diagnosed in one or more first-degree relatives with an HNPCC-related tumor, with one of the cancers being diagnosed under age 50 years.
5. Colorectal cancer diagnosed in two or more first- or second-degree relatives with HNPCC-related tumors, regardless of age

*Colorectal, endometrial, stomach, small bowel, ovarian, pancreas, ureter and renal pelvis, biliary tract, and brain (usually glioblastoma) cancers, and sebaceous gland neoplasms (carcinomas, adenomas) and keratoacanthomas.
[†]MSI-H, microsatellite instability-high; tumors with changes in two or more of the five National Cancer Institute-recommended panels of microsatellite markers.
[‡]Presence of tumor-infiltrating lymphocytes, Crohn's-like lymphocytic reaction, mucinous/signet ring differentiation, or medullary growth pattern.
Source: Umar A, Boland CR, Terdiman JP, et al. Revised Bethesda Guidelines for hereditary nonpolyposis colorectal cancer (Lynch syndrome) and microsatellite instability. J Natl Cancer Inst 2004;96:261; with permission from Oxford University Press.

Those with germline mutations should have colonoscopy annually. If a cancer is found, subtotal colectomy with ileorectal anastomosis is the appropriate therapy, followed by annual surveillance of the rectal stump.

Patients who survive curative therapy for colorectal adenocarcinoma should undergo periodic colonoscopic surveillance. If complete colonoscopy was performed prior to surgery, then surveillance is recommended at 12 months to evaluate for anastomotic recurrence. Otherwise, colonoscopy is recommended within 3–6 months postoperatively. Subsequently, the surveillance program depends upon the findings. If no polyps are found, then surveillance is recommended in 3 years and then every 5 years thereafter. Rectal cancer surveillance may be considered every 3–6 months for the first 2 or 3 years after a low anterior resection. The high risk of developing colon cancer in patients with long-standing ulcerative colitis is discussed in Chapter 29.

Colonic Lymphoma

Clinical presentation, diagnostic investigation, and management

Primary colonic lymphomas comprise 0.9–1.2% of all colonic malignancies. There is an increased incidence among patients with rheumatoid arthritis, Sjögren syndrome, Wegener granulomatosis, systemic lupus erythematosus, congenital immune deficiency syndromes, and acquired immunodeficiency syndrome (AIDS), as well as in organ transplant recipients treated with immunosuppressive therapy.

Patients usually present with nonspecific abdominal pain, weight loss, constipation, and gastrointestinal hemorrhage. On colonoscopy, tumors appear as discrete masses or, less commonly, as diffuse infiltrative lesions. Most gastric and colonic lesions can be diagnosed by biopsy. Although the optimal treatment has not been defined, most regimens include chemotherapy and radiation therapy. Surgery may be effective for localized disease, but the overall 2-year survival rate is only 40%.

Key practice points

- Colorectal cancer is the second leading cause of cancer death. However, screening with FOBT or flexible sigmoidoscopy has been proven to improve patient outcomes, including cancer incidence and mortality.

- Colorectal neoplasia is common and usually asymptomatic, though most polyps never progress to cancer.

- Colonoscopy is the procedure of choice for the investigation of suspected neoplasia.

- Colorectal cancer screening is appropriate for average-risk individuals aged 50–75 years. Those aged 76–85 should not undergo routine screening. Those over 86 should not be screened.

- Individuals with a positive colorectal cancer screening test (e.g. FOBT, sigmoidoscopy, CT colonography) should undergo evaluation with colonoscopy.

CHAPTER 31

Anorectal Diseases

Anorectal disorders are common among patients presenting to gastroenterologists and can be challenging to manage. Often, management by both gastroenterologists and surgeons is required.

Hemorrhoids

Hemorrhoids result from dilation of the superior and inferior hemorrhoidal veins that form the physiological hemorrhoidal cushion. Internal hemorrhoids arise above the dentate line in three locations – right anterior, right posterior, and left lateral – and are covered by columnar epithelium. External hemorrhoids arise below the mucocutaneous junction and are covered by squamous epithelium. Skin tags are redundant folds of skin arising from the anal verge. They may be residua of resolved, thrombosed, external hemorrhoids. The pathogenesis of hemorrhoids is believed to involve deterioration of the supporting connective tissue of the hemorrhoidal cushion, causing hemorrhoidal bulging and descent. Although it is widely believed that constipation is an important risk factor for hemorrhoids, recent studies suggest a more prominent role for diarrheal disorders.

Clinical presentation, diagnosis, and management

Patients with internal hemorrhoids may exhibit gross but not occult bleeding (rarely requiring transfusion), discomfort, pruritus ani, fecal soiling, and prolapse. First-degree hemorrhoids do not protrude from the anus. Second-degree hemorrhoids prolapse with defecation but spontaneously reduce. Third-degree hemorrhoids prolapse and require digital reduction, and fourth-degree hemorrhoids cannot be reduced and are at risk of strangulation.

Yamada's Handbook of Gastroenterology, Third Edition. Edited by Tadataka Yamada and John M. Inadomi.
© 2013 John Wiley & Sons, Ltd. Published 2013 by John Wiley & Sons, Ltd.

Most patients with new-onset bleeding should be evaluated with sigmoidoscopy or colonoscopy to confirm that the source of hemorrhage is hemorrhoidal. Most first-degree and second-degree hemorrhoids can be managed with a high-fiber diet, adequate fluid intake, possible use of bulking agents, sitz baths twice daily, and good anal hygiene. Suppositories, ointments, and witch hazel may relieve discomfort in some cases. Rubber band ligation, injection sclerotherapy with sodium morrhuate or 5% phenol, liquid nitrogen cryotherapy, electrocoagulation, or photocoagulation with lasers or infrared light are effective in treating selected patients with bleeding or other symptoms caused by first-degree, second-degree, and selected third-degree internal hemorrhoids. Surgical hemorrhoidectomy is the treatment of choice for most third-degree hemorrhoids, all fourth-degree hemorrhoids, and other hemorrhoids refractory to nonsurgical therapy. In patients with high resting anal sphincter pressures, lateral internal sphincterotomy may achieve results comparable with those of rubber band ligation.

Thrombosis of an external hemorrhoid can produce severe pain and bleeding. Most thrombosed external hemorrhoids can be managed with sitz baths, bulking agents, stool softeners, and topical anesthetics; resolution occurs after 48–72 h. If surgical evacuation or excision is required, it should be performed within 48 h of symptom onset. Symptoms of skin tags include sensation of a growth and difficulty with anal hygiene. Treatment is conservative and surgical resection is rarely needed.

Anorectal Varices

Anorectal varices are unrelated to hemorrhoids and are a consequence of portal hypertension in 45% of patients with cirrhosis.

Clinical presentation, diagnosis, and management

Anorectal varices appear as discrete, serpentine, submucosal veins that compress easily and extend from the squamous portion of the anal canal into the rectum. Massive, life-threatening bleeding may occur from the anal or rectal portion of the varix. Injection sclerotherapy, cryotherapy, rubber band ligation, and hemorrhoidectomy can be complicated by hemorrhage. Treatment by underrunning the variceal columns with an absorbable suture controls bleeding in most cases. Inferior mesenteric vein embolization and ligation have been used. Surgical or transjugular intrahepatic portosystemic shunting may ultimately be required.

Anal Fissure

An anal fissure is a painful linear ulcer in the anal canal, usually located in the posterior midline (90%) and less often in the anterior midline. Lateral fissures suggest a predisposing illness such as inflammatory bowel disease (usually

Crohn's disease), proctitis, leukemia, carcinoma, syphilis, or tuberculosis. Fissures are caused by traumatic tearing of the posterior anal canal during passage of hard stool. They may become chronic from high resting anal sphincter tone, which promotes a relative ischemia that prevents fissure healing. Reflex over-shoot anal contraction after defecation contribute to spasm and pain.

Clinical presentation, diagnosis, and management

Severe pain with scant red bleeding is the hallmark of an anal fissure. The fissure is best identified by simple inspection after spreading the buttocks. An acute anal fissure is a small, linear tear perpendicular to the dentate line. Chronic anal fissures appear as the triad of a fissure, a proximal hypertrophic papilla, and a sentinel pile at the anal verge. Patients usually respond to a high-fiber diet, the addition of bulking agents, stool softeners, topical anesthetics (e.g. benzocaine, pramoxine), and warm sitz baths. When these measures fail, agents that reduce anal pressure and increase anal blood flow, including topical nitroglycerin or diltiazem ointments, or intramuscular injection of botulinum toxin may promote fissure healing. Surgical lateral subcutaneous internal anal sphincterotomy may be necessary for some patients with chronic fissures.

Anorectal Abscess and Fistula

An anorectal abscess is an undrained collection of perianal pus, whereas an anorectal fistula is an abnormal communication between the anorectal canal and the perianal skin. Diseases associated with these disorders include hyper-tension, diabetes, heart disease, inflammatory bowel disease, and leukemia. Infection, most commonly with *Escherichia coli*, *Enterococcus* species, or *Bacteroides fragilis*, results from obstruction of anal glands as a result of trauma, anal eroticism, diarrhea, hard stools, or foreign bodies. Abscess and fistula formation may occur without primary glandular infection in patients with Crohn's disease, anorectal malignancy, tuberculosis, actinomycosis, lymphogranuloma venereum, radiation proctitis, leukemia, and lymphoma. Abscesses are classified by site of origin and potential pathways of extension. Fistulae are divided into intersphincteric, trans-sphincteric, suprasphincteric, and extrasphincteric types.

Clinical presentation, diagnosis, and management

Swelling and acute pain, exacerbated by sitting, movement, and defecation, are the main symptoms of an anorectal abscess. Malaise and fever are common. A foul-smelling discharge suggests that the abscess is spontaneously draining through the primary anal orifice. Inspection reveals erythema, warmth, swelling, and tenderness, although intersphincteric abscesses may produce only localized tenderness. Anal ultrasound and magnetic resonance imaging (MRI) can determine the location of an abscess relative to the sphincters. Anorectal abscesses require surgical drainage to prevent necrotizing infection, which carries a 50% mortality rate. Superficial perineal or ischiorectal abscesses may be drained under local anesthesia but other abscesses require surgery in an operating room. Antibiotics usually are not necessary and may mask signs of underlying suppurative infection. Broad-spectrum antibiotics are indicated for patients with diabetes, immunosuppression, leukemia, valvular heart disease, or extensive soft tissue infection. Warm sitz baths, stool-softening agents, and analgesics can minimize disease recurrence postoperatively.

Anorectal fistulae produce chronic, purulent drainage, pain on defecation, and pruritus ani. Examination may reveal a red, granular papule that exudes pus. Patients who are neutropenic may exhibit point tenderness and poorly demarcated induration. These patients have high mortality rates from disseminated infection. Multiple perineal openings suggest the possibility of Crohn's disease or hidradenitis suppurativa. Anoscopy and sigmoidoscopy are performed to locate the primary orifice at the level of the dentate line and to exclude proctitis. MRI findings predict the clinical outcome. The presence of an anorectal fistula is an indication for surgery, which involves removing the primary orifice and opening the fistulous tract with conservation of the external sphincter. Patients with Crohn's disease who have chronic fistulae may benefit from immunosuppressive therapy or antibiotics such as metronidazole or ciprofloxacin. Anti-tumor necrosis factor antibody therapy (e.g. infliximab) is effective against many refractory anal fistulae secondary to Crohn's disease. Local surgery or diversion of the fecal stream is necessary in some cases. Postoperative care is the same as that for anorectal abscesses.

Rectal Prolapse

Rectal prolapse is protrusion of the rectum through the anal orifice. The prolapse may be complete (all layers visibly descend), occult (internal intussusception without visible protrusion), or mucosal (protrusion of distal rectal tissue but not the entire circumference). Rectal prolapse in children may be idiopathic or secondary to spina bifida, meningomyelocele, or cystic fibrosis. In adults, the condition is associated with poor pelvic tone, chronic straining, fecal incontinence, pelvic trauma, and neurological disease. Defects that result from rectal prolapse include weakened endopelvic fascia, levator ani diastasis, loss of the normal horizontal rectal position, an abnormally deep pouch of Douglas, a redundant rectosigmoid colon, a weak anal sphincter, denervation of the striated muscle, and loss of the anocutaneous reflex. Disturbed sphincter function and innervation may explain the frequent reports of fecal incontinence after surgical correction of rectal prolapse.

Clinical presentation, diagnosis, and management

Patients report prolapse of tissue as well as defecatory straining, incomplete evacuation, tenesmus, and incontinence. On examination, the prolapse may be obvious when the patient is asked to sit and strain. Endoscopy or barium enema radiography excludes malignancy but may reveal a concomitant solitary rectal ulcer. Defecography is the best test to demonstrate occult prolapse. Persistently prolapsed tissue must be promptly reduced manually with or without intravenous sedation to avoid strangulation, ulceration, bleeding, or perforation. Complete rectal prolapse should be treated surgically (anterior sling rectopexy or Ripstein procedure, abdominal proctopexy with or without sigmoid resection). Perineal exercises or buttock strapping can be suggested to patients who refuse or who cannot undergo surgery. Perineal or extra-abdominal rectosigmoidectomy or diverting colostomy may be performed for elderly or debilitated patients. Occult prolapse is treated surgically if incontinence or solitary rectal ulcer is present; otherwise, conservative therapy is recommended.

Anal Stenosis

Anal stenosis results from malignancy (anal carcinoma, rectal carcinoma, invasion by urogenital malignancy) or benign conditions (prior rectal surgery, trauma, inflammatory bowel disease, laxative abuse, chronic diarrhea, radiation injury, tuberculosis, actinomycosis, lymphogranuloma venereum, congenital causes).

Clinical presentation, diagnosis, and management

Patients present with small-caliber stools, painful or resistant defecation, and bleeding. Mild strictures may respond to periodic dilation and dietary fiber supplementation; severe stenosis may require surgical anoplasty with or without lateral internal sphincterotomy.

Solitary Rectal Ulcer

Solitary rectal ulcer results from prolonged straining and difficulty initiating defecation. Ninety percent of patients have associated rectal prolapse, which is likely to be an important pathogenic factor. Patients also have higher anal pressures and thicker rectal walls that lead to increased transmural pressures during defecation.

Clinical presentation, diagnosis, and management

Patients present with fecal mucus and blood, altered bowel habits, and anorectal pain. On sigmoidoscopy, a variety of findings are seen that range from localized erythema or nodularity to multiple shallow ulcers. Typically, lesions are noted on the anterior rectal wall 7–10 cm from the anal verge. Conservative management with treatments to reduce straining and improve bowel habits is initiated. Refractory cases may benefit from surgical rectopexy or biofeedback therapy.

Fecal Incontinence

Fecal incontinence is the loss of rectal contents against one's wishes. Women, elderly individuals, and institutionalized persons are affected most often. Traumatic obstetric and surgical injuries, rectal or hemorrhoidal prolapse, and neuropathic disease may impair anal sphincter function and lead to incontinence (Table 31.1). Traumatic or neuropathic injury that leads to abnormal straightening of the

Table 31.1 Causes of fecal incontinence

Diarrhea
Fecal impaction
Irritable bowel syndrome
Anal diseases
    Anal carcinoma
    Congenital abnormalities
    Protruding internal hemorrhoids
    Rectal prolapse
    Perianal infections
    Fistulae
    Injury (e.g. surgical, obstetric, accidental)

Rectal diseases
    Rectal carcinoma
    Rectal ischemia
    Proctitis (e.g. inflammatory bowel disease, radiation therapy, infection)

Neurological diseases
    Central nervous system (e.g. cerebrovascular accident, dementia, toxic or metabolic disorders, spinal cord injury or tumors, multiple sclerosis, tabes dorsalis)
    Peripheral nervous system (e.g. diabetes, cauda equina lesions)

Miscellaneous
    Childbirth injury
    Chronic constipation
    Descending perineum
    Advanced age

anorectal angle can also cause incontinence. Other factors that predispose to fecal incontinence include loss of anal or rectal sensation secondary to neuropathy; poor rectal distension with ulcerative proctitis, radiation proctitis, or ischemia; and overwhelming diarrhea. Hypersensitivity to distension and abnormal rectal motility probably account for the incontinence often seen in patients with irritable bowel syndrome.

Clinical presentation

Partial incontinence is defined as minor soiling and poor flatus control. The elderly and those with internal anal sphincter deficiency, fecal impaction, and rectal prolapse are prone to partial incontinence. Some "leakers" have near normal sphincter pressures and experience soiling secondary to hemorrhoids or fissures. Major incontinence is the frequent loss of large amounts of stool. It is caused by neurological disease, traumatic injury, and surgical damage. Examination may reveal anal deformity, tumors, infections, fistulae, prolapsing hemorrhoids, loss of anal tone, and absence of the anal wink. The anorectal angle and puborectalis function are crudely assessed by palpating this muscle in the posterior midline during rest and voluntary squeeze.

Diagnostic investigation

Several tools assess the mechanisms of continence. Sigmoidoscopy excludes malignancy and proctitis. Anorectal manometry defines resting and maximal anal pressures, rectal compliance, and rectal sensitivity to distension. Advances in manometric technology include ambulatory monitoring and topographic characterization of sphincter pressures. Rectal compliance and sensitivity are quantified using rectal balloon inflation. Miniature probes measure thermal and electrical sensitivity of the anal canal. Electromyography assesses external sphincter and puborectalis muscle activity. Anorectal ultrasound and endoanal MRI measure sphincter muscle thickness and detect muscle defects from trauma or surgical injury. Defecography demonstrates the evacuation of a simulated barium stool and provides static and dynamic measurements of the anorectal angle, pelvic floor, and puborectalis function. Continence is tested by measuring leakage of rectally infused saline or resistance to evacuation of a solid object.

Management

Fecal incontinence often responds to a combination of interventions. Fiber therapy or opiate antidiarrheals are indicated for treating diarrhea. Anticholinergics may blunt the gastrocolonic response and reduce meal-associated incontinence. Fecal impactions are removed with enemas or by manual disimpaction. For individuals who fail these conservative measures, anal biofeedback produces success rates as high as 70% in appropriate patients. With this technique, the patient associates external anal contractions with visual cues such as manometric contractions or electrical discharges on electromyography. Similarly, biofeedback can be used to improve rectal sensation in patients with underlying neuropathy. Conditions that respond poorly to biofeedback therapy include severe organic disease with reduced rectal sensation, irritable bowel syndrome, anterior rectal resection, and prior posterior anal sphincterotomy.

Surgery is generally reserved for patients with major incontinence. Prior anal injury may be repairable with external anal sphincter repair; posterior proctopexy may be performed for complex sphincter injury, pelvic neuropathy, and loss of the normal anorectal angle. Anterior reefing procedures may be useful for women with anterior sphincter defects. Gracilis muscle transposition with or without electrical stimulation may benefit a patient with a destroyed sphincter or a congenital pelvic floor abnormality. Artificial sphincters may be implanted. Recently, sacral nerve stimulators have shown promise in reducing incontinent episodes in a range of clinical conditions. As a last resort, placing a colostomy should be considered.

Pruritus Ani

Clinical presentation

Pruritus ani is an itchy sensation of the anus and perianal skin that may result from perianal disease (fissures, fistulae, hemorrhoids, malignancy) or from residual fecal material. *Candida albicans* and dermatophyte infections appear as localized erythematous rashes but may also be present on apparently normal skin. Pinworm (*Enterobius vermicularis*) causes nocturnal pruritus ani in children and in adults exposed to infected children. Scabies (*Sarcoptes scabiei*) and pubic lice produce pruritus ani that may be associated with genital itching. Sexually transmitted diseases associated with the condition include herpes simplex, gonorrhea, syphilis, condyloma acuminatum, and molluscum contagiosum. Generalized skin conditions (e.g. psoriasis) as well as local irritants, allergens, and chemicals may produce perianal itching. Clinical experience suggests that certain dietary products such as coffee, cola, beer, tomatoes, chocolate, tea, and citrus fruits may be causative. Idiopathic pruritus ani results from a combination of perianal fecal contamination and trauma.

Diagnosis and management

Most cases of pruritus ani can be successfully managed. If identified, dermatological, infectious, and anorectal disorders should receive specific treatment (Table 31.2). A diagnosis of pinworms can be confirmed by detecting eggs on adhesive cellophane tape applied to the perianal skin early in the morning. Foods that predispose to

Table 31.2 Causes of pruritus ani

Anorectal diseases
  Diarrhea
  Fecal incontinence
  Hemorrhoids
  Anal fissures
  Fistulae
  Rectal prolapse
  Anal malignancy

Infections
  Fungal (e.g. candidiasis, dermatophytes)
  Parasitic (e.g. pinworms, scabies)
  Bacterial (e.g. *Staphylococcus aureus*)
  Venereal (e.g. herpes, gonorrhea, syphilis, condyloma acuminatum)

Local irritants
  Moisture, obesity, perspiration
  Soaps, hygiene products
  Toilet paper (e.g. perfumed, dyed)
  Underwear (e.g. irritating fabric, detergent)
  Anal creams and suppositories
  Dietary (e.g. coffee, beer, acidic foods)
  Medications (e.g. mineral oil, ascorbic acid, quinidine, colchicine)

Dermatological diseases
  Psoriasis
  Atopic dermatitis
  Seborrheic dermatitis

diarrhea or pruritus should be eliminated. The key to management in most cases rests on keeping the anal area clean and dry while minimizing trauma induced by wiping and scratching. The perianal skin should be cleansed with a moistened pad after defecation. Witch hazel or lanolin preparations can soothe irritated tissues. The area should be dried with a blow dryer or with a soft tissue using a blotting motion. Thin cotton pledgets may be needed for those with fecal discharge. Excess perspiration can be controlled with baby powder and loose cotton clothing. Healing can be facilitated by applying 1% hydrocortisone cream twice daily for no more than 2 weeks (because of atrophic effects on the skin) and zinc oxide ointment. Nocturnal pruritus may benefit from oral antihistamines (e.g. diphenhydramine). Intractable symptoms may respond to intracutaneous injections of methylene blue.

Rectal Foreign Bodies and Trauma

A variety of foreign bodies can become lodged in the rectum after insertion for medical treatment, concealment, assault, and eroticism. Foreign bodies are classified as low-lying if they are in the rectal ampulla and high-lying if they are at or proximal to the rectosigmoid junction. Rectal trauma may result from penetrating injury (e.g. gunshot), blunt trauma (e.g. motor vehicle collisions), impalement (e.g. assault), sexual activities (e.g. fist fornication), and iatrogenic injury (e.g. endoscopy, enemas, surgery).

Clinical presentation, diagnosis, and management

Anteroposterior and lateral radiographs may define the location of a foreign body and detect pneumoperitoneum, if present. Small, low-lying objects can be removed through an anoscope, whereas larger objects (e.g. vibrators) may require regional anesthesia, anal dilation, and a grasping forceps. Large, bulky items may be removed by inflating Foley catheters in the colon proximal to the object, followed by gentle traction on the catheters for careful extraction. High-lying foreign bodies are removed using spinal anesthesia and the lithotomy position. Gentle pressure on the abdomen pushes the object within the reach of forceps directed through a rigid sigmoidoscope. Laparotomy is indicated for objects that cannot be delivered distally, if abdominal distress develops, or if broken glass is present. Surgical procedures required for some cases of major rectal trauma include a diverting colostomy, presacral drain placement, rectal irrigation, and sphincter preservation.

Anal Malignancies

Several histological types of anal carcinoma have been described, including squamous cell (70–80%), basaloid or cloacogenic (20–30%), mucoepidermoid (1–5%), and small cell anaplastic (<5%) types. Patients present at a mean age of 60. Risk factors include receptive anal intercourse in men, genital or anal warts in both sexes, smoking, human immunodeficiency virus (HIV) infection, multiple sexual partners, cervical dysplasia, and immunosuppression. Human papilloma virus infection, particularly type 16, also plays a causal role. Anal adenocarcinoma may arise in anorectal fistulae. Extramammary Paget disease is a perianal glandular tumor that appears in the seventh decade as an erythematous, well-demarcated eczematoid plaque. Anal melanomas typically are large (>4 cm), nonpigmented in one-third of cases, and tend to metastasize early. Survival rates are poor. Basal cell carcinoma of the anus is characterized by rolled skin edges with central ulceration. Bowen disease is a slow-growing, squamous cell carcinoma *in situ* that manifests as red-brown scaly or crusted plaques.

Clinical presentation, diagnosis, and management

Bleeding, pain, pruritus, or palpable lymphadenopathy may be the presenting symptoms of anal cancer, although many patients are asymptomatic until the disease is detected in routine examination. At presentation, 15–30% of patients have lymph node involvement, and 10% have liver or lung metastases. The diagnosis is made by biopsy. Lesions arising from the anal canal are more aggressive, whereas those originating from the anal margin are more differentiated and less malignant. Findings that confer a poor prognosis include squamous cell tumors larger than 2 cm, basaloid or anaplastic carcinomas, sphincteric invasion, and nodal spread. Radiation therapy plus chemotherapy with 5-fluorouracil and mitomycin C cause complete tumor regression in most cases of small, non-infiltrating anal cancers, with a 5-year survival rate of 70% and preservation of sphincter function. Cisplatin-based regimens may prove superior to those containing mitomycin. Wide local excision remains a therapeutic option for some patients, although anal canal adenocarcinoma typically recurs despite resection. Surgical treatment of extramammary Paget disease includes wide local excision or radical abdominoperitoneal resection with ipsilateral groin dissection for advanced disease with nodal involvement. Surgery rarely cures anal melanoma. Resection or radiation therapy provides excellent results in treating basal cell carcinoma. Resection cures Bowen disease.

Proctalgia Fugax and Levator Ani Syndrome

Proctalgia fugax is characterized by sudden, brief episodes of severe rectal pain and is associated with irritable bowel syndrome and psychogenic disorders. In most cases, the cause is unknown. A familial internal anal sphincter myopathy has been described that causes proctalgia fugax and difficulty with defecation. The levator ani syndrome refers to aching rectal pain due to tenderness and spasm of the levator ani muscle group (ileococcygeus, pubococcygeus, puborectalis).

Clinical presentation, diagnosis, and management

Attacks of proctalgia fugax are described as intense stabbing or aching midline pain above the anus, lasting seconds to minutes, associated with an urge to expel flatus, a desire to lie on one side with hips flexed, cold sweats, syncope, and priapism. Often the attacks occur at night. Frequently, no clear precipitating cause is identified. Unproven local therapies include rectal massage, firm perineal pressure, and warm soaks or baths. Anecdotal reports claim that various medications, including amyl nitrate, nitroglycerin, salbutamol, clonidine, and diltiazem, reduce symptoms.

The pain of the levator ani syndrome is more chronic, aching, and pressure-like than that of proctalgia fugax. Defecation and prolonged sitting precipitate the pain. On examination, palpable tenderness and spasm of the levator muscles may be elicited. Treatment includes reassurance, local heat, rectal massage, muscle relaxants, electrogalvanic stimulation, and biofeedback training.

Miscellaneous Conditions

Coccygodynia is a sharp or aching pain in the coccyx that may radiate to the rectal region or buttocks and can be caused by traumatic arthritis, dislocation or fracture, difficult childbirth, or prolonged sitting. Manipulating the coccyx on examination reproduces the pain. Therapies include warm soaks, analgesics, local corticosteroid injection, and, rarely, coccygectomy. Other causes of anorectal pain include cauda equina tumors, pelvic tumors, perianal endometriosis, intermittent enteroceles, and retrorectal tumors and cysts.

Pilonidal disease is an acquired condition of the midline coccygeal skin in which small skin pits precede development of a draining sinus or abscess. In contrast to anorectal fistula or hidradenitis suppurativa, there is no communication with the anorectum. Patients, usually young men, present with a painful swelling and drainage. Definitive treatment usually is surgical. Squamous cell carcinoma may complicate the course of pilonidal disease.

Hidradenitis suppurativa is a suppurative condition of apocrine glands in the axilla and inguinoperineal regions that manifests in adolescence and young adulthood. Risk factors include obesity, acne, perspiration, and mechanical trauma. Repeated inflammation and healing produce fibrosis and draining sinus tracts, including anal and rectal fistulae. Warm, wet compresses are applied, and antibiotics are administered topically and systemically, but surgery is usually necessary.

Society guidelines

American Society for Gastrointestinal Endoscopy. The role of endoscopy in patients with anorectal disorder. Gastrointest Endosc 2010:72:1117–1123. vwww.asge.org/clinicalpractice/clinical-practice.aspx?id=352#lower

---

Key practice points

- Chronic anal fissure should be initially treated with topical nitrate or calcium channel blocker, or botulinum toxin injection.
- Lateral internal sphincterotomy is indicated for patients with chronic anal fissure in whom botulinum toxin injection fails.
- Those with symptomatic internal hemorrhoids (except fourth degree) in whom conservative management fails should be treated with band ligation.
- Solitary rectal ulcer may not be solitary or ulcerated – presentation ranges from localized erythema or nodularity to multiple shallow ulcers.

CHAPTER 32

Pancreatitis

Acute Pancreatitis

Clinical presentation

Acute pancreatitis is a clinical syndrome of sudden-onset abdominal pain and elevations in the levels of serum pancreatic enzymes caused by an acute necro-inflammatory response in the pancreas. The differential diagnosis for the etiology of acute pancreatitis is provided in Table 32.1. In the United States, more than 80% of acute pancreatitis cases are caused by binge drinking of ethanol or by biliary stones. In urban settings, most cases are associated with alcohol use whereas in suburban or rural settings, gallstones tend to be the predominant cause.

The initial symptom of acute pancreatitis is almost always abdominal pain, which is described as a deep, visceral pain that develops over several hours in the epigastric and umbilical region. Pain persists for hours to days and may radiate to the middle to lower back. Patients often are restless. Increased pain when supine prompts many patients to sit leaning forward in an effort to minimize discomfort. However, 5% of patients with acute pancreatitis present without abdominal pain.

Nausea and vomiting are present in most patients. Low-grade fever is commonly observed in uncomplicated pancreatitis but high fever and rigors suggest coexisting infection. In some cases of severe pancreatitis, the diagnosis is overlooked because of the patient's inability to report pain because of delirium, hemodynamic instability, or extreme respiratory distress.

Physical examination

Physical examination of a patient with pancreatitis may reveal several findings. Abdominal tenderness with guarding is common and usually most pronounced in the epigastric region. Bowel sounds are diminished as a result of superimposed

Yamada's Handbook of Gastroenterology, Third Edition. Edited by Tadataka Yamada and John M. Inadomi.

Table 32.1 Differential diagnosis of acute pancreatitis

Ethanol

Gallstones
   Choledocholithiasis
   Biliary sludge
   Microlithiasis

Mechanical/structural injury
   Sphincter of Oddi dysfunction
   Pancreas divisum
   Trauma
   Following endoscopic retrograde cholangiopancreatography
   Pancreatic malignancy
   Peptic ulcer disease
   Inflammatory bowel disease

Medications
   Azathioprine/6-mercaptopurine
   Dideoxyinosine
   Pentamidine
   Sulfonamides
   L-Asparaginase
   Thiazide diuretics

Metabolic
   Hyperlipidemia
   Hypercalcemia

Infectious
   Viral
   Bacterial
   Parasitic

Vascular
   Vasculitis
   Atherosclerosis

Genetic mutations
   Cationic trypsinogen (hereditary) (serine protease-1, PRSS1)
   Serine protease inhibitor, Kazal-type 1 (SPINK1)
   Cystic fibrosis transmembrane conductance regulator (CFTR)

Miscellaneous
   Scorpion bite
   Idiopathic pancreatitis
   Cystic fibrosis
   Coronary bypass
   Tropical pancreatitis

ileus. Tachycardia may be secondary to severe pain but hypovolemia is common, and severe cases may be complicated by hypotension from extravasation of fluids or hemorrhage in the retroperitoneum. Rare patients present with periumbilical (Cullen sign) or flank (Grey Turner sign) ecchymoses. Ethanol-induced pancreatitis is occasionally accompanied by signs or symptoms of alcoholic liver disease, including jaundice, hepatomegaly, ascites, and encephalopathy. It is estimated that 1% of alcoholics will have both pancreatitis and liver disease. Gallstone pancreatitis may be accompanied by jaundice caused by a retained common bile duct stone, although any severe cause of pancreatitis may be associated with jaundice that is caused by biliary obstruction from an edematous pancreas or associated fluid collection.

Diagnostic investigation

Laboratory studies

Elevated serum amylase and lipase levels are the most common abnormalities seen in laboratory studies of patients with acute pancreatitis and result from increased release and decreased renal clearance of the enzymes. Elevations greater than fivefold are virtually diagnostic of pancreatitis but disease severity does not correlate with the degree of enzyme elevation. Total serum amylase is composed of pancreatic and salivary isoforms. Salivary amylase levels increase with salivary gland disease, chronic alcoholism without pancreatitis, cigarette smoking, anorexia nervosa, esophageal perforation, and several malignancies. The pancreatic amylase isoform may also be elevated in cholecystitis, intestinal perforation, renal failure, and intestinal ischemia. Five percent to 10% of episodes of acute pancreatitis produce no increases in serum amylase and lipase levels, which are most common in underlying chronic alcoholic pancreatitis, long-term glandular destruction, and fibrosis with loss of functional acinar tissue. Hyperamylasemia has been reported in up to 40% of patients with AIDS yet clinical disease occurs in less than 10%. Macroamylasemia is characterized by persistent elevation of serum amylase levels because of decreased renal excretion of a high molecular weight macroamylase. The disorder is benign. Differentiation from pathological hyperamylasemia relies on calculating the amylase-to-creatinine clearance ratio (ACCR):

$$(\text{serum creatinine} \times \text{urine amylase}) / (\text{urine creatinine} \times \text{serum amylase}) \times 100$$

An ACCR less than 1% suggests macroamylasemia.

Serum lipase is reportedly a more specific marker of pancreatitis but mild elevations are observed in other conditions (e.g. renal failure and intestinal perforation). In pancreatitis, lipase levels may remain elevated for several days after amylase levels have normalized. Therefore, if the diagnosis is delayed, hyperlipasemia may be the only abnormal laboratory finding. A lipase-to-amylase ratio higher than 2 is reportedly specific for alcoholic pancreatitis; however, this should not replace the history and physical examination as the primary means for discerning the cause of pancreatitis.

Patients often have other laboratory abnormalities. Leukocytosis can result from inflammation or infection. An increased hematocrit may signal decreased plasma volume caused by extravasation of fluid; a decreased hematocrit may be caused by retroperitoneal hemorrhage. Pancreatic necrosis develops in about half of the patients whose hematocrit is higher than 44% when admitted to the hospital or if the hematocrit fails to decrease 24 h after admission. Electrolyte disorders are common, particularly hypocalcemia, which in part is caused by sequestration of calcium salts as saponified fats in the peripancreatic bed. Patients with underlying liver disease or choledocholithiasis may have abnormal liver chemistry levels. Bilirubin levels higher than 3 mg/dL suggest a biliary cause of pancreatitis.

Imaging studies

Ultrasound is the most sensitive noninvasive means for detecting gallstones, biliary tract dilation, and gallbladder sludge. Intralumenal gas may obscure images of the pancreas in 30–40% of patients, making ultrasound an insensitive technique for detecting the changes associated with pancreatitis. Computed tomographic (CT) scanning is superior to ultrasound for imaging the peripancreatic bed. In mild cases, the pancreas may appear edematous or enlarged. More severe inflammation may extend into surrounding fat planes, producing a pattern of peripancreatic fat stranding. CT scanning also is optimal for defining inhomogeneous pancreatic phlegmons with ill-defined margins or well-defined pseudocysts. A dynamic arterial phase CT scan can identify areas of tissue necrosis, which are at risk of subsequent infection. The magnitude of pancreatic necrosis predicts the prognosis. Given its high cost and the limited yield in evaluating mild disease, CT scanning should be reserved for patients with severe disease. Once pancreatitis has resolved, CT scanning may have a role in excluding pancreatic cancer as a cause of pancreatitis in older patients. Magnetic resonance cholangiopancreatography, which is considerably more expensive than ultrasound or CT scanning, has a sensitivity higher than 90% for detecting bile duct stones. Endoscopic ultrasound is a sensitive test for detecting persistent biliary stones and can be used to distinguish patients who may benefit from treatment with endoscopic retrograde cholangiopancreatography (ERCP). Endoscopic ultrasound also is useful for detecting small pancreatic or ampullary tumors, pancreas divisum, and chronic pancreatitis.

Endoscopic retrograde cholangiopancreatography is primarily a therapeutic tool in acute biliary pancreatitis; it has no role in diagnosing acute pancreatitis. After an acute attack has resolved, ERCP should be considered if the cause of the pancreatitis is unclear.

Management

Prognosis

The most common prognostic criteria used to assess acute pancreatitis are the Ranson criteria, which are observations made at admission and at 48 h after admission, and the simplified Glasgow criteria, which are variables measured at any time during the first 48 h after admission (Table 32.2). The prognostic accuracy of the two scales is similar. Although the Ranson criteria were developed to assess alcoholic pancreatitis, they are frequently applied to pancreatitis from other causes. If two signs or fewer are present, mortality is less than 1%; three to five signs predict a mortality rate of 5%; and six or more signs increase the mortality rate to 20%. Other factors associated with a poor prognosis include obesity and extensive pancreatic necrosis. A CT-based scoring system, measurement of serum levels of the trypsinogen activation peptide, and the APACHE II score have also been used to assess the severity of acute pancreatic damage.

Complications

Patients with severe pancreatitis may develop peripancreatic fluid collections or pancreatic necrosis; either can become infected. The role of prophylactic antibiotics in patients with severe pancreatitis is controversial, although two

Table 32.2 Prognostic criteria for acute pancreatitis

Ranson criteria	Simplified Glasgow criteria
At admission	**Within 48 h of admission**
Age >55	Age >55
Leukocyte count >16,000/µL	Leukocyte count >15,000/µL
Lactate dehydrogenase >350 IU/L	Lactate dehydrogenase >600 IU/L
Glucose >200 mg/dL	Glucose >180 mg/dL
Aspartate aminotransferase >250 IU/L	Albumin <3.2 g/dL
	Calcium <8 mg/dL
	Arterial PO$_2$ <60 mmHg
	Serum urea nitrogen >45 mg/dL
48 h after admission	
Hematocrit decrease >10%	
Serum urea nitrogen increase >5 mg/dL	
Calcium <8 mg/dL	
Arterial PO$_2$ <60 mmHg	
Base deficit >4 meq/L	
Estimated fluid sequestration >6 L	

Adapted from Agarwal N, Pitchumoni CS, Sivaprasad AV. Evaluating tests for acute pancreatitis. Am J Gastroenterol 1990;85:356, and Marshall JB. Acute pancreatitis: a review with an emphasis on new developments. Arch Intern Med 1993;153:1185.

meta-analyses have concluded that prophylaxis decreases sepsis and mortality in patients with necrosis. If administered, imipenem-cilastatin, cefuroxime, and a combination of a quinolone with metronidazole are most effective for preventing infectious complications. Infections in the first 1–2 weeks usually involve peripancreatic fluid collections or pancreatic necrosis and are characterized by florid symptoms. More indolent courses are characteristic of pancreatic abscesses, which can arise several weeks after a bout of pancreatitis in well-defined pseudocysts or areas of resolving pancreatic necrosis. Gram stain and culture of fluid obtained by CT-guided aspiration is mandatory if infection is suspected. Polymicrobial, Gram-negative enteric bacteria, and anaerobic organisms are most often identified. Infected necrotic tissue and pancreatic abscesses require immediate surgical debridement, although some well-defined abscesses may be drained percutaneously. Sterile pancreatic necrosis should be managed with supportive medical care unless symptomatic or if significant clinical deterioration occurs.

Pseudocysts develop in 10% of patients with acute pancreatitis, most commonly in those with alcoholic pancreatitis. Pseudocysts can persist for several weeks, causing pain, compressing adjacent organs, and eroding into the mediastinum. Cysts more than 5–6 cm in diameter have a 30–50% risk of complications, including rupture, hemorrhage, and infection. Although most pseudocysts spontaneously resolve or decrease in size, persistent (>6 weeks) large cysts or rapidly expanding cysts should be drained using surgical, endoscopic, or percutaneous procedures. Percutaneous drainage may be complicated by formation of a pancreaticocutaneous fistula. Administration of the somatostatin analog octreotide may lower the risk of fistula formation by decreasing pancreatic secretions. Endoscopic drainage may be achieved by transpapillary stent placement or transgastric placement of a cystenterostomy. The use of endoscopic ultrasound in endoscopic drainage can decrease the risk of hemorrhage and free perforation. Rarely, pseudocysts may erode into the splenic artery and present as hemosuccus pancreaticus, a life-threatening event.

Pancreatitis may be complicated by several pulmonary processes. Mild hypoxemia is present in most patients with pancreatitis. Chest radiography may demonstrate increased interstitial markings or pleural effusions, which usually are left-sided and small but occasionally are large enough to compromise respiration. The interstitial edema occurs in the setting of normal cardiac function; the etiology is unclear. Severe adult respiratory distress syndrome requires artificial respiratory support. Multisystem organ failure develops in about 50% of patients with pancreatic necrosis and is an independent predictor of mortality.

Other systemic complications of severe pancreatitis include stress gastritis, renal failure, coagulopathy, hypocalcemia, delirium, and disseminated fat necrosis (involving bones, joints, and skin). Extension of the inflammatory process into the peripancreatic bed may produce splenic vein thrombosis, which may be complicated by development of splenomegaly, gastric varices, and gastrointestinal hemorrhage.

Therapy

Therapy for most cases of acute pancreatitis is supportive, although severe cases may require massive volume repletion with crystalloids and colloids. Early enteral feeding is recommended in patients with severe acute pancreatitis; compared to parenteral nutrition, it is less expensive and decreases infectious complications. Total parenteral nutrition should be considered for patients with pronounced ileus. Nasogastric suction is useful primarily for intractable vomiting but it is not needed in all cases. There is no evidence to support the routine use of antibiotics or somatostatin. The decision to reinitiate feeding should not be based on serum enzyme levels but rather on the clinical status of the patient. Resolution of pain and emergence of hunger reliably indicate that the patient is ready to eat in patients with mild acute pancreatitis.

Gallstone pancreatitis is managed differently from acute pancreatitis of other causes. Urgent ERCP with sphincterotomy and stone extraction reduces the complication rate and shortens the hospital stay for patients with severe gallstone pancreatitis. These procedures should be reserved for patients with severe disease or for those who fail to improve with conservative treatment. ERCP does not significantly worsen pancreatitis. Patients with mild gallstone pancreatitis should be treated conservatively; ERCP is performed after recovery to assess for retained bile duct stones. The risk of recurrent gallstone pancreatitis is up to 33%; therefore, all patients should undergo expeditious and definitive surgical therapy. For patients who are poor operative risks, endoscopic sphincterotomy without cholecystectomy is an acceptable therapeutic option.

Key practice points: acute pancreatitis

- Elevations of amylase and/or lipase greater than five times the upper limit of normal are virtually diagnostic of pancreatitis but disease severity *does not* correlate with the degree of enzyme elevation.
- Bilirubin levels higher than 3 mg/dL suggest a biliary cause of pancreatitis.
- Ultrasound is the most sensitive noninvasive means for detecting gallstones, biliary tract dilation, and gallbladder sludge.
- The severity of acute pancreatitis needs to be determined based upon clinical, laboratory, and radiological risk factors as well as the application of a severity grading system (Ranson criteria, APACHE II score, CT severity score, etc.).
- Early enteral feeding should be initiated in patients with severe acute pancreatitis.

Chronic Pancreatitis

Clinical presentation

Chronic pancreatitis causes irreversible morphological and functional damage to the pancreas. In many cases, there are intermittent flares of acute pancreatitis. The clinical distinction between acute recurrent pancreatitis, with restoration of

Table 32.3 Causes of chronic pancreatitis

Ethanol (70%)
Idiopathic (including tropical) (20%)

Other (10%)
   Hereditary
   Hyperparathyroidism
   Hypertriglyceridemia
   Obstruction
   Trauma
   Cystic fibrosis
   Autoimmune pancreatitis
   Pancreas divisum

normal pancreatic function and structure between attacks, and chronic pancreatitis may be difficult. Ethanol use accounts for most cases of chronic pancreatitis in the United States whereas in Asia and Africa, malnutrition is the major cause (Table 32.3). The prevalence of chronic pancreatitis in autopsy series is 0.04–5.0%, although it may be as high as 45% among alcoholics. Most cases are probably subclinical; only 5–10% of heavy ethanol users develop clinical pancreatitis.

Abdominal pain and malabsorption are the most common clinical features of chronic pancreatitis. Pain, which is present in 85% of patients, is likely to be caused by noxious stimulation of peripancreatic afferent nerves or increased intraductal pressure. Morphological studies show that the pancreatic nerves are larger and more numerous in patients with chronic pancreatitis. Pain typically is felt in the upper quadrants and may radiate to the back. It often is less intense while sitting forward. Patients may report steady, unremitting pain or several days of pain with pain-free intervals. Food ingestion increases the intensity of pain, leading to a fear of eating (sitophobia), which is the main cause of weight loss in early chronic pancreatitis.

Malabsorption in late chronic pancreatitis results from inadequate secretion of pancreatic enzymes. Maldigestion is the physiological defect that occurs when the exocrine function is less than 10% of normal. Steatorrhea is the initial manifestation of malabsorption; azotorrhea occurs in more advanced disease. Because the mucosal absorptive capacity is intact, voluminous diarrhea is unusual; most patients complain of bulky or greasy stools. A pattern of steatorrhea and weight loss in the absence of abdominal pain is common in idiopathic chronic pancreatitis.

Most patients eventually develop symptomatic hyperglycemia. Although insulin often is required to control symptoms, most patients are not prone to ketosis. Patients with ethanol-induced chronic pancreatitis may have symptoms of liver disease, including ascites, encephalopathy, variceal bleeding, and jaundice. Jaundice can also result from compression or stricturing of the intrapancreatic portion of the common bile duct.

Physical examination findings may be normal or there may be marked abdominal tenderness. Patients may have stigmata of chronic alcoholism including gonadal atrophy, gynecomastia, and palmar erythema. A midline mass suggests the presence of a pseudocyst or complicating neoplasm. Patients rarely have pancreatic ascites. Marked deficiencies of fat-soluble vitamins (A, D, E, and K) are seldom seen.

Diagnostic investigation

Laboratory studies

The findings of laboratory evaluation are often normal in chronic pancreatitis. Patients rarely exhibit hyperbilirubinemia and abnormal liver chemistry levels as a result of concurrent alcoholic liver disease or common bile duct stricture. Acute flares of pancreatitis may be accompanied by leukocytosis. Macrocytic anemia occurs in the rare patient with vitamin B_{12} deficiency. Coagulopathy may result from vitamin K malabsorption or alcoholic liver disease. Because azotorrhea occurs only in advanced disease, serum albumin levels usually are normal despite profound weight loss. Serum amylase and lipase levels may be slightly elevated but marked elevations, as observed in acute pancreatitis, are unusual. If exocrine function is severely impaired, serum lipase levels may be low, whereas serum amylase levels usually are normal in this setting because salivary amylase production is normal.

Assessment of pancreatic exocrine function

Numerous methods for assessing pancreatic enzyme output are available. The simplest tests are those that detect increased fat in the stool, which develops if exocrine secretion is less than 10% of normal. Steatorrhea may be detected by qualitative fecal fat tests (Sudan stain) or quantitative 72-h fecal fat measurements. In severe cases, the amount of fat excreted in the feces may approach the amount of fat ingested, which is indicative of profound reductions in pancreatic enzyme output. Such high degrees of steatorrhea are rarely observed with mucosal disease of the small intestine.

Pancreatic exocrine function is more accurately assessed by pancreatic stimulation tests after injecting secretin or cholecystokinin (CCK), or after ingesting a high protein meal, with simultaneous collection of pancreatic secretions through a catheter positioned in the distal duodenum. The collected fluid is assayed for bicarbonate (for secretin stimulation) or lipase and trypsin (for CCK stimulation). Chronic pancreatitis is characterized by decreased secretory output in response to these stimulants. Pancreatic stimulation tests may yield false-positive results in diabetes mellitus and cirrhosis, and after Billroth II gastrojejunostomy. Incomplete duodenal recovery of pancreatic juice or gastric acid inactivation of enzymes may lead to underestimation of pancreatic function. The sensitivity of pancreatic function tests for detecting chronic pancreatitis is 70–95%, which includes most patients with only mild-to-moderate pancreatic insufficiency.

The findings from a Schilling test are abnormal in chronic pancreatitis because of impaired cleavage of R protein, which prevents the binding of vitamin B_{12} to intrinsic factor. Expanding this test to include vitamin B_{12} bound to intrinsic factor can differentiate the maldigestion of R protein from the malabsorption of the vitamin B_{12}–intrinsic factor complex. Ingestion of the triglyceride ^{14}C-olein with subsequent measurement of breath $^{14}CO_2$ excretion assesses triglyceride digestion and absorption.

Structural studies

Confirming the diagnosis of chronic pancreatitis usually requires imaging studies of the pancreas. Abdominal radiography demonstrates the diagnostic finding of pancreatic calcifications in 30–40% of patients with chronic pancreatitis. This obviates the need for more expensive imaging procedures. Ultrasound has a sensitivity of 70% and a specificity of 90% for detecting chronic pancreatitis. If abdominal radiography and ultrasound fail to confirm the diagnosis, a CT scan demonstrates the architectural changes of chronic pancreatitis with a sensitivity of 80% and specificity of 90%. Findings may include duct dilation, calcifications, and cystic lesions. CT scans can also be useful in differentiating chronic pancreatitis from pancreatic carcinoma, and can reveal splenomegaly and venous collaterals resulting from splenic vein thrombosis.

Endoscopic retrograde pancreatography (ERP) provides the most detailed anatomical assessment of the pancreatic ducts. The main pancreatic duct is normal in early pancreatitis but the side branches may be dilated. Patients at this stage often have normal secretory function but occasionally the exocrine function is reduced out of proportion to the ERP findings. With more advanced disease, dilation and an irregular contour of the main pancreatic duct may be observed. Although pancreatic cancer may produce a discrete stricture of the main pancreatic duct, chronic pancreatitis often leads to multiple ductal strictures and filling defects as a result of stone formation. Brush cytology specimens obtained under fluoroscopic guidance may be used to distinguish benign strictures from malignant strictures. Endoscopic ultrasound (EUS) is also sensitive for diagnosing chronic pancreatitis. Findings on EUS that suggest the diagnosis of chronic pancreatitis include pancreatic duct stones, parenchymal calcifications, visible side branches irregular main pancreatic duct, echogenic main pancreatic duct wall, hyperechoic strands and foci, hypoechoic lobules, and cysts. Several reports suggest that this technique is equivalent to ERP; both tests exhibit sensitivities and specificities higher than 90%. Unlike ERP, EUS has no risk of inducing pancreatitis. EUS-guided fine needle aspiration can differentiate chronic pancreatitis from malignancy.

Endoscopic retrograde pancreatography and EUS are costly, invasive procedures that should be used only when less invasive procedures fail to substantiate the diagnosis of chronic pancreatitis or if a diagnostic finding such as a stricture, ductal dilation, or intraductal calculus will alter management. Advances in magnetic resonance (MR) imaging and MR cholangiopancreatography allow detailed examination of the pancreatic and biliary ducts without exposure to radiation or the use of oral or intravenous contrast agents. These techniques also can be used to direct endoscopic therapy.

Management and course

Medical therapy

Medical therapy for chronic pancreatitis focuses on relief of pain and repletion of digestive enzymes. If the patient has symptoms of maldigestion, pancreatic enzyme supplements should be taken before all meals. Steatorrhea usually is more difficult to treat than azotorrhea. At least 25,000–30,000 units of lipase per meal are necessary to provide adequate lipolysis; therefore, patients will need to take 2–10 pills with each meal, depending on the preparation.

Analgesics remain the primary means of controlling the pain of chronic pancreatitis. An initial trial of acetaminophen or nonsteroidal anti-inflammatory drugs (NSAIDs) is preferable. Patients should be cautioned about excessive doses of acetaminophen. Severe cases require opiate analgesics. Concerns over addiction should not interfere with the goal of pain relief; a strong patient–physician relationship may prevent abuse of prescribed narcotics.

The somatostatin analog octreotide inhibits pancreatic secretion and has visceral analgesic effects; thus, it might be expected to decrease pain in chronic pancreatitis. Octreotide may also have a role in managing refractory pancreatic fistulae or pseudocysts.

Nonmedical therapy

A small percentage of patients are refractory to medical measures and require more invasive procedures to control pain. Although celiac plexus neurolysis has been effective for pain control in patients with pancreatic adenocarcinoma, results in patients with chronic pancreatitis have been disappointing. Most patients experience only transient relief. Endoscopic pancreatic stone extraction, occasionally performed in conjunction with extracorporeal shock wave lithotripsy, reduces pain in 50–80% of cases. Patients with tight strictures may obtain pain relief after endoscopic balloon dilation and stent placement.

For severe debilitating pain unresponsive to medical therapy, surgical therapy is a legitimate means of restoring the quality of life to a patient with chronic pancreatitis. Patients with dilation of the main pancreatic duct are optimal candidates for pancreaticojejunostomy (modified Puestow procedure), a procedure with initial success rates of 80%. Unfortunately, many patients develop recurrent pain several years postoperatively. Patients without significant ductal dilation may require partial or subtotal pancreatectomy according to the extent of parenchymal disease. One-half of patients experience pain relief. Ketosis-prone diabetes invariably complicates subtotal pancreatectomy. Pancreatic islet cell autotransplantation at the time of the operation may prevent postoperative diabetes.

Complications

Patients with chronic pancreatitis who report severe refractory pain or worsening of pain should be evaluated for the development of a pseudocyst. Ultrasound detects many pseudocysts but a CT scan is the definitive diagnostic procedure. Pseudocysts in chronic pancreatitis usually are found in the body of the gland. They may rupture, bleed, or become infected; the risk of these complications is much lower than the corresponding risk of complications from acute pseudocysts. Cysts larger than 6 cm rarely resolve and require internal drainage using surgical or endoscopic techniques. EUS can be used to direct endoscopic drainage of mature cysts that impinge on the gastric or duodenal walls. Percutaneous CT-guided catheter drainage has proved successful in some cases, although a persistent pancreaticocutaneous fistula may develop.

Key practice points: chronic pancreatitis

- Serum amylase and lipase levels may be slightly elevated but marked elevations, as observed in acute pancreatitis, are unusual.

- The classic triad for diagnosing chronic pancreatitis includes pancreatic calcifications, steatorrhea, and diabetes mellitus but this triad is usually seen only in advanced disease.

Case studies

Case 1

A 45-year-old man presents to the emergency department with a 2-day history of severe periumbilical abdominal pain that was rapid in onset and has become progressively worse. The pain radiates to his back. He has developed severe nausea and vomiting. He denies any alcohol consumption. He does report having had intermittent episodes of right upper quadrant abdominal pain for the past year that would often occur after meals but would always resolve. On physical exam his heart rate is 120, blood pressure is 130/80, respiratory rate is 22, and temperature is 37.5 °C. The patient is alert and appears uncomfortable. Eyes show mild scleral icterus. Abdomen is tender to palpation in the periumbilical region and bowel sounds are absent. Labs are notable for a WBC 22 thousand, hematocrit (HCT) 56%, BUN 25 mg/dL, glucose 220 mg/dL creatinine 1.3 mg/dL, AST 330, ALT 370, total bilirubin 3.2, amylase 2120, and lipase 1950.

Abdominal ultrasound demonstrates a dilated common bile duct but visualization of the head of the pancreas is obscured by bowel gas. The patient is aggressively hydrated with 4 L of normal saline over a period of 8 h. A diagnosis of severe acute gallstone pancreatitis is made and the patient has early ERCP performed, at which time a 1 cm gallstone is found to be impacted at the ampulla of Vatter and is removed after performing a sphincterotomy.

Discussion: gallstone pancreatitis

- Gallstone pancreatitis should be suspected based on history of right upper quadrant abdominal pain, elevated liver function tests (especially bilirubin), and finding of dilated bile duct on ultrasound imaging.
- Early intervention with ERCP (within 24–48 h) is indicated in patients with severe acute pancreatitis or evidence of cholangitis.

Case 2

A 55-year-old man presents with 4–5 loose, oily stools per day and notes a 30 lb weight loss over the past year. He has a long history of heavy alcohol consumption; however, his alcohol consumption has decreased due to worsening abdominal pain. He has chronic midepigastric abdominal pain that is worse after meals. He has had a 30 lb unintentional weight loss over the past year which he attributes to decreased oral intake because of abdominal pain. He was also diagnosed with diabetes 1 year ago. On physical examination he has a scaphoid abdomen and has tenderness to palpation in the midepigastric region. Labs are significant for a 24-h fecal fat collection that weighs 350 g and has 35 g of fat. An abdominal radiograph demonstrates diffuse calcifications of the pancreas (Figure 32.1). The patient is prescribed pancreatic enzyme replacement therapy for his steatorrhea. He achieves some pain relief with pancreatic enzymes but continues to experience significant epigastric pain. He is prescribed amitriptyline 10 mg po before bed, which further controls his pain.

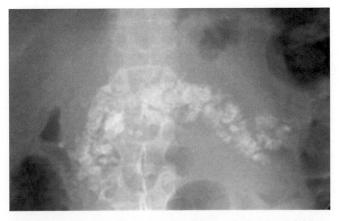

Figure 32.1 Abdominal radiograph demonstrating diffuse calcifications of the pancreas.

Discussion: chronic pancreatitis

- The classic triad to diagnose chronic pancreatitis includes steatorrhea, pancreatic calcifications, and diabetes. This triad of symptoms occurs in advanced chronic pancreatitis where <10% of the gland remains functional.

- Management of chronic pancreatitis is based on symptoms. Steatorrhea can be managed with a low-fat diet and pancreatic enzymes. Pain management can be challenging and should be performed in a stepwise fashion, beginning with pancreatic enzyme therapy, nonopioid analgesics, low-dose tricyclic antidepressants for neuropathic pain modulation, and then opioid analgesics. For patients with severe chronic abdominal pain requiring long-term narcotic use, a chronic pain specialist should be involved in the patient's management.

CHAPTER 33

Pancreatic Adenocarcinoma

Ductal Adenocarcinoma

Pancreatic ductal adenocarcinoma is the fourth leading cause of cancer motality in the United States and has a 5-year survival rate of less than 5%. Gastroenterologists play a critical role in the diagnosis and management of patients with this disease.

Clinical presentation

Most patients experience abdominal pain that often radiates to the back. The indolent onset of the pain contrasts with the acute severe pain of acute pancreatitis and cholangitis. Careful questioning of the patient often reveals that pain developed up to 3 months before the onset of jaundice. The pain of pancreatic cancer results from ductal obstruction or malignant perineural invasion. It usually is poorly localized and constant. Persistent severe pain often reflects unresectability and is associated with perineural invasion. As with other forms of pancreatic pain, the severity may be increased by lying supine and decreased by leaning forward while sitting.

Seventy percent of pancreatic adenocarcinomas occur in the head of the pancreas, and virtually all of these lesions produce obstructive jaundice. Cancers in the body or tail of the gland only rarely cause jaundice because of the anatomical spacing between the tumors and the common bile duct that courses posterior to the head of the pancreas. Jaundice in patients with tumors in the pancreatic body or tail usually results from adenopathy in the porta hepatis or extensive liver metastasis. Pruritus and pale-colored stools are common with jaundice, owing to impaired bile excretion caused by an extrahepatic biliary obstruction.

The loss of more than 10% of body weight almost invariably occurs with pancreatic cancer. Weight loss usually results from anorexia and inadequate

---

Yamada's Handbook of Gastroenterology, Third Edition. Edited by Tadataka Yamada and John M. Inadomi.

caloric intake. Sixty percent of patients with pancreatic adenocarcinoma have delayed gastric emptying, most often in the absence of mechanical gastroduodenal obstruction. Gastroparesis may be secondary to infiltration of the local splanchnic neural network and disruption of the neurohumoral mechanisms responsible for co-ordinated gastroduodenal motility. Reduced secretion of pancreatic enzymes with consequent maldigestion can also contribute to weight loss. Maldigestion is particularly prominent with tumors of the pancreatic head because obstruction of the pancreatic duct in this location results in nearly total loss of pancreatic enzyme secretion.

Diabetes mellitus is present in more than 60% of patients with pancreatic adenocarcinoma. Most patients first experience glucose intolerance within 2 years of the diagnosis of pancreatic cancer, which suggests that the malignancy causes diabetes. Enhanced secretion of islet amyloid peptide from the islets of Langerhans adjacent to the tumor is the purported cause. Elevated serum levels of this peptide produce marked insulin resistance and relative glucose intolerance.

Acute pancreatitis is the initial manifestation in 5–10% of pancreatic tumors. Adenocarcinoma of the pancreas should be considered in any older adult with acute pancreatitis unrelated to gallstones or ethanol. Duodenal obstruction caused by local invasion of the pancreatic mass occurs in 10% of patients. Obstruction is rarely a presenting feature, and it is almost always a preterminal event. Other uncommon complications include gastric variceal hemorrhage resulting from splenic vein thrombosis, major depression, and migratory superficial thrombophlebitis (Trousseau syndrome).

The physical examination of patients with pancreatic adenocarcinoma often reveals jaundice and evidence of significant weight loss. The chest and extremities may have extensive excoriations and lichenification from constant scratching because of the effects of jaundice. Tumors in the body and tail may be detected as palpable masses because they grow to enormous size before causing symptoms. With long-standing biliary obstruction, the gallbladder may become markedly distended and palpable, defining the classic Courvoisier sign.

Diagnostic investigation

Laboratory studies

At the time of clinical presentation, patients often have several laboratory abnormalities but none is specific for the diagnosis of pancreatic adenocarcinoma. Serum amylase and lipase levels may be mildly elevated but this finding is not universal, and normal levels should not preclude further testing. There may be mild elevations of liver chemistry levels and disproportionate increases in alkaline phosphatase levels. Hematological abnormalities include anemia caused by nutritional deficiencies or blood loss and thrombocytopenia caused by splenomegaly associated with splenic vein thrombosis. The tumor markers carcinoembryonic antigen (CEA) and CA19-9 are elevated in 75–85% of patients with pancreatic adenocarcinoma. Assays of these serum markers lack the specificity necessary for a reliable diagnosis and the search for better diagnostic markers is ongoing.

Imaging studies

Ultrasound has a sensitivity of 70% for identifying pancreatic cancer but overlying intralumenal gas and excess adipose tissue often compromise image quality. Even if examination of the pancreas is incomplete, ultrasound may demonstrate ancillary findings of pancreatic cancer, including dilation of the biliary tract and enlargement of the gallbladder. Computed tomography (CT) is superior to ultrasound and provides a sensitivity of 80% for detecting pancreatic masses. CT can define the tumor stage using dynamic contrast-enhanced imaging and can identify unresectable lesions with a positive predictive value of 98%. False-positive results may occur in the presence of focal pancreatitis or if normal anatomical variants are mistaken for tumors. Spiral or helical CT represents an advance in tomographic technology; image resolution is improved and imaging during the arterial and venous phases of contrast enhancement is possible. Ongoing studies should clarify whether spiral CT is superior to standard dynamic CT for detecting and staging pancreatic masses. Ultrasound and CT are used to guide needle biopsy of a pancreatic mass; however, anecdotal reports of tumor seeding along the needle track have prompted concern about performing these procedures in patients with potentially resectable tumors.

Endoscopic retrograde cholangiopancreatography (ERCP) has a sensitivity and specificity of 90% in diagnosing pancreatic malignancy. Abrupt obstruction of both a dilated common bile duct and a dilated pancreatic duct is termed the double-duct sign. This finding is virtually diagnostic of pancreatic cancer and is usually indicative of an advanced tumor in the pancreatic head. Less advanced lesions and cancers in the body or tail more often produce discrete pancreatic duct strictures. Cytological samples of a pancreatic stricture can be obtained at the time of ERCP but the yield is limited and the sensitivity is only 30–40%.

Endoscopic ultrasound (EUS) has a sensitivity of 90% for detecting pancreatic tumors. It is more sensitive than CT or ultrasound for detecting tumors smaller than 2 cm. EUS is the most accurate imaging test for staging the local extent of pancreatic tumors and is particularly useful for detecting invasion of the major splanchnic vessels. EUS-guided fine needle aspiration (FNA) of the mass can establish a cytological diagnosis of adenocarcinoma, with a sensitivity of 80–90%. Because the needle track is confined to the area of surgical resection, there is no concern for tumor seeding outside the field of resection.

Management and course

Staging

Curative surgical resection provides the only chance for long-term survival to patients with pancreatic adenocarcinoma. Unfortunately, more than 85% of patients have unresectable disease at presentation. Preoperative staging of pancreatic cancer is essential to establish the prognosis and to plan the optimal treatment strategy. As with many other cancers of the gastrointestinal tract, pancreatic tumors are staged on the basis of the TNM classification system (Table 33.1). The staging system continues to evolve and now allows for attempted curative resection in patients with superior mesenteric and even portal vein invasion (T3). Only those primary tumors involving the celiac axis and superior mesenteric artery (T4) are deemed unresectable. Most tumors involving the major splanchnic vessels cannot be resected for cure. Because splenectomy and hence splenic vein resection are often performed at the time of pancreatic cancer resection, invasion of the splenic vein does not preclude complete excision of the tumor. Although metastasis to regional lymph nodes (N1) does not preclude complete surgical excision, patients with these tumors have an unfavorable prognosis relative to patients without lymph node metastasis.

Several complementary procedures are used to define the stage of pancreatic cancer. Contrast-enhanced CT scanning is the best noninvasive means for detecting liver metastasis. Invasion of the large splanchnic vessels can be detected with a sensitivity of 30–50%. Angiography detects vascular invasion with a sensitivity of 75%. EUS has emerged as the most accurate means of detecting vascular

Table 33.1 TNM classification of pancreatic cancer

Primary tumor (T)	
T1	Tumor ≤2 cm, limited to pancreas
T2	Tumor ≥2 cm, limited to pancreas
T3	Tumor extends beyond the pancreas but does not involve the celiac axis or the superior mesenteric artery
T4	Tumor involves the celiac axis or superior mesenteric artery (unresectable primary tumor)
Regional lymph nodes (N)	
N0	No regional lymph node metastasis
N1	Regional lymph node metastasis
Distant metastasis (M)	
M0	No distant metastasis
M1	Distant metastasis

Reproduced with permission from the *AJCC Cancer Staging Manual*, 7th edition.

invasion, with a sensitivity and specificity approaching 90%. As with angiography, EUS is not a reliable method for detecting distant metastatic disease so the optimal staging strategy combines CT and EUS studies. Magnetic resonance imaging has been refined to improve the definition of the vascular anatomy of the peripancreatic bed. Ongoing studies will define the staging role of this imaging method.

Surgical therapy

Surgical exploration to perform curative resection should be attempted in all patients who have apparently resectable disease. An initial staging laparoscopy should be part of the planned resection to inspect the peritoneum and liver for evidence of distant metastases not detected on CT scans. Even when all staging procedures, including laparoscopy, indicate a resectable tumor, unresectable disease is found in 10–20% of patients after surgical dissection. Cancers localized to the pancreatic head require a pancreaticoduodenectomy – the Whipple procedure. Lesions in the body or tail can be treated with distal pancreatectomy. Alternative procedures, including total pancreatectomy and the pylorus-sparing Whipple procedure, have no proven advantage relative to standard operations In the past, operative mortality rates for curative resection averaged 10–20% but specialized centers are reporting mortality rates of 2–5%.

The poor overall prognosis for pancreatic cancer is underscored by 5-year survival rates of 10–25% for patients who undergo surgical resection. The long-term survival of patients with T1 cancers is only 35–40%; most deaths result from recurrent disease. Unfortunately, survival for 5 years does not guarantee a cure from this disease; 40% of these persons eventually die of recurrent pancreatic adenocarcinoma. Lymph node metastasis, poorly differentiated histology, and tumors larger than 2.5 cm are all associated with a poor prognosis.

Palliative therapy

Because most patients with pancreatic cancer have unresectable disease at presentation and have an expected survival of 6 months, palliation of symptoms is the primary goal. Correction of nutritional deficiencies and control of pain can be achieved with supportive measures. Malabsorptive symptoms can be alleviated with adequate pancreatic enzyme supplementation. Adequate protein and caloric intake may require enteral nutrition, given the high rate of malnutrition in these patients. NSAIDs and acetaminophen may be adequate for pain control but if pain is severe, narcotics should be administered. Narcotics may have constipating effects, necessitating the concomitant use of osmotic or stimulant laxatives. For relief of tumor-associated refractory pain, surgical or radiologically guided percutaneous injection of alcohol into the celiac ganglion is 90% effective.

Obstructive jaundice and pruritus may be treated by surgical biliary bypass or by endoscopic or percutaneous placement of a biliary stent. Endoscopic stent placement and surgical bypass are more than 90% successful in relieving biliary obstruction but surgical therapy is associated with longer hospitalizations, higher morbidities, and higher periprocedural mortality rates. Percutaneous stent placement for distal common bile duct malignant strictures has higher morbidity and mortality relative to endoscopic stent placement because of the hemorrhage and bile leaks associated with transhepatic puncture. Therefore, endoscopic placement is preferred. Unfortunately, 40% of biliary stents become obstructed with debris and sludge 5–6 months after placement. As a prophylactic measure, plastic stents often are replaced every 3–6 months to prevent cholangitis secondary to stent occlusion. Expandable metallic biliary stents have shown lower occlusion rates, and should be considered in patients who are not candidates for surgical resection.

In contrast to biliary obstruction, symptomatic duodenal obstruction is best managed surgically. This complication occurs in 10% of patients with pancreatic cancer. Gastrojejunostomy is the procedure of choice. Unfortunately, duodenal obstruction is often preterminal, and surgical intervention may be contraindicated because of the overall poor clinical status of the patient.

The role of chemotherapy and radiation therapy for patients with pancreatic cancer is limited. Combined radiation and chemotherapy may prolong survival by 2–4 months but there is often significant therapeutically induced toxicity. The chemotherapeutic agent gemcitabine slightly improves survival, reduces pain, and improves the quality of life.

Key practice points: pancreatic cancer

- Pancreatic cancer often presents as advanced disease due to lack of symptoms in early disease. Symptoms include abdominal pain radiating to the back, unintentional weight loss, and jaundice.
- CT scan should be performed for staging to evaluate for metastatic disease.
- If the tumor appears to be resectable but there appears to be possible vascular involvement, EUS should be performed for local staging.
- EUS-guided fine needle aspiration is the optimal modality for obtaining tissue diagnosis if indicated.
- Placement of a metal biliary stent should be considered for patients with unresectable tumors causing biliary obstruction.

Other Malignant and Premalignant Diseases of the Pancreas

Cystic neoplasms

Cystic neoplasms of the pancreas may be benign or malignant. These lesions must be differentiated from the pseudocysts that often complicate the course of acute and chronic pancreatitis. Cystadenomas are classified as mucinous, also termed macrocystic adenomas, and serous, also termed microcystic adenomas. The distinction is critical because serous cystadenomas have almost no malignant potential whereas mucinous cystadenomas have a high incidence of progression to cystadenocarcinoma. Both lesions occur more commonly in women; serous lesions usually are diagnosed in elderly patients, and mucinous lesions usually are diagnosed in middle-aged patients. Because mucinous lesions are larger, abdominal pain, weight loss, and vomiting are common presenting symptoms. Serous lesions are usually smaller than 4–6 cm and contain many small cysts smaller than 1–2 cm in diameter. One-third of serous lesions exhibit a characteristic stellate "sunburst" calcification, sometimes evident on abdominal radiography. In contrast, mucinous cystadenomas contain a few large cysts, and a curvilinear calcification of the cyst capsule may occur.

Despite these characteristic anatomical features, distinguishing the two neoplasms on the basis of imaging alone is difficult. CEA levels and K-RAS mutations are useful in establishing the diagnosis of mucinous cystic neoplasms but they are unable to identify presence of malignancy or risk for malignant progression. Asymptomatic serous lesions require no further therapy but all mucinous lesions should be referred for consideration of surgical resection or monitored closely. In comparison with the poor survival rate of ductal adenocarcinoma, patients with mucinous cystadenomas and cystadenocarcinomas have a 5-year survival rate higher than 50% after surgical resection.

Solid pseudopapillary neoplasms

Solid pseudopapillary neoplasms arise from the epithelium of ductules, usually in the tail of the pancreas. Most patients are adolescent girls or women in their early 20s. Tumors are often larger than adenocarcinomas and frequently exhibit a cystic appearance on CT or ultrasound studies as a result of liquefaction necrosis. Despite their large size, many tumors remain localized. Resection is associated with long-term survival.

Intraductal papillary mucinous neoplasms

Intraductal papillary mucinous neoplasms (IPMNs) are premalignant ecstatic/cystic lesions involving the pancreatic duct. They are typically classified as either main duct or side branch type. Main duct IPMN often is associated with significant dilation of the main pancreatic duct upstream of the lesion. The risk of malignancy in main duct IPMN is approximately 70% whereas the risk of malignancy in side branch IPMN is approximately 25%. Patients present with abdominal pain, weight loss, and steatorrhea. By endoscopic examination, the ampulla of Vater may be seen to release copious amounts of viscous mucus into the duodenum and have a characteristic "fish mouth" appearance. Papillary projections of dysplastic mucosa and intraductal collections of mucinous debris often produce diffuse filling defects on ERCP. At presentation, patients may have coexisting adenocarcinoma. Surgical excision is curative if the lesion is detected before carcinoma develops.

Key practice points: pancreatic cysts and ipmns

- Cysts and IPMNs are often asymptomatic at presentation and are often identified incidentally.
- Cysts and IPMNs should be evaluated with EUS fine needle aspiration for cyst fluid analysis (CEA and amylase) and cytology.
- Mucinous cyst adenomas and IPMNs have risk of malignancy.
- Main duct IPMN has a 70% risk of malignancy and should be surgically resected.

Case studies

Case 1

A 65-year-old woman presents to her physician with new-onset jaundice. She denies any abdominal pain. She does report a 10 lb unintentional weight loss over the past 3 months. She denies any nausea, vomiting, or fevers. Physical examination is unremarkable. Labs are notable for a total bilirubin 6.0 mg/dL, AST 230 U/L, ALT 180 U/L, WBC 5.0, and HCT 35%. A CT scan demonstrates a 3 cm ill-defined mass in the head of the pancreas, dilated common bile duct and intrahepatic ducts, and a dilated main pancreatic duct. There is no evidence of metastatic disease but the mass appears to be adjacent to the portal vein. EUS FNA is then performed that demonstrates the portal vein to be free from the tumor. FNA of the mass is performed, confirming the diagnosis of pancreatic adenocarcinoma. The patient has an ERCP to place a plastic biliary stent to relieve the biliary obstruction. The patient is later taken to surgery for a Whipple resection.

Discussion: pancreatic cancer

- Pancreatic head masses often present with painless jaundice.
- A CT scan should be performed to evaluate for a pancreatic head mass.
- EUS FNA is the best method to obtain tissue to confirm the diagnosis of pancreatic cancer. Tissue diagnosis is recommended since benign inflammatory masses from autoimmune pancreatitis may also present as a pancreatic head mass causing biliary obstruction and do not require resection.
- Resection of a pancreatic head mass requires a Whipple resection (pancreaticoduodenectomy).

Case 2

A 50-year-old woman is involved in a car accident and has a CT scan performed in the emergency department due to complaints of abdominal pain. There is no evidence of abdominal trauma on CT scan but a 3 cm pancreatic cyst is incidentally identified. The patient is then referred for further evaluation with EUS FNA which demonstrates a 3 cm cystic lesion without any septae or associated masses. The pancreatic duct and parenchyma are normal in appearance. FNA is performed on the cyst, revealing a clear, nonviscous fluid. Fluid analysis demonstrates a CEA <0.5 ng/dL, amylase 40 U/L, and cytology does not show any atypical cells. The patient is informed that the cyst is likely to be a benign serous cystadenoma.

Discussion: pancreatic cyst

- Pancreatic cysts are often incidentally identified on cross-sectional imaging.
- Certain pancreatic cysts have malignant potential; therefore, evaluation with EUS FNA is necessary to obtain high-resolution imaging of the cyst and adjacent tissue to evaluate for a possible mass and to aspirate the fluid from the cyst for biochemical analysis (CEA, amylase, and possibly K-RAS mutation analysis).
- IPMNs and mucinous cystadenomas have malignant potential. Serous cystadenomas are benign.

CHAPTER 34

Structural Anomalies, Tumors, and Diseases of the Biliary Tract

Biliary Cysts

Biliary cysts can occur throughout the biliary tract, involving the intrahepatic and extrahepatic bile ducts. Biliary cysts can lead to biliary complications, with some cysts having an increased risk of malignancy.

Clinical presentation

Patients with type I choledochal cysts typically present in infancy with jaundice and failure to thrive, although 20% of patients present after age 2 with intermittent abdominal pain and recurrent jaundice. Patients rarely remain asymptomatic. Cirrhosis and portal hypertension are frequent complications, particularly if the cysts present in infancy. Patients with type II cysts classically present with obstruction of the common bile duct. Seventy-five percent of patients with choledochoceles (type III cysts) present after age 20 with pain and obstructive jaundice. Pancreatitis is a complication in 30–70% of cases of choledochocele. Patients with type IV and type V cysts typically have recurrent cholangitis, liver abscesses, and portal hypertension. Caroli disease may be associated with medullary spongy kidney, which should be distinguished from autosomal dominant polycystic kidney disease. The latter disease is characterized by hepatic cysts, which are pathologically distinct from biliary cysts. Unlike biliary cysts, hepatic cysts do not communicate with the biliary tract. See Figure 34.1 for classification of biliary cysts.

Diagnostic investigation

Imaging with ultrasound or computed tomography (CT) may detect biliary cysts. However, direct visualization of the biliary system with endoscopic

Yamada's Handbook of Gastroenterology, Third Edition. Edited by Tadataka Yamada and John M. Inadomi.

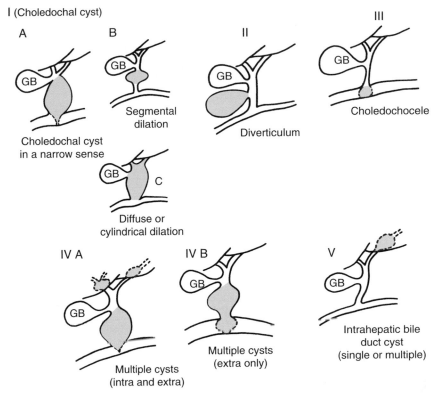

Figure 34.1 Today's classification of biliary cysts based on location. Hatched areas represent cystic dilations. (Source: Yamada T et al. (eds) *Textbook of Gastroenterology*, 5th edn. Oxford: Blackwell Publishing Ltd, 2009.)

retrograde cholangiopancreatography (ERCP) or percutaneous transhepatic cholangiography (PTC) has long been the standard for diagnosing biliary cysts. Advances in magnetic resonance imaging have made magnetic resonance cholangiopancreatography (MRCP) useful for diagnosis. Because the test is noninvasive, MRCP has replaced ERCP and PTC for initial evaluation of these patients. ERCP and PTC offer a therapeutic advantage over MRCP if stones or potentially malignant disease are suspected. Endoscopic ultrasound can provide detailed images of cyst structure, and intraductal ultrasound can evaluate malignant transformation.

Management and course

Small intraduodenal choledochoceles are best treated by endoscopic sphincterotomy but all other biliary cysts require surgical therapy. For extrahepatic cysts, excision and drainage is preferable to drainage alone because of the risks of recurrent cholangitis and malignant transformation. Resection is the preferred treatment for localized intrahepatic cysts The patient with diffuse intrahepatic cysts may require hepatic transplantation if hepatic failure or portal hypertension develops. Chronic antibiotic therapy may reduce the risk of recurrent cholangitis, particularly in Caroli disease.

In addition to cholangitis, pancreatitis (type III), biliary cirrhosis, and liver abscesses may complicate the course of disease in patients with biliary cysts. Cyst rupture during pregnancy or labor has prompted the recommendation that pregnant women with symptomatic cysts deliver by cesarean section. The most feared complication is malignant degeneration. This risk is particularly high for adult patients, as 15% develop carcinoma. Carcinoma may occur throughout the biliary tract and pancreas, including the gallbladder and sites uninvolved by the cysts. The prognosis of these tumors is dismal. Almost all patients die soon after diagnosis.

Primary Sclerosing Cholangitis

Primary sclerosing cholangitis (PSC) is a disorder of the bile ducts involving chronic inflammation leading to structuring of bile ducts and liver fibrosis. Patients with PSC have a high prevalence of ulcerative colitis (up to 90%). PSC may eventually lead to end-stage liver disease.

Clinical presentation

The onset of PSC is insidious, and it can be diagnosed when asymptomatic elevations in serum liver biochemistry values are detected. Alternatively, symptomatic patients may have progressive fatigue, pruritus, weight loss, and jaundice for an average of 2 years before a diagnosis is made. Cholangitis is uncommon and often indicates the presence of superimposed choledocholithiasis or bile duct carcinoma. Patients with associated inflammatory bowel disease are more likely to have both intrahepatic and extrahepatic ductal disease. Isolated involvement of the extrahepatic ducts is more common in patients without inflammatory bowel disease (38%) than in patients with inflammatory bowel disease (7%). A small percentage of patients with PSC have other associated immune disorders (e.g. Sjögren syndrome, hereditary acquired immunodeficiency syndromes, or the antiphospholipid antibody syndrome) (Table 34.1). PSC should be differentiated from other causes of chronic cholestasis, including primary biliary cirrhosis, autoimmune hepatitis, and recurrent pyogenic cholangitis (oriental cholangiohepatitis).

Table 34.1 Disorders associated with primary sclerosing cholangitis

Disorder	Prevalence (%)
Inflammatory bowel disease	
Chronic ulcerative colitis	50–75
Crohn's disease	<5
Immunodeficiency syndromes	
Angio-immunoblastic lymphadenopathy	Rare
Acquired immunodeficiency syndrome	Rare
Familial immunodeficiency syndromes	Rare
Miscellaneous	
Recurrent pancreatitis	4–25
Antiphospholipid antibody syndrome	Rare
Sjögren syndrome	Rare
Rheumatoid arthritis	Rare
Retroperitoneal fibrosis	Rare

Diagnostic investigation

Most patients have at least a twofold elevation of alkaline phosphatase levels, which is out of proportion to the elevations of serum bilirubin levels. Aminotransferase levels are only mildly increased. The standard technique for diagnosis is ERCP, which is preferred over PTC because of the technical difficulties of cannulating strictured intrahepatic ducts. The characteristic cholangiographic features include multifocal strictures, usually in the intrahepatic and extrahepatic ducts, with intervening normal or dilated ductal segments that produce a "string of beads" pattern. This pattern is not specific for PSC and may be seen in patients with metastatic cancer to the liver, primary biliary cirrhosis, allograft ischemic injury, and the diffuse form of cholangiocarcinoma. Differentiating cholangiocarcinoma from PSC can be difficult, especially because bile duct cancer is a potential complication of PSC. Magnetic resonance imaging is used more often in the initial evaluation of patients with suspected PSC. Liver biopsy is required for staging disease severity and determining prognosis but it is rarely diagnostic.

Management and course

Primary sclerosing cholangitis usually follows a slow, progressive course. A small subset of patients has stable disease for decades, but over years, most patients with PSC progress to portal hypertension and death caused by liver failure. The 5-year survival rate is 60–70%. Patients who present with symptomatic disease have significantly worse prognoses. Cholangiocarcinoma complicates the course of disease in 7–15% of patients with PSC; it can be difficult to diagnose in view of the cholangiographic abnormalities observed in PSC. The mean age at diagnosis of cholangiocarcinoma in these patients is 42, compared with the mean age of 66 for the general population.

The treatment of PSC patients is primarily supportive. Orthotopic liver transplantation is reserved for patients with end-stage disease, recurrent cholangitis despite medical therapy, or uncontrolled peristomal variceal bleeding. No immunosuppressive regimen has been demonstrated to slow the progression of the disease. Although ursodeoxycholic acid (ursodiol) may relieve pruritus and improve biochemical profiles, it fails to halt disease progression. Prophylactic colectomy in patients with ulcerative colitis does not alter the natural course of PSC nor does it prevent the complication of cholangiocarcinoma. Dominant symptomatic strictures may be treated with endoscopic balloon dilation and stenting. Surgical resection and biliary reconstruction may be necessary for selected patients with refractory strictures or for those who may have bile duct carcinoma.

Carcinoma of the Bile Ducts

Cholangiocarcinoma is an aggressive malignancy that arises from the epithelial cells of the bile duct. It can involve the intrahepatic or extrahepatic bile ducts and often leads to biliary obstruction.

Clinical presentation

Nonspecific symptoms of anorexia and weight loss are common in patients with cholangiocarcinoma. Jaundice develops if the extrahepatic ducts become obstructed. Pain and cholangitis are not typical symptoms unless the patient has had prior surgery or superimposed choledocholithiasis. Fifty percent of extrahepatic tumors involve the hilum of the right and left hepatic ducts (i.e. Klatskin tumor), and the other 50% involve the common hepatic duct or common bile duct. Ten percent of tumors spread diffusely throughout the biliary tract and may mimic PSC. Bile duct tumors tend to invade locally, and patients generally do not present with widely metastatic disease.

Diagnostic investigation

Initially, ultrasound should be used to evaluate patients suspected of having bile duct tumors. Intrahepatic bile duct dilation with no evidence of extrahepatic dilation suggests an extrahepatic bile duct tumor. A CT scan is more accurate in defining distal common bile duct lesions and is more sensitive than ultrasound in detecting intrahepatic lesions. The definitive imaging procedure is cholangiography by PTC or ERCP. Contrast-enhanced CT, angiography, and magnetic resonance imaging can define vascular invasion.

Histological confirmation of malignancy can be obtained by transhepatic or endoscopic cytological brushings. These tests have sensitivities of only 30–50% but show specificities approaching 100%. Because of this, cytology is useful if results are positive but of little value if negative. The addition of forceps biopsy to cytological testing increases the diagnostic yield to 70%. Many tumors are well differentiated and occur in PSC, making diagnosis very difficult without surgical resection.

Management and course

Surgical resection is the only option for long-term survival. At diagnosis, 20–30% of proximal duct tumors and 60–70% of distal duct tumors are resectable. Involvement of both the right and left hepatic lobes or invasion of the portal vein or hepatic artery indicates unresectability. The median survival time for patients who successfully undergo resection with tumor-free margins is 3 years, compared with 1 year for patients who have unresectable tumors.

Jaundiced patients with unresectable tumors should be considered for palliative biliary-enteric anastomosis. If the patient is a poor operative candidate, placement of a biliary stent during ERCP or PTC usually provides adequate drainage. Radiation therapy may also palliate symptoms and improve survival. Hepatic transplantation prolongs survival but the high incidence of recurrent disease in these patients suggests that transplantation should be done only in the setting of a research protocol.

Carcinoma of the Gallbladder

Gallbladder cancer is rare in the United States, with less than 5,000 cases annually. However, it is an aggressive malignancy associated with a poor prognosis.

Clinical presentation

The signs and symptoms of gallbladder carcinoma are nonspecific. Only 10–20% of patients have the diagnosis established preoperatively. Pain is the most common complaint but the pattern is variable. Jaundice occurs in

30–60% of patients and is a poor prognostic sign, usually indicative of an unresectable tumor. Other symptoms include nausea, vomiting, anorexia, and weight loss. Cholecystenteric fistulae are rare complications of gall-bladder tumors.

Management and course

Most patients with gallbladder tumors have stage IV or unresectable disease. The median survival time for these patients is 5 months. Patients with noninvasive stage I tumors limited to the gallbladder can be cured by simple cholecystectomy. Stage II and stage III tumors have a small chance of cure with a radical cholecys-tectomy, which involves wedge resection of the liver and regional lymphadenec-tomy. The role of chemotherapy and radiation therapy for treating gallbladder tumors has not been defined.

Key practice points: diseases of the biliary tract

- MRCP is the diagnostic method of choice for imaging suspected choledochal cysts.
- Most patients with PSC have at least a twofold elevation of alkaline phosphatase levels, which is out of proportion to the elevations of serum bilirubin levels.
- Cytological and histological diagnosis of bile duct carcinoma can be challenging.

Case studies

Case 1

A 67-year-old man presents to his physician with new-onset jaundice. He also reports a 10 lb unintentional weight loss. He denies any abdominal pain or fevers. Physical exam demonstrates the man to be jaundiced with scleral icterus. Otherwise his exam is unremarkable. Labs demonstrate a bilirubin of 9.3 mg/dL, AST 360 U/L, ALT 390 U/L, and WBC 7.5 thousand. CT scan demonstrates an ill-defined mass in the hilum of the liver with markedly dilated intrahepatic bile ducts. There is no evidence of portal vein or hepatic artery involvement. The patient is given antibiotics and ERCP is performed, demonstrating a stricture involving the common hepatic duct with no visualization of the right hepatic ducts and dilation of the left intrahepatic bile ducts. Brushings and biopsies of the stricture are obtained, followed by placement of a plastic biliary stent into the left hepatic system. Histology confirms the diagnosis of cholangiocarcinoma. Since the disease appears localized, the patient is referred to surgery for consideration of resection.

> ### Discussion: cholangiocarcinoma
>
> - The presentation of cholangiocarcinoma is often painless jaundice.
> - CT scan findings of a cholangiocarcinoma will show a hypodense lesion with upstream biliary dilation.
> - On ERCP, if both the left and right hepatic ducts are obstructed, unilateral drainage is often sufficient to normalize bilirubin and aminotransferases. If contrast is injected into the dilated system, a stent must be placed into the system to prevent cholangitis.
> - Systemic antibiotics should be administered prior to ERCP.

Case 2

A 45-year-old man with ulcerative colitis and long-standing PSC presents with worsening jaundice and pruritus. He has been feeling more lethargic and fatigued. He reports a 10 lb unintentional weight loss over the last 3 months. He denies abdominal pain, nausea, or vomiting. On exam he appears jaundice and fatigued. His abdomen is soft and nontender. Labs are notable for a bilirubin of 6.4 mg/dL, AST 260 U/L, ALT 285 U/L, alkaline phosphatase 370 U/L. Antibiotics are given prior to undergoing ERCP, which demonstrates a dominant stricture involving the common hepatic duct. Brushings and biopsies of the stricture do not demonstrate any evidence of malignancy. The stricture is balloon dilated without placement of a biliary stent.

> ### Discussion: primary sclerosing cholangitis
>
> - Patients with primary sclerosing cholangitis can present with a dominant stricture that can appear similar to cholangiocarcinoma. Biopsies and brushings of dominant strictures should be performed.
> - Symptomatic dominant strictures can be treated with endoscopic therapy including balloon dilation and/or short-term stenting.

CHAPTER 35

Biliary Tract Stones and Postcholecystectomy Syndrome

Gallstones

Gallstone-related conditions are among the most common gastrointestinal disorders requiring hospitalization. Prevalence varies widely among ethnic groups. Pima Indians, Chileans, and whites in the United States manifest the highest rates. Asians in Singapore and Thailand have exceptionally low incidences of gallstone disease. The composition of stones also varies among cultures. Cholesterol stones account for 75% of gallstones in western countries, whereas pigment or bilirubinate stones predominate in Africa and Asia. Gallstones are more prevalent in females across all age and ethnic groups.

Clinical presentation

Gallbladder stones produce a wide spectrum of clinical presentations, including episodic biliary colic, acute cholecystitis, and chronic cholecystitis. Passage of a gallstone through the common bile duct may lead to acute cholangitis or acute pancreatitis. Despite the high incidence of these complications in the general population, more than two-thirds of patients with gallstones will never develop symptoms.

Biliary colic

Most patients with symptomatic cholelithiasis present with biliary colic. This is a visceral pain that is caused by transient gallstone obstruction of the cystic duct. The pain typically is severe and episodic and lasts 30 min to several hours. The term biliary colic is a misnomer because the pain is steady and does not fluctuate in intensity. It is usually epigastric and is often referred to the right shoulder or interscapular region. During attacks, patients are restless and may have associated diaphoresis and vomiting. The interval between attacks is highly variable and may be days to years. There is no convincing evidence that ingesting fatty foods precipitates an attack of biliary colic.

Yamada's Handbook of Gastroenterology, Third Edition. Edited by Tadataka Yamada and John M. Inadomi.
© 2013 John Wiley & Sons, Ltd. Published 2013 by John Wiley & Sons, Ltd.

Acute cholecystitis

When a biliary colic attack lasts longer than 3 h or if localized right upper quadrant tenderness and fever develop, the diagnosis of acute cholecystitis should be entertained. The pain of acute cholecystitis may wane but the tenderness usually increases. A Murphy sign, the abrupt cessation in inspiration in response to pain on palpation of the right upper quadrant, is a classic finding observed in 60–70% of patients. High fever, hemodynamic instability, and peritoneal signs suggest gallbladder perforation, which is a complication in 10% of patients with acute cholecystitis. Ten percent to 15% of patients develop jaundice, which is a symptom that may be caused by gallstone obstruction of the common bile duct or by Mirizzi syndrome, which is an obstruction of the common hepatic duct caused by edema and inflammation at the origin of the cystic duct. Most patients with acute cholecystitis have had previous attacks of biliary pain.

Chronic cholecystitis

Patients with chronic cholecystitis usually have gallstones and have had repeated attacks of biliary pain or acute cholecystitis, which results in a thickened and fibrotic gallbladder. It is uncommon for the gallbladder to be palpable during an attack of pain. In fact, patients may have few symptoms referable to the gallbladder itself, presenting instead with complications such as cholangitis and gallstone pancreatitis.

Acalculous cholecystitis

There is no evidence of cholelithiasis in 5–10% of patients with acute cholecystitis. Acalculous cholecystitis occurs in critically ill patients, often with multiorgan failure, extensive burn injuries, major surgery, and trauma. Perforation is more common and the course is more fulminant.

Diagnostic investigation

Laboratory studies

Most patients with acute cholecystitis exhibit leukocytosis with a left shift. Some may have elevations in aminotransferases, alkaline phosphatase, bilirubin, or amylase caused by choledocholithiasis or cystic duct edema with resulting biliary obstruction. Patients with uncomplicated biliary colic usually have normal biochemical profiles.

Structural studies

Ultrasound is highly sensitive and specific for diagnosing cholelithiasis. In uncomplicated biliary colic, gallstones may be the only finding. Thickening of the gallbladder wall is a nonspecific finding commonly observed in acute and chronic cholecystitis. Pericholecystic fluid and intramural gas are specific ultrasonographic features of acute cholecystitis. Dilation of the intrahepatic or extrahepatic ducts suggests choledocholithiasis; however, ultrasound is insensitive for imaging common bile duct stones. ^{99m}Tc-labeled iminodiacetic scintigraphy can confirm a diagnosis of acute cholecystitis. The tracer is injected intravenously and excreted in bile. Failure to image the gallbladder within 90 min suggests cystic duct obstruction. The gallbladder cannot be visualized in 85% of patients with acalculous cholecystitis. Computed tomography (CT) may be beneficial in evaluating patients with complicated disease (e.g. perforation or gangrene).

Management and course

Most patients with gallstones remain asymptomatic but over a 20-year period, 15–25% of these asymptomatic patients develop symptoms. Once symptoms occur, there is a high risk of recurrent attacks of pain and complications such as cholecystitis, pancreatitis, and cholangitis.

Although there are many nonsurgical alternatives, cholecystectomy is the definitive treatment for symptomatic cholelithiasis. Laparoscopic cholecystectomy is favored because there are fewer wound-related complications, shorter hospital stays, and more rapid recoveries. However, the technique results in a 2–3% incidence of bile duct injuries, a higher incidence than with open cholecystectomy. Open cholecystectomy is preferred if acute cholecystitis is evident, if extensive scarring from prior abdominal surgery exists, if exploration of the common bile duct is planned, or if visualization by laparoscopy is inadequate.

Given the overall benefits of surgical therapy, dissolution therapy with chenodeoxycholic acid or ursodeoxycholic acid should be reserved for patients who are at high risk of surgery. Because of its superior side-effect profile, ursodeoxycholic acid is preferred. Small (<1.5 cm diameter) noncalcified stones that float on oral cholecystography are suitable for dissolution. Candidate patients should demonstrate adequate gallbladder filling and emptying by oral cholecystography. Dissolution often requires longer than 6 months of therapy. Response rates range from 60% to 70%. There are frequent recurrences after therapy is discontinued. Direct-contact dissolution therapy with mono-octanoin and methyl-*tert*-butyl ether is often successful in days to weeks but it has a high rate of complications and thus remains experimental.

Extracorporeal shock wave lithotripsy is 90% successful in achieving stone fragmentation and clearance of solitary, small, radiolucent stones. Most patients also require dissolution therapy. As with dissolution therapy, it may take months of extracorporeal shock wave lithotripsy to clear the gallbladder of stones. About 20% of patients experience biliary colic for several weeks after fragmentation.

Key practice points: gallstones

- Gallbladder perforation is a complication in 10% of patients with acute cholecystitis.
- Ultrasound is highly sensitive and specific for diagnosing cholelithiasis.
- Cholecystectomy is the definitive treatment for symptomatic cholelithiasis.
- Dissolution therapy with ursodeoxycholic acid should be reserved for patients who are at high risk of surgery. Small (<1.5 cm diameter) noncalcified stones that float on oral cholecystography are suitable for dissolution therapy.

Choledocholithiasis

In the United States, most bile duct stones are cholesterol stones that have migrated from the gallbladder. Ten percent to 15% of patients who undergo cholecystectomy have concomitant bile duct stones, and 1–4% exhibit residual postoperative choledocholithiasis, even after the common bile duct is explored. Conversely, more than 80–90% of patients with choledocholithiasis have gallbladder stones. The incidence of choledocholithiasis increases with age; one-third of octogenarians who undergo cholecystectomy have coexistent bile duct stones. The prevalence of choledocholithiasis and intrahepatic stones is higher in Asian societies. These populations have higher incidences of pigment stones, which usually are formed *de novo* in the bile ducts.

Clinical presentation

Unlike with gallbladder stones, most patients with bile duct stones develop symptoms. Some remain asymptomatic for decades while others present suddenly with potentially life-threatening cholangitis or pancreatitis. Patients with choledocholithiasis often present with biliary colic indistinguishable from the pain of cystic duct obstruction. The pain is steady, lasts for 30 min to several hours, and is located in the epigastrium and right upper quadrant.

Cholangitis is the result of superimposed infection in the setting of a biliary obstruction. The Charcot classic triad of right upper quadrant pain, fever, and jaundice may be present in only 50–75% of patients with acute cholangitis. Ten percent of episodes are marked by a fulminant course with hemodynamic instability and encephalopathy. Reynolds pentad refers to the constellation of the Charcot triad plus hypotension and confusion.

Diagnostic investigation

Laboratory studies

Immediately after an attack, levels of serum aminotransferases are often elevated because of hepatocellular injury. Alkaline phosphatase levels are often elevated, mildly in asymptomatic patients, and not more than five times higher than normal in symptomatic patients. Most symptomatic patients have hyperbilirubinemia; the bilirubin level is in the range of 2–14 mg/dL. Higher elevations of alkaline phosphatase or bilirubin levels suggest malignant obstruction of the biliary tree.

Structural studies

In contrast to gallbladder stones, bile duct stones are not readily detected by ultrasound; the sensitivity is less than 20%. The technological advances of helical CT scanning have led to improved accuracy in sensitivity and specificity of 80–85% in detecting bile duct stones. Endoscopic retrograde cholangiopancreatography (ERCP) is the procedure of choice for evaluating patients with suspected choledocholithiasis. ERCP has a sensitivity of 90% for diagnosing choledocholithiasis and has the advantage of facilitating therapeutic sphincterotomy and stone extraction. Endoscopic ultrasound can detect 95% or more of common bile duct stones but current instruments cannot extract stones. Magnetic resonance (MR) cholangiography has a sensitivity similar to ERCP for detecting bile duct stones. It may be used in the initial evaluation of patients for whom the index of suspicion for stones is only low or moderate, to avoid unnecessary exposure to the risks of ERCP.

There is no consensus on the optimal evaluation of choledocholithiasis in patients undergoing elective cholecystectomy for gallstone disease. If open cholecystectomy is planned, intraoperative cholangiography and common bile duct palpation can be used. If stones are found, the common bile duct should be explored and stones should be extracted. Several alternative strategies are available to patients undergoing planned laparoscopic cholecystectomy. One strategy involves minimal preoperative assessment, including ultrasound and CT scanning. An intraoperative cholangiogram is performed during the laparoscopic procedure. Those patients with documented intraductal stones undergo stone extraction laparoscopically or by open cholecystectomy. Alternatively, ERCP with endoscopic sphincterotomy could be performed postoperatively. A second strategy identifies patients preoperatively at high or low risk of coexisting choledocholithiasis on the basis of the biochemical profile and the presence or absence of biliary tract dilation on ultrasound. Patients at high risk undergo preoperative endoscopic ultrasonography or ERCP; those with confirmed biliary stones undergo endoscopic stone extraction. When the stones are cleared from the bile duct, the patient then proceeds to laparoscopic cholecystectomy. Patients with a low risk of choledocholithiasis undergo laparoscopic cholecystectomy with intraoperative cholangiography, as previously described. Benefits and risks are associated with each strategy; the approach is largely determined by the resources available at individual institutions.

Management and course

Common bile duct stones, even if asymptomatic, require therapy because of the high complication rate (e.g. cholangitis and pancreatitis). Secondary biliary cirrhosis may develop in cases of persistent biliary obstruction (i.e. >5 years). In such cases, reversal of portal hypertension and cirrhosis has been reported, suggesting that even late efforts to relieve obstruction are warranted. Definitive therapy involves common bile duct exploration and stone extraction but this procedure increases the operative mortality rate of a cholecystectomy from 0.5% to 3–4%. The perioperative mortality rate for patients younger than age 60 is 1.5%, whereas the risk for patients older than 65 is 5–10%.

On the basis of this high mortality rate, endoscopic sphincterotomy and stone extraction represent a favorable approach, especially in older patients. The risk of recurrent symptoms is high if patients have intact gallbladders; therefore, cholecystectomy should be performed. In elderly patients with severe comorbid illness, however, the surgical risks may outweigh the risk of recurrent gallstone symptoms. Endoscopic sphincterotomy alone may be an acceptable therapy for these patients. If bile duct stones cannot be extracted endoscopically, long-term internal stenting is also a therapeutic option for this high-risk group.

Young, healthy patients who have minimal operative risk factors may be treated with primary cholecystectomy and common bile duct exploration with stone extraction. The choice of endoscopic versus surgical removal of bile duct stones in this group may be determined by local expertise and resources. It is worth noting that even after surgical common bile duct exploration, 1–4% of patients have retained common bile duct stones.

Patients presenting with cholangitis or pancreatitis are treated initially with conservative measures, including parenteral fluid repletion, bowel rest, and parenteral antibiotics (for cholangitis). In patients with severe pancreatitis that progresses or fails to improve within 48 h and in patients with severe cholangitis, emergency ERCP with possible stone extraction reduces morbidity and mortality. Patients who do not pass their stones by ERCP or who have superimposed cholecystitis require emergency surgical intervention.

Key practice points: choledocholithiasis

- The Charcot classic triad consists of right upper quadrant pain, fever, and jaundice and is present in 50–75% of patients with acute cholangitis.
- ERCP is the procedure of choice for evaluating patients with suspected choledocholithiasis.
- Common bile duct stones, even if asymptomatic, require therapy because of the high complication rate (e.g. cholangitis and pancreatitis).

Postcholecystectomy Syndrome

After cholecystectomy, 20–40% of patients experience abdominal discomfort, and 2–10% have debilitating pain. Patients who do not have gallstones confirmed on surgical pathological examination are more likely to remain symptomatic after cholecystectomy. Most of these patients have functional abdominal pain but a small percentage of patients with the postcholecystectomy syndrome have symptoms originating from the biliary tract. Possible causes include retained common bile duct stones, postoperative bile duct strictures, biliary tumors, and sphincter of Oddi (SO) dysfunction. SO dysfunction is primarily a disease of women who have undergone prior cholecystectomy. The disorder is uncommon and accounts for only 5–10% of patients who present with postcholecystectomy pain. SO dysfunction is also the putative cause in 10–20% of patients with idiopathic pancreatitis.

Clinical features

Patients with SO dysfunction may manifest idiopathic pancreatitis or recurrent abdominal pain after cholecystectomy. The pain is similar to biliary colic; it is localized to the epigastrium and right upper quadrant and often radiates to the scapula.

Diagnostic investigation

Given the confounding possibility that either sludge or small gallbladder stones are the cause of symptoms, SO dysfunction can be diagnosed reliably only in patients who have undergone prior cholecystectomy. Liver chemistry profiles are obtained during an attack of pain and ultrasound is performed to exclude biliary dilation. ERCP is necessary to exclude alternative diagnoses, such as retained common bile duct stones or postoperative biliary strictures. ERCP can also assess the drainage capability of the biliary tree. The results of laboratory testing, ultrasound, and ERCP can be used to classify patients into groups with distinct probabilities of the presence of physiological SO dysfunction. Type I describes patients with biliary pain, liver chemistry values elevated to at least twice normal on two occasions, dilated common bile ducts, and delayed contrast drainage from the common bile duct during ERCP. Type II is defined by biliary pain with one or two of the above criteria, and type III includes patients with biliary-type pain but none of the other features described. The incidence of manometrically confirmed SO dysfunction is nearly 100% in type I, 50% in type II, and 25% in type III patients.

If ERCP demonstrates biliary dilation and delayed common bile duct contrast drainage (>45 min) in a patient with liver chemistry abnormalities during two previous episodes of pain, a presumptive diagnosis of SO dysfunction can be made and the patient can be treated at the time of ERCP with endoscopic sphincterotomy. Papillary stenosis rather than sphincter dyskinesia is the mechanism of dysfunction in most type I patients. SO manometry is indicated to confirm high sphincter pressures in type II and type III patients. It is performed by passing a manometry catheter into the common bile duct through a duodenoscope. The catheter is slowly withdrawn across the sphincter as basal and phasic pressures are recorded. Although many manometric abnormalities have been observed in patients with SO dysfunction, an elevated basal sphincter pressure (>40 mmHg) is the only criterion that predicts a therapeutic response to endoscopic sphincterotomy. A basal pressure higher than 40 mmHg is essential, therefore, to diagnosing SO dysfunction in type II and type III patients.

Management and course

Pharmacological therapy for SO dysfunction has been disappointing, mostly because of its inefficacy in treating the papillary stenosis variant of the abnormality and the high incidence of side-effects. The mainstay of therapy is disruption of the sphincter mechanism. Surgical sphincterotomy has a high success rate but this approach has been supplanted by endoscopic sphincterotomy, which has become the standard therapy for SO dysfunction. Sphincterotomy alleviates abdominal pain in 90% of patients with manometrically confirmed SO dysfunction. Although results of longer follow-up periods are required, 5% of patients develop restenosis.

Endoscopic sphincterotomy carries a significant complication rate, especially for patients with SO dysfunction. The incidence of post-ERCP pancreatitis in these patients is 10–20%. The incidence is higher in patients without common bile duct dilation. A temporary pancreatic duct stent, which is typically left in place for 1–5 days following the procedure, reduces the risk of ERCP-related pancreatitis in individuals with SO dysfunction. Hemorrhage and perforation are less common complications.

Key practice points: postcholecystectomy syndrome

- After cholecystectomy, 20–40% of patients experience abdominal discomfort, and 2–10% have debilitating pain.
- Papillary stenosis is the mechanism of dysfunction in most type I patients. Sphincterotomy is indicated in these patients without the need for manometry.
- SO manometry is indicated to confirm high sphincter pressures in type II and III patients.
- Endoscopic sphincterotomy carries a significant complication rate in patients with SO dysfunction.

Miscellaneous Complications of Biliary Tract Stones

Bile duct strictures

Trauma and the chronic inflammatory response induced by biliary stones can result in benign strictures of the extrahepatic bile ducts. Other common causes of benign strictures include surgical trauma, chronic pancreatitis, parasitic infection, and sclerosing cholangitis. Patients may present with cholangitis, painless jaundice, or asymptomatic elevations of alkaline phosphatase levels. Diagnosis requires direct bile duct visualization by ERCP or percutaneous transhepatic cholangiography. Given the inadequate long-term efficacy of biliary stenting, surgical decompression is the treatment of choice for benign strictures. Failure to relieve the obstruction predisposes the patient to cholangitis, stone formation, and secondary biliary cirrhosis.

Biliary fistula

The most common cause of biliary fistula formation is surgical trauma during cholecystectomy. Hepatobiliary scintigraphy can detect bile leaks and fistulae with more than 90% sensitivity. Most leaks respond to endoscopic therapy using biliary sphincterotomy and/or stenting. Most spontaneous biliary-enteric fistulae are produced by gallstones; alternative causes include malignancy, peptic ulcer disease, and penetrating trauma. Patients with gallstone-induced fistulae can be asymptomatic, or they may present with nonspecific symptoms of anorexia, weight loss, and malabsorption. Gallstone ileus results when a large gallstone (>3 cm) passes into the gut through a cholecystenteric fistula and causes lumenal obstruction in the distal ileum. Biliary fistulae can often be detected on abdominal radiographs or upper gastrointestinal barium radiographs as air or barium in the biliary tree. Treatment requires surgical excision of the fistula, cholecystectomy, and extraction of all bile duct stones.

Hematobilia

Hemorrhage from the biliary tract is a rare complication of gallstones. The more common causes are penetrating trauma or iatrogenic trauma from a liver biopsy. In the United States, hepatobiliary tumors and aneurysms are possible causes, whereas parasitic diseases are possible causes in Asian societies. Diagnosis requires upper gastrointestinal endoscopy to exclude other sources of upper gastrointestinal hemorrhage. Angiography can confirm the site of bleeding. Angiographic embolization is the preferred initial treatment of hepatic causes of hematobilia. Surgical intervention is recommended to treat hemorrhage from the extrahepatic biliary tree.

Oriental cholangiohepatitis (recurrent pyogenic cholangitis)

In selected regions of South East Asia, the most common presentation of gallstone disease is a syndrome characterized by intrahepatic bile duct stones, ductal dilation and stricturing, and recurrent cholangitis, known as oriental cholangiohepatitis or recurrent pyogenic cholangitis. It occurs primarily in patients older than 50 and is associated with malnutrition and low socio-economic status. There are inconsistent associations with infections caused by *Clonorchis sinensis* and *Ascaris lumbricoides* but the pathogenetic role of these parasites remains unclear.

The stones in this disease are pigmented calcium bilirubinate stones that preferentially involve the left intrahepatic ducts. Patients typically present with relapsing cholangitis and hepatic abscesses. Ultrasound is of limited value because echogenic material often fills the intrahepatic ducts. The diagnosis relies on cholangiography. The primary treatment is surgical and often requires hepatic resection and extensive biliary reconstruction to relieve any obstruction and clear the ductal system of stones. Most patients require reoperation, although long-term prophylactic antibiotics may reduce the frequency of infectious complications.

Case studies

Case 1
A 45-year-old woman presents to the emergency department with complaints of right upper quadrant (RUQ) abdominal pain, nausea, vomiting, jaundice, and fever. She has no other significant past medical history. On physical exam she has a temperature of 38.7°C, pulse 110, blood pressure 100/50, and respiratory rate 18. She appears uncomfortable and jaundiced. The abdomen is obese and tender to palpation in the RUQ with a positive Murphy sign. Labs demonstrate an elevated total bilirubin of 4.0 mg/dL and alkaline phosphatase of 260 U/L. Ultrasound exam demonstrates dilation of the biliary system proximal to the cystic duct take-off and a stone impacted in the neck of the gallbladder. ERCP demonstrates obstruction of the common hepatic duct and an impacted stone in the cystic duct as well as multiple stones within the common bile duct. A sphincterotomy is performed and the intraductal stones are removed. The patient is diagnosed with type I Mirizzi syndrome (compression of the common hepatic duct by a stone impacted in the cystic duct) and taken to surgery for cholecystectomy.

Discussion: Mirizzi syndrome

- Mirizzi syndrome describes a condition in which the common bile duct is obstructed due to extrinsic compression from an impacted stone in the cystic duct or neck of the gallbladder.
- Typical symptoms in Mirizzi syndrome include jaundice, right upper quadrant abdominal pain, and fever.
- Lab abnormalities include elevated total bilirubin and alkaline phosphatase.
- Diagnosis can be suspected on ultrasound or CT scan; however, definitive diagnosis requires cholangiography.
- Surgery is the definitive therapy for Mirizzi syndrome.

Case 2

A 40-year-old woman presents to the gastrointestinal clinic with a 3-month history of intermittent severe right upper quadrant abdominal pain typically lasting approximately 1–2 h per episode. The pain is not exacerbated by eating. She denies any nausea or vomiting. The patient had similar symptoms in the past and underwent cholecystectomy 2 years prior. The patient had a severe episode 2 days ago and presented to the emergency department at that time. Labs from the emergency department visit demonstrated an elevated AST, ALT, and total bilirubin. An ultrasound performed during the visit to the emergency department demonstrated a dilated common bile duct at 9 mm without any evidence of intraductal stones. The patient has had two similar previous episodes where she presented to the emergency department and was noted to have elevated AST/ALT/bilirubin and dilated bile duct on ultrasound examination. Physical exam is unremarkable except for tenderness to deep palpation in the RUQ. The patient is diagnosed with type I sphincter of Oddi dysfunction (SOD) and undergoes ERCP with biliary sphincterotomy.

Discussion: sphincter of Oddi dysfunction

- SOD is divided into biliary and pancreatic types.
- Biliary SOD presents with biliary-type pain, abnormal liver enzymes, and dilation of the common bile duct.
- Biliary SOD is classified into three types (all with biliary-type pain):
  - type I – abnormal liver tests *and* a dilated common bile duct
  - type II – abnormal liver tests *or* a dilated common bile duct
  - type III – normal liver tests and normal-caliber common bile duct.
- Patients with SOD should be evaluated and managed at a center familiar with treating this disorder due to the risk of ERCP-related pancreatitis in this population of patients.

CHAPTER 36
Diseases of the Abdominal Cavity

Diseases of the abdominal cavity include a vast array of disorders, such as structural anomalies, hernias, abscesses, fistulae, and retractile mesenteritis.

Developmental Abnormalities of the Abdominal Cavity

Omphalocele and gastroschisis

The embryonic celomic cavity is too small to accommodate the intestines until the 10th gestational week, when they re-enter the abdomen. Omphalocele occurs when the viscera herniate through the umbilical ring and persist outside the body, covered by a membranous sac. At least 50% of infants with omphalocele have associated abnormalities of the skeletal, gastrointestinal, nervous, or genitourinary systems. Gastroschisis is a condition in which the peritoneal sac has ruptured *in utero* and the viscera are in free contact with the exterior.

Clinical presentation, diagnosis investigation, and management

The diagnosis of omphalocele or gastroschisis is obvious from examination at birth. It also can be diagnosed prenatally by ultrasound examination. Immediate treatment of these conditions is required to prevent dehydration, visceral desiccation, sepsis, and death. Antiseptic solutions are applied to the sac in infants with omphalocele. With gastroschisis, the viscera are wrapped in a silicone sheet, which is sutured to the abdominal wall until growth of the infant permits reduction of the hernia and closure of the defect. Amnion inversion is an alternative therapy for high-risk infants. Despite aggressive intervention, the mortality rate for these abnormalities is 40–50%. Many infants who survive exhibit slow recovery of bowel function.

Yamada's Handbook of Gastroenterology, Third Edition. Edited by Tadataka Yamada
and John M. Inadomi.
© 2013 John Wiley & Sons, Ltd. Published 2013 by John Wiley & Sons, Ltd.

Diaphragmatic hernias

Congenital diaphragmatic hernias are common defects that occur in weak areas of the diaphragm. Anteromedial diaphragmatic hernias through the sternocostal area (i.e. hernia of Morgagni) contain the stomach, colon, or omentum. Posterolateral diaphragmatic hernias through the lumbocostal area (i.e. hernia of Bochdalek) are large and are associated with hypoplasia of the ipsilateral lung (usually on the left) due to displacement of the thoracic contents by the bowel (Figure 36.1).

Clinical presentation, diagnosis investigation, and management

Anterior diaphragmatic hernias usually are small and rarely cause significant symptoms. Chest radiographs show an air shadow lateral to the xiphoid. Anterior hernias are corrected surgically with minimal morbidity and mortality. Posterolateral diaphragmatic hernias produce respiratory distress, mediastinal displacement, and nausea and vomiting as a result of intestinal obstruction. Respiratory sounds may be absent on the affected side, heart sounds may be audible in the right side of the chest, and bowel sounds may be audible in the left hemithorax. The abdomen may be scaphoid. Chest radiographs show left thoracic air–fluid levels, mediastinal displacement, and loss of the diaphragmatic line. Upper gastrointestinal radiography using water-soluble contrast may reveal intestinal loops in the thorax. Mortality from congenital diaphragmatic hernias results from respiratory insufficiency, malnutrition, failure to thrive, and intestinal strangulation. Mortality depends upon the age of the patient, associated malformations and the degree of lung hypoplasia, with mortality rates as high as 50% for emergency surgery in the first week of life. Extracorporeal membrane oxygenation may reduce the pulmonary consequences of this condition.

Umbilical hernias

Umbilical hernias are caused by congenitally large umbilical rings or by rings that are distended by high intra-abdominal pressures. Predisposing factors include prematurity, Down syndrome, gargoylism, amaurotic family idiocy, cretinism, and Beckwith–Wiedemann syndrome.

Clinical presentation, diagnosis investigation, and management

Most umbilical hernias reduce and heal spontaneously; strangulation complicates 5% of cases. Surgery before age 3 is indicated only for large, symptomatic hernias or in the event of incarceration or strangulation. If the hernia does not spontaneously improve by 3–4 years of age, elective surgery is performed.

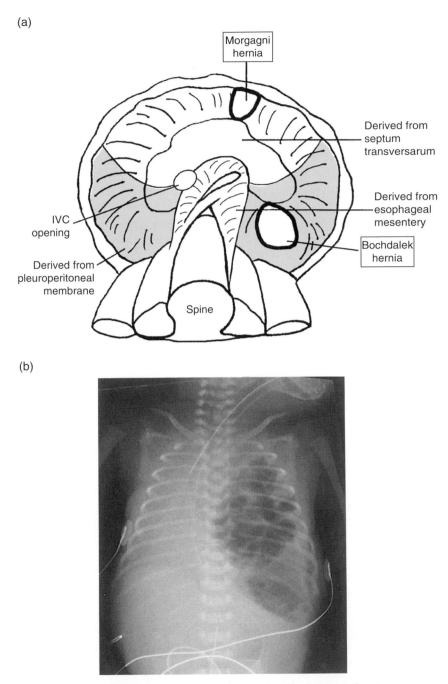

Figure 36.1 Development of the diaphragm and congenital diaphragmatic hernia.
(a) Abdominal surface of the diaphragm and the derivation of the components during
development. The pleuroperitoneal membranes, the septum transversum, and the esophageal
mesentery form the diaphragm. A Bochdalek hernia forms when there is a posterolateral defect.
Morgagni hernias are less common and are present anteriorly. (b) Chest radiograph of a child
with a congenital posterolateral (Bochdalek) diaphragmatic hernia on the left. The mediastinum
is displaced to the right by the intestinal loops present in the left chest. (Source: Yamada T et al.
(eds) *Textbook of Gastroenterology*, 5th edn. Oxford: Blackwell Publishing Ltd, 2009.)

Hernias in Adults

Epigastric hernias

Epigastric hernias occur in the midline of the abdominal wall between the umbilicus and the xiphoid in a small area of congenital weakness of the linea alba that may contain incarcerated preperitoneal fat. Multiple hernias are reported in 20% of cases.

Clinical presentation, diagnosis investigation, and management

Although most epigastric hernias are asymptomatic, some produce symptoms ranging from a small, painless nodule to acute obstruction of the small intestine. Pain that is exacerbated by exertion and relieved by reclining is characteristic. Raising the head from the examining table may increase pain. The diagnosis, which may be difficult in obese patients with small hernias, is made by palpation of a tender mass on physical examination. Surgery is indicated for epigastric hernias.

Umbilical hernias

Umbilical hernias in adults occur in multiparous women, obese individuals, and up to 40% of cirrhotic patients with ascites. Intestinal or omental incarceration and strangulation complicate 20–30% of cases, especially if the umbilical ring is small. Other complications in cirrhotic patients with ascites are hernia ulceration and perforation, which may be further complicated by peritonitis (often caused by *Staphylococcus aureus*) or renal failure.

Clinical presentation, diagnosis investigation, and management

Large umbilical hernias are obvious from physical examination. If the diagnosis is not self-evident, abdominal radiographs may demonstrate an intestinal loop outside the abdominal wall. Umbilical hernias are treated surgically. Preoperative control of ascites is important to avoid failure of the repair.

Groin hernias

Groin hernias represent 85% of all hernias (Table 36.1). There are three clinically relevant types: indirect inguinal hernias (through the internal inguinal ring into the inguinal canal), direct inguinal hernias (superior to the inguinal ligament

Table 36.1 Epidemiology of groin hernias*

Hernia type	Occurrence (%)
Inguinal	80
Indirect	(48)
Direct	(24)
Both	(8)
Femoral	5
Inguinal and femoral	2
With a sliding component	12
Sigmoid	(8)
Cecum	(4)
Other	2

*Groin hernias account for 85% of all hernias.

(a)   (b)

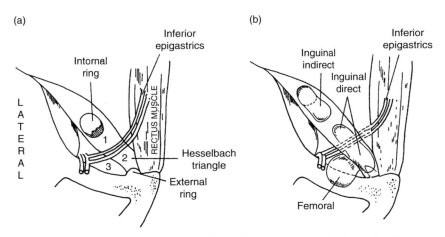

Figure 36.2 The right inguinal region. (a) Schematic anatomy showing internal and external rings and Hesselbach triangle. Spaces where hernias occur include Hesselbach triangle (2), the inguinal canal (1, 2), and the femoral space (3). (b) The most common groin hernias are direct and indirect hernias above the inguinal ligament and femoral hernias below the inguinal ligament. (Source: Yamada T et al. (eds) *Textbook of Gastroenterology*, 5th edn. Oxford: Blackwell Publishing Ltd, 2009.)

but not through the inguinal canal), and femoral hernias (inferior to the inguinal ligament and medial to the epigastric vessels) (Figure 36.2). Most inguinal hernias occur in males, with a male-to-female ratio of about 7/1, whereas there is a female predominance by 2/1 in the incidence of femoral, umbilical, and incisional hernias. Although femoral hernias are more common in women than in men, indirect inguinal hernias are the most common hernias in women. Most groin hernias contain ileum, omentum, colon, or bladder. An indirect inguinal hernia containing a Meckel diverticulum is known as a Littre hernia. Inguinal hernias are thought to originate from a patent processus vaginalis in conjunction with conditions associated with increased intra-abdominal pressure such as chronic cough, pregnancy, massive ascites, and extreme athletics.

Clinical presentation, diagnosis investigation, and management

A patient with a groin hernia presents with an inguinal mass that appears with increased intra-abdominal pressure. Pain usually is mild; local pain or colicky abdominal pain is suggestive of incarceration or strangulation. The diagnosis of hernias of the groin is made on physical examination by inserting a finger through the external inguinal ring into the inguinal canal to the internal ring. Indirect hernias are felt exiting the internal ring at the examiner's fingertip, whereas direct hernias are palpated laterally along the side of the finger. Femoral hernias are felt below the inguinal ligament in the femoral region. Strangulation affects 5% of indirect hernias, and 20–30% of femoral hernias strangulate, whereas direct hernias rarely develop this complication. Laparoscopy may visualize the site of herniation and the area of bowel that is trapped. Traditional or laparoscopic surgery is indicated for groin hernias.

Pelvic hernias

Pelvic hernias involve bowel herniation through the obturator foramen, the greater or lesser sciatic foramina, or the perineal muscles. Pelvic hernias are rare; obturator hernias are the most prevalent pelvic hernias. Obturator hernias usually contain ileum and are more common in women.

Clinical presentation, diagnosis investigation, and management

Patients with obturator hernia often have a history of transient attacks of acute intestinal obstruction. Diagnosis usually is made at laparotomy because the obturator is not easily palpated in the thigh. On rectal or vaginal examination, however, a soft, tender, anterolateral, fluctuating mass may be palpated. The Howship–Romberg sign (medial thigh pain radiating to the knee or hip) is present in 50% of patients. An abnormal gas shadow in the intestine may be detected on radiographs of the obturator foramen. A computed tomographic (CT) scan may be diagnostic if there is hernia incarceration. Pelvic hernias are treated surgically.

Lumbar hernias

Lumbar hernias are congenital or they are acquired through flank or rib trauma, through iliac crest fracture, or by removal of a fragment of the iliac crest for bone grafting. Lumbar herniation in the posterior abdominal wall may be superior (bounded by the 12th rib, internal oblique, and sacrospinalis) or inferior (bounded by the iliac crest, latissimus dorsi, and external oblique).

Clinical presentation, diagnosis investigation, and management

Lumbar hernias can be asymptomatic or they can produce lumbar pain referred to the back or pelvis. Surgery is indicated because these hernias generally increase in size.

Spigelian hernias

A spigelian hernia is a small protrusion through the external oblique fascia lateral to the rectus abdominis muscle, below the arcuate line of Douglas. Spigelian hernias are rare and usually occur in elderly persons.

Clinical presentation, diagnosis investigation, and management

Patients present with discomfort from straining or coughing. Sensation of a mass may be reported. A gas shadow may be seen on radiographs of the abdominal wall, whereas upper gastrointestinal contrast radiography may demonstrate bowel lumen outside the abdominal cavity. Surgery is mandatory.

Traumatic diaphragmatic hernias

Penetrating or blunt trauma may produce diaphragmatic tears. The most common injury is a tear from the esophageal hiatus to the left costal attachment, with herniation of the stomach, spleen, colon, and left hepatic lobe into the thorax.

Clinical presentation, diagnosis investigation, and management

Diaphragmatic injury produces upper abdominal pain referred to the left shoulder and scapula. Visceral herniation causes nausea and vomiting, central abdominal pain and diaphoresis from traction of the mesentery and blood vessels, and respiratory distress from lung compression and mediastinal deviation. In rare cases, symptoms are mild and the hernia remains undiagnosed for years. Chest radiographs, upper gastrointestinal contrast radiographs, ultrasound, and CT scans may demonstrate abdominal viscera in the thorax. The disorder requires immediate surgical repair.

Internal hernias

An internal hernia is the protrusion of an intraperitoneal viscus into a compartment within the abdomen. Paraduodenal hernias originate from a defect in midgut rotation and may involve bowel herniation into the left fossa of Landzert or the right fossa of Waldeyer. Herniation of the cecum and terminal ileum through the foramen of Winslow into the lesser sac is facilitated by a large foramen and abnormal colonic mobility. The small intestine is involved in 70% of cases and the colon in 25%. Pericecal hernias are characterized by passage of the ileum through the ileocecal fossa into the right paracolic gutter. Loops of small intestine rarely become incarcerated in the intersigmoid fossa, which is a pocket between the two sigmoid loops. About 5–10% of internal hernias in adults occur through defects in the mesentery and omentum. These are the most common type of internal hernias in infants and often are associated with an atretic segment of the intestine.

Clinical presentation, diagnosis investigation, and management

Internal hernias produce recurrent nausea, vomiting, and pain from intermittent obstruction of the small intestine. The diagnosis relies on abdominal radiography or laparotomy. Arteriography is also useful for diagnosis because it can demonstrate blood vessel displacement or reversal of their course. Radiographs of left paraduodenal hernias show encapsulated small intestine with superior displacement of the stomach and inferomedial displacement of the left colon, whereas right paraduodenal hernias displace the right colon anteriorly. Radiographs of hernias through the foramen of Winslow reveal gas-distended bowel loops in the lesser sac and anterior displacement of the stomach and colon. Intersigmoid hernias produce retrograde ileal filling that can be seen by barium enema radiography. Therapy for internal hernias is surgical.

Iatrogenic hernias

Iatrogenic hernias result from surgically created weak areas and abnormal foramina in the abdominal cavity. A retroanastomotic hernia is herniation of the intestine through a mesenteric space left open during construction of an anastomosis (e.g. Billroth II). Incisional hernias are caused by defective abdominal muscle suturing, defects at exteriorized drain sites, vertical laparotomies, multiple incisions (e.g. laparoscopic surgery), infraumbilical incisions, malnutrition, anemia, and wound hematomas or infections.

Clinical presentation, diagnosis investigation, and management

Retroanastomotic hernias are frequently acute and cause intestinal obstruction. Upper gastrointestinal barium radiography is diagnostic. Immediate surgical treatment is mandatory. Incisional hernias are detected by physical examination. Operative correction is generally required.

Abscesses

Abscesses are fluid collections that contain necrotic debris, leukocytes, and bacteria. The usual causes are operative complications, trauma, visceral perforation, pancreaticobiliary disease, and genitourinary infection. Sources of bacterial contamination include exogenous seeding from penetrating trauma, hematogenous or lymphatic spread from adjacent or distant sites, and local spread from gastrointestinal perforation.

Most intra-abdominal abscesses are contaminated by multiple microbes, including Gram-negative facultative organisms (*Escherichia coli* and *Klebsiella*, *Enterobacter*, *Proteus*, and *Pseudomonas* species) and anaerobes (e.g. *Bacteroides fragilis*), although prior antibiotics may influence the bacteriological spectrum in some cases, leading to fungal infection. Abscesses can develop almost anywhere in the peritoneal cavity. Initially localized inflammatory processes such as appendicitis and diverticulitis may produce localized abscesses in the lower abdomen if perforation occurs after the inflammatory reaction is walled off. If perforation occurs before a localized inflammatory process develops, generalized peritonitis may result. Abscess formation in dependent areas in the recumbent patient, such as the subdiaphragmatic, subhepatic, and pelvic spaces, is associated with generalized peritonitis.

Clinical presentation

Patients with intra-abdominal abscesses present with intermittent fever, abdominal pain, anorexia, and malaise. Subphrenic abscesses may produce shoulder pain, cough, and hiccups. Abscesses adjacent to the bladder or rectum may produce urinary or fecal urgency, respectively. Physical findings are variable, ranging from point tenderness and a focal mass to advanced sepsis with obtundation and hypotension. Bowel sounds may be reduced or absent, and rectovaginal examination may reveal a localized mass or tenderness. Involvement of the psoas muscle may cause pain on flexion of the hip (psoas sign). Even if the physical examination is unrevealing, clinicians must maintain a high degree of suspicion with all patients at risk of abscess formation. After surgery, incisional pain and the effects of analgesics often mask detection of an intra-abdominal abscess. Factors associated with poor outcome in patients with intra-abdominal abscesses include advanced age, associated organ failure, a recurrent or persistent abscess, and multiple abscesses. Complications of abscesses include sepsis, secondary abscesses caused by direct extension or hematogenous spread, bowel obstruction or fistula formation, and blood vessel erosion with massive hemorrhage.

Diagnostic investigation

Blood testing can suggest but not confirm the presence of an abscess. A complete blood count may show mild anemia or leukocytosis. Liver chemistry values may reveal hyperbilirubinemia secondary to the effects of bacteremia. Peripancreatic abscesses can produce hyperamylasemia. Blood cultures may be positive for one or more organisms, usually Gram-negative bacilli or anaerobes.

A CT scan is the imaging test of choice for most patients because it is positive in 90% of cases. Abscesses on CT scans appear as well-defined fluid collections. Ultrasound may be useful in selected regions, including the right upper quadrant, retroperitoneum, and pelvis, but lumenal gas may obscure visualization of other intra-abdominal sites. Endoscopic ultrasound (EUS) is useful for diagnosing pancreatic abscesses and pseudocysts, and it can detect associated varices and direct subsequent therapy. In selected cases, EUS-guided aspiration can be used to treat abscesses inaccessible by CT or in patients who are poor candidates for surgery.

Management

The mainstay of treating intra-abdominal abscess is drainage (typically percutaneously or surgically). Requirements for optimal percutaneous catheter drainage include:
- an abscess that can be approached adequately via a safe percutaneous route
- an abscess that is unilocular
- an abscess that is not vascular and the patient has no coagulopathy
- joint radiological, surgical and medical evaluation with adequate back-up for any complications
- the possibility of dependent drainage for the percutaneously placed drain.

When these criteria are met, percutaneous drainage is successful in 80–90% of cases. Patients whose abscesses are drained by any method but who do not respond within 4 days should be restudied with a CT scan or ultrasound, and repeat percutaneous drainage or surgery should be considered. Antibiotics are adjunctive therapy for intra-abdominal abscesses and should be administered prophylactically prior to catheter manipulation. Antibiotic therapy should be broad enough to treat Gram-negative and -positive aerobes and anaerobes. The duration of antibiotic therapy should be determined by the patient's condition and the results of blood and tissue cultures.

Key practice points

- A high degree of suspicion is warranted for patients at risk of abscess formation because the physical exam is often unrevealing.
- Factors associated with poor outcome in patients with intra-abdominal abscesses include advanced age, associated organ failure, a recurrent or persistent abscess and multiple abscesses.
- A CT scan is the imaging test of choice for intra-abdominal abscesses.
- Drainage is the mainstay of treatment for intra-abdominal abscesses.

Fistulae

Fistulae are abnormal communications from a hollow organ (gut, biliary tract, pancreatic duct, urinary tract) to another hollow organ or the skin. Fistulae develop in response to surgery, the use of prosthetic mesh to close abdominal wall defects, radiation therapy, inflammatory bowel disease, trauma, and malignancy (Table 36.2). Rarely, fistulae develop when abscesses erode into the adjacent bowel.

Clinical presentation

The most common presentations of abdominal fistulae include enteric drainage through the skin and signs and symptoms of an intra-abdominal abscess. High-output fistulae (>500 mL per day) that involve the proximal gut produce significant fluid and electrolyte abnormalities, including metabolic acidosis from duodenal fistulae and hypochloremic, hypokalemic metabolic alkalosis from gastric fistulae. Fluid loss may be so severe as to cause dehydration, hypotension, and renal failure. Skin irritation may result from exposure to activated digestive enzymes. Malnutrition may result from protein and nutrient loss from the fistula, decreased oral intake, and the increased energy demands of the underlying illness. Malnutrition can significantly increase morbidity and mortality rates associated with fistulae. The presence of multiple, recurrent, or complex fistulae should suggest Crohn's disease. Recurrent urinary tract infection or pneumaturia suggests an enterovesical fistula, whereas diarrhea and malnutrition may be the presenting symptoms of a patient with an enteroenteric fistula that bypasses significant segments of gut. Fistulae are often mistaken for wound infections until fecal contents are identified on the dressings.

Table 36.2 Etiological classification of enteric fistulae

Congenital
Tracheo-esophageal fistula
Patent vitelline duct

Postoperative
Inadvertent injury
Failure of anastomosis
Proximity of drain

Posttraumatic
Direct injury
Open abdominal wound

Inflammatory
Crohn's disease
Adjacent abscess

Postirradiation
Spontaneous
Postoperative

Malignant
Adherence of tumor to adjacent bowel or abdominal
wall with subsequent tumor necrosis

Diagnostic investigation

Various studies may be needed to diagnose the presence of a fistula accurately. The course of enterocutaneous fistulae can be defined by careful injection of a radiographic contrast medium into the skin opening. Persistently positive urine cultures for enteric organisms may suggest an enterovesical fistula. Upper or lower gastrointestinal contrast radiography may demonstrate disease that leads to fistula formation but rarely defines the fistula itself. Cystoscopy is the most helpful test for diagnosing enterovesical fistulae. Gastrointestinal contrast radiographs usually demonstrate enteroenteric fistulae, whereas endoscopy is not often helpful. CT scanning and ultrasound may rarely detect fistulae but can be helpful in defining predisposing factors such as intra-abdominal abscess cavities.

Management

The goals of treating an abdominal fistula include correction of fluid and electrolyte abnormalities, drainage of associated abscesses, protection of the skin, nutrient repletion, reduction of fistula drainage, and treatment of the underlying disease.

For high-output fistulae, daily adjustments in replacement fluids may require direct measurement of the electrolyte composition in the fistula fluid. Effective drainage of associated abscesses is achieved by placement of sump drains. Skin can be protected with stoma appliances, similar to those used for surgically placed ileostomies or colostomies. The choice of enteral versus parenteral nutrition in patients with gastrointestinal fistulae must be individualized. Enteral feedings may increase fluid output from proximal fistulae of the small intestine, rendering parenteral nutrition more useful. In contrast, patients with fistulae of the distal small intestine or colon may be adequately nourished by enteral feedings without increasing fistulous output. Somatostatin and its analog, octreotide, reduce pancreatic and intestinal secretion and have been proposed for patients with intestinal or pancreatic fistulae. Most trials showed a reduction in the time to closure of fistulae, although only one showed a significant improvement in the spontaneous closure rate.

Factors that predict an unfavorable response to conservative management of fistulae include malignancy, inflammatory bowel disease, foreign bodies, poorly drained abscesses, distal gut obstruction, disruption of more than 50% of the bowel wall, a fistula tract less than 2.5 cm from the skin or more than 2 cm long, age older than 65, fistula output of more than 500 mL per day, chronicity, and localization to the distal small intestine and colon. Aggressive medical management with parenteral nutrition, skin care, evacuation of associated abscesses and control of infection results in spontaneous closure in 60–75% of cases. Endoscopic obliteration with fibrin sealant has been used with variable success in patients with upper gastrointestinal tract fistulae. Surgery is considered for fistulae that persist after 4–6 weeks. Use of anti-TNF therapy is associated with Crohn's fistulae closure rates approaching 60%.

Mesenteric Panniculitis and Retractile Mesenteritis

Mesenteric panniculitis is a nonspecific inflammation of the adipose tissue of the mesentery. Possible etiologies include trauma, infection, autoimmunity, abdominal malignancy, or ischemia but the cause is often unknown. It can be part of the generalized Weber–Christian disease. Pathological features include a thickened mesentery, usually a solid mass, representing excess growth of fat and subsequent degeneration, fat necrosis, xanthogranulomatous inflammation (macrophages, histiocytes, lymphocytes, foreign body giant cells), fibrosis, and calcification. If mesenteric panniculitis progresses to retractile mesenteritis, the thickened mesentery becomes fibrotic. Fat necrosis may produce mesenteric pseudocysts.

Clinical presentation, diagnosis investigation, and management

Symptoms of mesenteric panniculitis include abdominal cramps, weight loss, nausea, vomiting, and low-grade fever. Sixty percent of the abdominal masses are palpable. Radiographic findings include displacement and extrinsic compression of bowel, stretching of the vasa recta and vascular encasement on angiography, and an inhomogeneous mass on CT scans. Retractile mesenteritis produces similar symptoms, as well as obstruction of the small intestine, mesenteric thrombosis, lymphatic obstruction with ascites, steatorrhea, and protein-losing enteropathy. The prognoses for these conditions depend on the underlying disease. Biopsy should be considered to rule out malignancy. In patients with symptomatic progressive sclerosing or retractile mesenteritis, improvement has been reported with use of progesterone, prednisone and azathioprine or with cyclophosphamide. However, the data are insufficient to determine the efficacy of these medical therapies in this usually self-limiting disease. Surgical resection usually is not possible, though bypass may be considered for symptomatic relief in cases of obstruction.

CHAPTER 37

Viral Hepatitis

Hepatitis is a nonspecific clinicopathological term that encompasses all disorders characterized by hepatocellular injury accompanied by histological evidence of a necroinflammatory response. Hepatitis is classified into acute hepatitis, defined as self-limited liver injury of less than 6 months' duration, and chronic hepatitis, in which the inflammatory response persists after 6 months. These two fundamental forms of hepatitis can be further subdivided on the basis of the underlying disease process or cause. Five viruses have been associated with acute and chronic hepatitis, namely hepatitis A, B, C, D, and E (Table 37.1). Hepatitis B and C may manifest as both acute and chronic hepatitis. Others, such as viral hepatitis A, are strictly acute.

Hepatitis A

Epidemiology

Hepatitis A virus (HAV) causes 200,000 cases of acute hepatitis annually. It is transmitted primarily by fecal–oral routes. Epidemics can be traced to contaminated water or food. HAV is rarely acquired by parenteral exposure. About 30% of the population of the United States has serum IgG antibody to HAV, which suggests prior exposure. Significant racial and ethnic differences in the prevalence of antibody to HAV are likely to reflect both country of origin and socio-economic status. In developing countries, essentially all children are exposed to the virus, which often produces subclinical illness in this age group. Risk factors for acquiring HAV include male homosexuality, household contact with an infected person, travel to developing countries, and contact with children in day care. Outbreaks have also been associated with the consumption of raw shellfish, frozen strawberries, salads, and raw onions.

Yamada's Handbook of Gastroenterology, Third Edition. Edited by Tadataka Yamada and John M. Inadomi.
© 2013 John Wiley & Sons, Ltd. Published 2013 by John Wiley & Sons, Ltd.

Table 37.1 Human hepatitis viruses

Virus	Genome	Genome size (kb)	Envelope	Classification family	Genus
HAV	RNA positive sense, single-stranded, linear	7.5	–	Picornaviridae	Hepatovirus
HBC	DNA partially double-stranded, circular	3.2	+	Hepadnaviridae	
HCV	RNA positive sense, single-stranded, linear	9.6	+	Flaviviridae	Hepacivirus
HDV	RNA positive sense, single-stranded, linear	1.7	+	Unclassified (viroid)	Deltavirus
HEV	RNA positive sense, single-stranded, linear	7.5	–	Unclassified	Togavirus-like and alphavirus-like

Source: Yamada T et al. (eds) *Textbook of Gastroenterology*, 5th edn. Oxford: Blackwell Publishing Ltd, 2009.

Pathogenesis

Hepatitis A virus is an RNA virus that produces hepatocellular injury by mechanisms that remain poorly understood. Both direct cytopathic and immunologically mediated injury seem probable but neither has been proven. After exposure, there is a 2–6-week incubation period before symptom onset, although the virus may be detectable in the stool 1 week before clinically apparent illness. The immune response to HAV begins early and may contribute to hepatocellular injury. Immunological clearance of HAV is the rule and unlike hepatitis viruses B and C, HAV never enters a chronic phase. By the time symptoms are manifest, patients invariably have IgM antibodies to HAV (anti-HAV IgM), which typically persist for 3–6 months. IgG antibodies to HAV (anti-HAV IgG) also develop and provide life-long immunity against reinfection.

Clinical course

Many patients with HAV infection, in particular 80–90% of children, are asymptomatic. Only 5–10% of patients with serological evidence of prior HAV infection recall an episode of jaundice. Factors that contribute to subclinical versus clinical infection remain unclear.

The syndrome of acute hepatitis caused by HAV is clinically indistinguishable from other viral causes of acute hepatitis. Patients usually present with a nonspecific prodrome of fatigue, anorexia, nausea, headache, myalgias, and arthralgias. This may be followed by jaundice and right upper quadrant pain. Some patients may experience pruritus but this rarely requires treatment. Vomiting is common and may lead to fluid and electrolyte imbalance. Physical signs include icterus and tender hepatomegaly. The spleen is palpable in a minority of patients. A prolonged form of HAV infection is characterized by pruritus, fever, weight loss, serum bilirubin >10 mg/dL and a clinical course lasting a minimum of 12 weeks. It is seen more often in older individuals. A relapsing variant characterized by initial clinical improvement followed by recrudescent symptoms 5–10 weeks after recovery affects 20% of patients, and the clinical course is rarely protracted, lasting no longer than 12 weeks. Resolution of HAV infection with complete recovery, except in the rare cases of fulminant hepatitis (~1%), is the rule.

Diagnostic and serological studies

Elevations in levels of aminotransferases usually occur 1–2 weeks before the onset of symptoms and persist for up to 4–6 weeks. The alanine aminotransferase (ALT) level usually is higher than the aspartate aminotransferase (AST) level; absolute values often exceed 1000 IU/L. The level of enzyme elevation does not correlate with disease severity. Asymptomatic cases may have serum AST or ALT levels in the thousands. Serum bilirubin levels usually peak 1–2 weeks after symptoms appear but they rarely exceed 15–20 mg/dL. HAV infection occasionally produces a cholestatic pattern of liver biochemical abnormalities with a disproportionate elevation in the alkaline phosphatase level. Other laboratory abnormalities include relative lymphocytosis with a normal total leukocyte count.

Diagnosis relies on detecting anti-HAV IgM in the serum. Because this IgM component of the humoral immune response lasts only 3–6 months, its presence implies recent or ongoing infection (Figure 37.1). Liver biopsy is not necessary if the findings from serological testing are positive and is performed only if the diagnosis is in doubt. Although there are no distinguishing features of any form of viral hepatitis, patchy necrosis and lobular lymphocytic infiltrates are typical findings. Occasionally, ultrasound scanning may be necessary to exclude biliary obstruction, particularly in patients with the cholestatic variant of HAV infection. This test may confirm hepatomegaly and reveal an inhomogeneous liver parenchyma but findings usually are nonspecific.

Management

Hepatitis A virus is self-limited, and symptoms resolve in most cases over the course of 2–4 weeks. There is no specific treatment, and patients should be encouraged to maintain fluid and nutritional intake. Ten percent of patients require hospitalization for intractable vomiting, worsening laboratory values, or comorbid illnesses. The overall mortality rate for hospitalized patients is less than 1%.

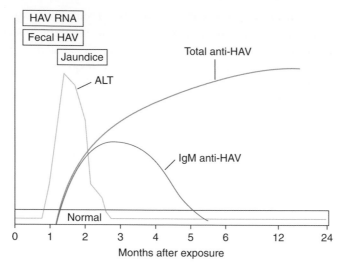

Figure 37.1 Typical serological course of acute hepatitis A virus (HAV) infection. ALT, alanine aminotransferase; IgM, immunoglobin M. (Source: Yamada T et al. (eds) *Textbook of Gastroenterology*, 5th edn. Oxford: Blackwell Publishing Ltd, 2009.)

Deaths are mainly the result of the rare case of fulminant hepatitis, which is characterized by signs of hepatic failure, including encephalopathy. These patients are typically older and may have chronic hepatitis C infection, and should be referred to liver transplant centers for management and potential transplantation.

Prevention

Infection with HAV can be prevented by either passive or active immunization. Patients exposed to feces of HAV-infected individuals should be given immunoglobulin (0.02 mL/kg) within 2 weeks of exposure. Travelers to endemic areas may be given immunoglobulin, which provides protection for about 3 months, or the formalin-inactivated hepatitis A vaccine, which provides long-term immunity to more than 90% of persons, beginning 1 month after the first dose of the two-dose regimen.

Hepatitis B

Epidemiology

Hepatitis B virus (HBV) is an important cause of acute and chronic hepatitis. In regions of Africa, Asia, and the Mediterranean basin where HBV is endemic, there are high rates of chronic HBV infection. Worldwide, there are 400 million HBV carriers. In the United States during the 1990s, HBV accounted for more than 175,000 cases of acute hepatitis annually, and 5% of these entered a chronic phase. In contrast, perinatal transmission of HBV leads to chronic HBV infection in more than 90% of cases. About 0.3% of the population in the United States suffers chronic infection with HBV. Although 30–50% of infections with HBV have no identifiable source, the main route of transmission is percutaneous. The most common means of transmission are sexual contact with an infected individual, intravenous drug use, and vertical transmission from mother to child. Several epidemiological surveys have emphasized the importance of contact transmission among individuals in the same household, even in the absence of intimate or sexual contact. The mechanism of this contact-associated transmission remains poorly defined. Blood transfusion is an unlikely source of HBV in western countries with the use of blood bank screening but poses a major risk in developing countries that do not screen blood or blood products for HBV.

Pathogenesis

Hepatitis B virus is a DNA virus that has seven genotypes, A–G, based on differences in sequence. One component of HBV is an envelope that contains a protein called hepatitis B surface antigen (HBsAg). Inside the envelope is a nucleocapsid that contains the hepatitis B core antigen (HBcAg), which is not detectable in serum. During viral replication, a third antigen, termed the hepatitis B e antigen (HBeAg), and HBV DNA are detectable in the serum. While in the replicative phase, HBV produces hepatocellular injury primarily by activating the cellular immune system in response to viral antigens on the surface of hepatocytes. The vigor of the immune response determines the severity of acute HBV hepatitis and the probability that the infection will enter a chronic phase. An exuberant response can produce fulminant hepatic failure, whereas a lesser response may fail to clear the virus.

After exposure to HBV, there is an incubation period of several weeks to 6 months before the onset of symptoms. HBsAg appears in the serum, followed shortly by HBeAg late in the incubation period. Detectable levels of HBeAg correlate with active viral replication, as does the quantity of HBV DNA. The first detectable immune response is antibody to HBcAg (anti-HBc), which is usually present by the time symptoms occur. As with HAV, the initial antibody response is primarily IgM, which persists for 4–6 months and is followed by a life-long IgG response. Antibodies to HBsAg (anti-HBs) develop in more than 90% of adult individuals with acute hepatitis. The appearance of anti-HBs, usually several weeks after the disappearance of HBsAg and resolution of symptoms, signifies recovery. Anti-HBs provides life-long immunity to reinfection, although titers may decrease to undetectable levels over the course of years.

Antibodies to HBeAg (anti-HBe) appear earlier than anti-HBs and usually signify the clearance of HBeAg and cessation of replication. In chronic HBV infection, the virus may be in a replicative phase characterized by the presence of HBsAg, HBeAg, and high levels of HBV DNA, along with an immune-mediated chronic inflammatory response. Alternatively, HBV may enter a nonreplicative state, formerly referred to as the carrier state, in which HBV is maintained by insertion into the host genome. In this phase, HBsAg persists but HBeAg disappears and anti-HBe appears. HBV DNA is present at low levels (fewer than 100,000 copies/mL). The inflammatory response in this nonreplicative state usually is minimal but due to integrated HBV DNA in the hepatocytes, the risk of hepatocellular carcinoma persists

Clinical course

Most acute HBV infections are asymptomatic, especially if acquired at a young age when chronicity is more likely. Thirty percent of infections with HBV in adults result in acute hepatitis, which is indistinguishable from other forms of acute viral hepatitis. The illness usually has a 1–6-month incubation period. Hepatitis may be preceded by a serum sickness syndrome characterized by fever, urticaria, arthralgias, and, rarely, arthritis. This syndrome is probably caused by immune complexes of HBV antigens and antibodies, which may also produce glomerulonephritis and vasculitis (including polyarteritis nodosa) in patients with chronic HBV infection. Patients with chronic HBV infection may have a history of a distant bout of acute hepatitis but a history of jaundice is unusual. Most patients with chronic HBV infection remain asymptomatic for years. When symptoms develop, they usually are nonspecific, including malaise, fatigue, and anorexia. Some patients exhibit jaundice and complications of portal hypertension, such as ascites, variceal hemorrhage, or encephalopathy. Physical examination in the chronic phase may be normal. Some patients may present with stigmata of cirrhosis and portal hypertension, including ascites, dilated abdominal veins, gynecomastia, and spider angiomata.

Diagnostic and serological studies

Diagnosis of acute hepatitis B is based on a typical serological pattern in acute hepatitis. Serum aminotransferase elevations in the thousands and other liver biochemical abnormalities are indistinguishable from alternative causes of acute viral hepatitis. Acute infection is diagnosed by the presence of IgM antibodies to HBcAg (anti-HBc IgM) and evidence of ongoing infection represented by HBsAg, HBeAg, and HBV DNA. In 5–10% of patients with acute hepatitis, the latter three markers may be cleared before clinical presentation, leaving anti-HBc IgM as the only indicator of recent infection. It is important to measure the anti-HBc IgM because the isolated presence of IgG antibodies to HBcAg (anti-HBc IgG) is the most common serological pattern in resolved HBV infection (Figure 37.2).

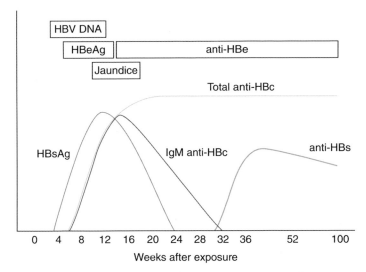

Figure 37.2 Typical serological course of acute hepatitis B virus (HBV) infection. HBeAg, hepatitis Be antigen; HBsAg, hepatitis surface antigen; IgM, immunoglobulin M. (Source: Yamada T et al. (eds) *Textbook of Gastroenterology*, 5th edn. Oxford: Blackwell Publishing Ltd, 2009.)

The timing of HBsAg disappearance is variable but it is absent in 80–90% of cases by 4 months after infection. Persistence of HBsAg beyond 6 months indicates chronic infection. Anti-HBs will appear several weeks after the disappearance of HBsAg. This antibody provides life-long immunity but titers may drop to undetectable levels over the course of years. As with acute HAV, liver biopsy for acute HBV is needed only if the diagnosis is not substantiated by serological testing.

Chronic HBV may produce several serological patterns based on the replicative state of the virus. The presence of HBsAg, HBeAg, and HBV DNA and the absence of anti-HBs and anti-HBe are characteristic of active viral replication. The presence of HBsAg and anti-HBe in the absence of HBeAg, along with low levels of HBV DNA, is representative of the nonreplicative or chronic inactive state. All patients with chronic HBV have anti-HBc IgG. A small number of patients may have low titers of anti-HBc IgM, particularly when the virus is transiting from the replicative phase to the nonreplicative phase. In addition, several mutations exist, including precore mutations that result in negative HBeAg in serum, positive anti-HBe but significant HBV DNA, as well as pre-S and polymerase mutations. The latter usually arise in response to therapy, such as the YMDD mutation that is associated with lamivudine resistance.

Biochemical variables and symptoms correlate poorly with the histological severity of liver damage. Liver biopsy provides important prognostic information in patients with chronic hepatitis B. Patients with active viral replication demonstrate a variable degree of chronic periportal inflammation. Extension of chronic inflammatory cells into the hepatic lobule is termed piecemeal necrosis, whereas inflammation and hepatocellular destruction extending from portal tract to portal tract is termed bridging necrosis. Patients in the nonreplicative phase usually have minimal to no inflammation. Variable stages of fibrosis or even cirrhosis can be present in any patient with chronic HBV. Determining the extent of inflammation and fibrosis is often critical in making therapeutic decisions for chronic HBV.

Management

Acute HBV hepatitis usually resolves clinically and biochemically over several weeks to months. As with other forms of acute viral hepatitis, treatment is supportive. One percent of cases follow a fulminant course that results in hepatic failure and encephalopathy. These patients should be referred to transplantation centers.

The risk that HBV infection will become chronic is in large part related to the patient's age at acquisition. Chronicity rates are 90% for infections acquired perinatally. The rate is lower in older children and is about 5% in adults. The mechanism of this variability in the ability of HBV to enter a chronic phase is probably related to changes in immune tolerance with aging. Once established, chronic HBV infection is usually life-long. Annually, up to 1% of chronic HBV carriers lose HBsAg and develop anti-HBs, suggesting complete viral eradication. Also each year, the replicative phase of the virus transforms into the nonreplicative phase in 1–10% of patients (i.e. HBeAg is lost and anti-HBe is gained). An acute clinical and biochemical flare of the infection often accompanies this seroconversion. The transition to a nonreplicative state does not indicate complete clearance of HBV. Many patients exhibit reactivation of replication with reappearance of HBeAg at some point in the future. Although cirrhosis may develop at any stage of chronic HBV infection, it usually requires many years of infection. The risk is greatest for patients with bridging necrosis and active viral replication. Because chronic HBV is indolent and produces minimal or no symptoms, complications of cirrhosis, including ascites, variceal hemorrhage, and encephalopathy, may be the initial manifestations of chronic HBV. The lifetime risk of hepatocellular carcinoma is about 20% in persons with chronic HBV infection; therefore, patients with HBV infection that lasts longer than 10 years should be screened every 6 months by imaging with ultrasound (or in some cases computed tomography or magnetic resonance imaging) with or without serum α-fetoprotein measurements, to facilitate early detection. The course of acute and chronic HBV infection can also be complicated by superinfection with hepatitis D virus.

Treatment

Treatment of acute HBV infection is rarely indicated, although it is at times attempted for fulminant infection. The goals of antiviral therapy include bringing the HBV DNA down to undetectable levels (<60 IU/mL). The options for treatment of chronic HBV include antiviral or immunomodulatory therapy with nucleoside analogs and interferon-α. Candidates for interferon therapy ideally have higher levels of serum liver enzymes, lower serum levels of HBV DNA, and genotype A disease. They should not have histological evidence of cirrhosis or decompensated liver disease. Interferon therapy consists of standard or pegylated interferon for 12 months. With this therapy, the virus in 30–50% of cases will transition from the active replicative phase to the nonreplicative phase (eAg clearance) and up to 15% of patients will experience HBsAg clearance with long-term follow-up. Side-effects are substantial; there is an almost universal occurrence of an influenza-like illness with myalgia, fever, chills, and headache. Other adverse reactions include depression, bone marrow suppression, alopecia, and autoimmune thyroiditis. Patients should be selected with this side-effect profile in mind, especially if there are pre-existing psychiatric conditions and cytopenias.

There are currently five oral agents that are approved by the Food and Drug Administration for treatment of chronic hepatitis B in the United States: lamivudine, adefovir, entecavir, telbivudine, and tenofovir. These medications can be used by individuals who are HBeAg positive or negative, including those with decompensated liver disease. Lamivudine has been associated with a high rate of viral resistance (50–70% at 3 years), as has adefovir, although to a lesser degree (11% at 3 years, 30% at 4.5 years). Resistance to telbivudine is also common after 1–2 years of monotherapy, with cross-resistance with lamivudine. Currently, entecavir and tenofovir are first-line agents, with similar and highly effective antiviral efficacy. These agents provide superior rates of biochemical and virological response, as well as marked improvements in histology over time, with vanishingly low rates of resistance in treatment-naïve patients.

Prevention

Prevention of HBV has widespread public health implications. A program of universal vaccination of infants with the recombinant hepatitis B vaccine is in place in the United States. This vaccine is also indicated for healthcare workers, patients on hemodialysis, intravenous drug users, persons who have household contact with HBV carriers, adolescents and individuals who are sexually active with more than one partner, and travelers who reside in an endemic area longer than 6 months. The three-dose regimen is given at time 0, 1 month, and 6 months. It is more than 90% effective in producing protective anti-HBs. Response rates may be lower in immunosuppressed individuals. Although titers may decrease over time, the protective effect is long-lived owing to the amnestic response at the time of exposure.

Postexposure prophylaxis requires the use of hepatitis B immune globulin (HBIG) (0.06 mg/kg) in addition to the recombinant vaccine. Those who have had sexual or parenteral exposure to persons with active HBV infection should receive HBIG within 2 weeks of exposure. Infants born to mothers with HBsAg should receive HBIG at birth and vaccination should be initiated. All exposed persons should receive the vaccine on the usual dosing schedule.

Hepatitis C

Epidemiology

Hepatitis C virus (HCV) is an RNA virus in the Flaviviridae family that has been classified into six genotypes, based on sequence variation. Because most infections with HCV assume a chronic phase, preventing transmission is critical. Along with human immunodeficiency virus (HIV), screening of the blood supply for antibodies to HCV has dramatically reduced the incidence of posttransfusion hepatitis to less than 1% of all transfusions. Most HCV infections in the United States result from intravenous drug use. Given that the main mode of transmission is parenteral, the epidemiology of HCV infection mirrors to some extent that of HBV and HIV infections; however, sexual and perinatal transmission are rare for HCV.

In most regions of the world, the prevalence of HCV antibodies ranges from 0.5% to 2%. Higher rates are observed in developing countries and lower socio-economic groups. Within the United States, there is variation among racial groups, with a 7–8% HCV positivity rate among inner-city African-American and Hispanic populations compared with 0.5% among inner-city whites. In the United States, 70% of HCV infections are caused by genotypes 1a and 1b; the remaining 30% of infections are caused by genotypes 2 and 3. Although parenteral exposure is the primary means of contracting HCV, 10% of cases still have no identifiable source of infection. Groups at high risk of infection with HCV include intravenous drug users and persons who required transfusions or other blood products prior to 1991 or in countries outside the United States. The risk of sexual transmission is poorly defined but appears to be 3–5% in long-standing monogamous relationships. The risk of vertical transmission from mother to fetus is 3–5%. The risk is higher (12–14%) if the mother is seropositive for HIV-1. Nosocomial infections from contaminated instruments or multidose vials, and needlestick injuries account for a small proportion of HCV infections.

Pathogenesis

Based on the observation that HCV infection follows a slightly more aggressive course with immunosuppression secondary to medications or HIV infection, HCV does not appear to rely solely on immune-mediated injury. Dual mechanisms of hepatocellular injury include a direct cytopathic effect of HCV, as well as injury from specific and nonspecific T-cell-mediated immunological injury. No protective antibodies to HCV have been demonstrated. In addition, the immune response in HCV infection is responsible for the syndrome of mixed cryoglobulinemia observed in a small fraction of chronic HCV infections. In this disorder, HCV antigens associated with monoclonal IgM and polyclonal IgG antibody complexes are deposited in the end organ and activate complement, producing dependent purpura, glomerulonephritis, arthritis, and vasculitis. The incubation period after exposure is usually 2–12 weeks; the average is 6–7 weeks. Similar to HBV infection, antibodies develop against several viral proteins and are detected by the enzyme-linked immunosorbent assay (ELISA) and the immunoblot assay (RIBA). Anti-HCVs may not be detectable for up to 2 months after the onset of acute hepatitis; however, HCV RNA is detectable within 1–3 weeks after the onset of acute infection. HCV antibodies are neither neutralizing nor protective, and 70–85% of HCV infections assume a chronic phase.

Clinical course

Most patients infected with HCV never develop a clinical syndrome of acute hepatitis. About 15–20% of patients develop malaise, fever, fatigue, nausea, vomiting, arthralgia, and right upper quadrant pain. Systemic symptoms may be followed by jaundice. HCV does not appear to be the agent responsible for the large number of cases of fulminant hepatic failure attributed to non-A and non-B hepatitis, and although fulminant HCV has been reported, it is exceedingly rare. After acute infection, 75–85% of adults and 55% of children with HCV infections enter a chronic phase. Spontaneous clearance of chronic HCV is rare. Many patients remain asymptomatic for years and are detected only during health screening or when donating blood. The most common symptoms of chronic HCV are nonspecific malaise, fatigue, and right upper quadrant abdominal discomfort. Some patients may remain asymptomatic even as the disease progresses to cirrhosis. Chronic HCV leads to cirrhosis in at least 20–25% of immunocompetent patients within 20 years of infection. The factors that influence the rate of progression to cirrhosis include gender, age at infection, coexisting liver disease and consumption of alcohol.

In recent years, much has been learned about a single nucleotide polymorphism (rs12979860 C/T) 3 kb upstream of the interleukin 28B (IL-28B) gene. This IL-28B polymorphism has been shown to be associated with the likelihood of spontaneous hepatitis C clearance as well as likelihood of treatment response, and possibly disease severity. The CC genotype is associated with greater spontaneous clearance and superior response rates to interferon-based treatment, with the TT genotype having the least favorable profile.

Diagnostic and serological studies

Patients with acute hepatitis caused by HCV usually have aminotransferase levels lower than 1000 IU/L; less than 10% have levels higher than 2000 IU/L. Serum bilirubin levels rarely exceed 10–15 mg/dL. Severe liver dysfunction with abnormal coagulation variables is uncommon. As with other forms of acute viral hepatitis, the cornerstone of diagnosis is serological testing. The main obstacle to diagnosing acute infection is the variable delay in the appearance of anti-HCV. Only 65% of patients have anti-HCV within 2 weeks of symptom onset but 90% are seropositive after 3 months. The remaining 10% usually develops anti-HCV over several months. The presence of virus can be assessed for using polymerase chain reaction (PCR) or branched DNA (bDNA) amplification methods. HCV RNA is detectable within 7–21 days of infection. For patients with established chronic HCV infection, quantitative HCV PCR does not correlate with disease severity or histology. It does help to predict the likelihood of response to antiviral therapy, and should be carefully monitored during HCV treatment. HCV genotype can be determined using genetic sequence detection techniques. Genotype does not correlate with disease severity but is used to determine the likelihood of treatment success and the appropriate treatment regimen. IL-28B gene polymorphism can be tested for to aid in prediction of antiviral treatment response.

Liver biopsy is generally not useful for diagnosing acute HCV infection but it is important in managing chronic HCV. In chronic HCV, there is a variable degree of periportal chronic inflammation, often with discrete lymphoid aggregates. The severity may vary from a minimal increase in periportal lymphocytes to the confluent destruction of hepatocytes in bridging necrosis. There is also a variable degree of fibrosis, ranging from no fibrosis to cirrhosis. The severity of histological injury correlates poorly with symptoms and elevations in levels of aminotransferases. Liver biopsy has been uniformly recommended by the National Institutes of Health and European consensus conferences for individuals being considered for antiviral treatment of HCV infection.

Management

With supportive therapy, most patients with acute HCV experience a gradual resolution of symptoms over weeks to months. The infection is self-limited in 15–30% of cases and the virus is cleared but in the remaining 70–85% of cases, the infection becomes chronic. Consideration should be given to treating patients with interferon-based therapy after 6 months of infection, as sustained virological response rates are very high with just 6 months of treatment in recently infected individuals. Chronic HCV infection is an indolent disease. There are often significant fluctuations in levels of serum aminotransferases. Complications generally occur more than 10 years after acquisition. Serial liver biopsy can provide information regarding the degree of fibrosis (stage) to aid in decision making regarding antiviral therapy. Cirrhosis occurs in 20–25% of patients within 20 years of onset. Once a patient develops cirrhosis, careful monitoring for complications of portal hypertension and hepatocellular carcinoma is indicated. Referral for liver transplantation should be considered as a patient experiences decompensation of their liver disease.

There have been many recent advances in the treatment of chronic hepatitis C. Much has been learned about the predictors of response to treatment, and the greatest predictors include the HCV genotype, the IL-28B genetic polymorphism, race, and the stage of fibrosis. Treatment itself has recently changed significantly, with the advent of two new direct-acting antiviral agents which were approved by the Food and Drug Administration in May 2011 for use in genotype 1 patients. Telaprevir and bocepravir are protease inhibitors intended for use with pegylated interferon and ribavirin. The addition of these medications to the previous standard of care has markedly improved rates of sustained virological response (SVR) from approximately 40% to almost 80% in treatment-naïve patients, and reduced the treatment duration for many from 48 weeks to 24 weeks. These protease inhibitors are not approved for use in genotype 2 patients, and are ineffective in genotype 3 patients. Fortunately, genotype 2 and 3 patients enjoy a high likelihood, approximately 80%, of achieving an SVR with a 6-month course of pegylated interferon and ribavirin. Once achieved, an SVR is associated with long-term clearance of the hepatitis C virus and can be regarded as a "cure," with positive impact on morbidity and mortality. Unfortunately, hepatitis C medications are often tolerated poorly, and patients with active psychiatric disorders and marked cytopenias generally are not candidates for interferon therapy because of the substantial risk of complications associated with therapy. The next big milestone in the treatment of hepatitis C will be the development of interferon-free treatment regimens.

Hepatitis D

The hepatitis D virus (HDV), also termed the delta agent, is a defective RNA virus that requires the presence of HBV to replicate. Only patients with acute or chronic HBV infection are susceptible to infection with HDV, occurring as either an acute coinfection or as superinfection. HDV is present worldwide, with high incidences in regions of Africa, South America, and the Mediterranean but a low incidence in the United States. Modes of transmission appear to be both parenteral and sexual. Diagnosis requires a high level of suspicion. Identification of HDV infection has improved as there is now a quantitative HDV RNA assay available, in addition to antibody testing. Infection with HDV in chronic HBV carriers may result in increased severity of hepatitis and clinical decompensation of patients with cirrhosis. Thus far, only interferon-α treatment has been shown to exert significant antiviral activity against HDV and has been linked to improved long-term outcomes. Recent data on the use of pegylated interferon confirm earlier findings, with pegylated interferon leading to SVR rates in about one-quarter of patients.

Hepatitis E

The hepatitis E virus (HEV) is an RNA virus epidemiologically and clinically similar to HAV. It is endemic in developing countries, especially Mexico, Africa, central Asia, and southern Asia. Reports in the United States are rare and usually represent infection acquired while traveling in endemic regions. Transmission is mainly by the fecal–oral route. Outbreaks are typically caused by contaminated water or food. The incubation period and clinical syndromes of acute hepatitis E are identical to those for HAV. For reasons that remain poorly defined, HEV infection in the third trimester of pregnancy is associated with a fulminant course in 15–25% of cases and has a high mortality rate. Diagnosis relies on detecting IgM antibodies to HEV. Detection of IgG antibodies to HEV signifies resolved infection and is associated with immunity. Treatment is supportive, and except for the high rate of fulminant hepatitis in pregnancy, full recovery from HEV infection is the rule. An exception to this rule is in the immunosuppressed patient who has undergone solid organ or bone marrow transplantation. There are multiple published reports of chronic hepatitis E in this population.

Key practice points

- Hepatitis A is an RNA virus spread primarily via fecal–oral contact. The majority of cases have only mild symptoms, although <1% will have a fulminant presentation. There are cases of prolonged cholestatic and relapsing variants but resolution of disease with complete recovery is the rule. Passive and active immunization is available for disease prevention.

- Hepatitis B is a DNA virus, with the most common modes of transmission including sexual, vertical and via intravenous drug use. Approximately 95% of adults recover without chronic infection, while >90% of perinatally exposed persons develop chronic infection. There are multiple phases of disease activity, depending on the replicative state of the virus. Treatment is rarely curative but rather aimed at viral suppression. Persons with chronic HBV infection are at increased risk for hepatocellular carcinoma, so screening for HCC is recommended. Effective vaccination is available.

- Hepatitis C is an RNA virus which is transmitted parenterally, largely via intravenous drug use. Sexual and perinatal transmission is rare. The majority of patients with acute HCV infection are asymptomatic. Seventy percent to 85% of HCV infections become chronic, and 20–25% of infected patients progress to cirrhosis over 20 years. Predictors of disease progression include older age at infection, coexisting liver disease, alcohol consumption, and possibly IL-28 genotype. Factors affecting response to interferon-based antiviral therapy include viral genotype, viral load, stage of fibrosis, race, and IL-28B genotype.

CHAPTER 38

Nonviral Hepatitis

While much of the burden of liver disease is caused by viral hepatitis, there are many nonviral etiologies of liver disease that must be considered. These include highly prevalent diseases, such as nonalcoholic fatty liver disease, and rare disorders such as Wilson disease and $\alpha 1$-antitrypsin deficiency. Autoimmune hepatitis, primary biliary cirrhosis, and primary sclerosing cholangitis are discussed in other chapters (39, 41).

Nonalcoholic steatohepatitis

A form of liver injury histologically indistinguishable from alcoholic hepatitis is often observed in patients who do not have histories of ethanol abuse. This syndrome has been termed nonalcoholic fatty liver disease (NAFLD), representing a spectrum of disease from simple steatosis to nonalcoholic steatohepatitis (NASH). NASH is characterized histologically by the presence of steatosis, inflammation, hepatocyte ballooning, Mallory hyaline and pericellular fibrosis. Nonalcoholic steatohepatitis is more common in obese patients and in those with hyperlipidemia, diabetes mellitus, or insulin resistance. Mild elevations in levels of serum aminotransferases are often observed, and nonspecific symptoms of fatigue, anorexia, and abdominal discomfort are present in a minority of patients.

There is no specific treatment for nonalcoholic steatohepatitis but clinicians advise weight loss for obese patients and aggressive treatment of hyperlipidemia and diabetes. Trials of ursodeoxycholic acid (ursodiol) have not provided data to support its use. Insulin-sensitizing agents including pioglitazone and metformin have provided encouraging data. The use of vitamin E has also shown potential benefit. Although reports suggest that up to 20% of cases progress to advanced fibrosis or cirrhosis, further clinical experience will help define the natural history of this disorder. The prevalence of NAFLD continues to rise, likely due to increasing rates of obesity and diabetes.

Yamada's Handbook of Gastroenterology, Third Edition. Edited by Tadataka Yamada and John M. Inadomi.
© 2013 John Wiley & Sons, Ltd. Published 2013 by John Wiley & Sons, Ltd.

Ischemic Hepatitis

An acute form of ischemic liver injury, termed ischemic hepatitis or shock liver, often complicates the course of critical illness. The portal vein provides about two-thirds of the hepatic blood supply; the residual one-third comes from the hepatic artery. Ischemic injury usually requires reduced flow in both systems. Most patients with ischemic hepatitis have circulatory shock from cardiovascular disease, sepsis, or profound hypovolemia.

In the hours to days after the hemodynamic insult, levels of serum aminotransferases, lactate dehydrogenase, and bilirubin increase to variable degrees. Severe injury is associated with aminotransferase levels in the several thousands and marked prolongation of prothrombin time. The treatment of ischemic hepatitis is largely supportive. Systemic hemodynamics should be optimized and any coexistent infections should be treated with broad-spectrum antibiotics. Despite apparent severe biochemical dysfunction, most of the laboratory abnormalities improve over 1–2 weeks with rapid declines in aminotransferases over the first 24–48 h. If the patient survives, liver function usually returns to normal. The overall prognosis usually is poor because of the underlying critical illness.

Wilson Disease

Incidence and epidemiology

Wilson disease, or hepatolenticular degeneration, is an autosomal recessive disorder caused by mutations in the *ATP7B* gene that lead to excessive accumulation of total body copper. It is a rare disorder with a worldwide incidence of 3 cases per 100,000 of population. Higher incidences may be noted in populations prone to inbreeding. The incidence of heterozygotes is 1 in 90. Abnormal copper metabolism is established from birth. Patients usually are diagnosed in adolescence, although rarely cases manifest after age 50.

Etiology and pathogenesis

The gene for Wilson disease is a copper-transporting P-type ATPase expressed exclusively in the liver. A defective structure or function of the transporter results in impaired biliary excretion and increased hepatic stores of copper. Free copper is also released into the serum and deposited in end organs. Accumulations in the brain, kidneys, bones, and eyes are responsible for the extrahepatic complications of Wilson disease.

Clinical presentation

Patients with Wilson disease almost universally present between ages 5 and 50; the second decade of life is the peak time of onset. Liver disease affects 50% of patients but the proportion who present with hepatic or neuropsychiatric symptoms varies with age. Potential hepatic manifestations include chronic active hepatitis with associated malaise, fatigue, and anorexia. Alternatively, patients present with complications of cirrhosis or a syndrome of fulminant hepatic failure with marked jaundice, encephalopathy, and hemolytic anemia. The diagnosis might be suggested by asymptomatic elevations of serum aminotransferase levels in an adolescent or young adult, often with a very low alkaline phosphatase level.

Because the primary metabolic defect is localized in the liver, all symptomatic patients with Wilson disease have some degree of liver disease but 50% of patients present with extrahepatic manifestations. In 40% of patients, neuropsychiatric complications dominate. For unclear reasons, Wilson disease never leads to sensory deficits but spasticity, choreiform movements, dysarthria, ataxia, and intention tremor result from copper accumulation in the lenticular nuclei. Patients also usually have subtle behavioral or psychiatric changes. The diagnosis should be suspected in adolescents with marked declines in scholastic or social performance. Patients with neuropsychiatric manifestations universally have Kayser–Fleischer rings, which are deposits of copper in the peripheral cornea. Other extrahepatic manifestations include Fanconi syndrome and proximal renal tubular acidosis, osteoporosis with spontaneous fractures, and copper-induced hemolytic anemia.

Diagnostic investigation

All siblings of Wilson disease patients should undergo diagnostic testing, in addition to young persons with abnormal liver chemistry profiles or clinical symptoms suggestive of Wilson disease. Screening for Wilson disease in a young patient with elevated levels of aminotransferases should include measurement of serum ceruloplasmin, which is decreased in more than 95% of homozygotes. Ceruloplasmin may also be low in 20% of heterozygotes and in patients with malnutrition, protein-losing enteropathy, and other forms of hepatic failure. Therefore, low ceruloplasmin levels should be confirmed by demonstrating 24-h urinary copper excretion of more than 100 mg. The diagnosis cannot be excluded on the basis of a normal ceruloplasmin level. If Wilson disease is strongly suspected, further diagnostic evaluation with 24-h urinary copper measurement should be performed with or without penicillamine challenge. Urinary copper also may be elevated in patients with cholestasis from other causes. Detection of Kayser–Fleischer rings may require slit-lamp examination. Although the presence of Kayser–Fleischer rings helps to confirm the diagnosis in the appropriate clinical setting, they may be absent in early Wilson disease. The standard for diagnosis is quantitation of hepatic copper levels in liver biopsy specimens. Histological findings include steatosis, glycogenated nuclei, and variable degrees of periportal mononuclear infiltrates and fibrosis. Genetic testing is not useful because of the large number of mutations described for the *ATP7B* gene.

Management and course

The critical factor in managing Wilson disease is establishing a definitive diagnosis early in its clinical course. Untreated, the disease is universally fatal. When treated, patients have a normal life expectancy but because treatment is life-long, the diagnosis should be established with certainty. The cornerstone of treatment has been copper chelation with oral penicillamine (1 g/day). The major obstacle is a 20% incidence of hypersensitivity reactions (e.g. neutropenia, thrombocytopenia, rash, and arthritis). Patients may require dose reduction because of drug-induced nephrotic syndrome. For hypersensitivity reactions other than neutropenia, a 2–3-week withdrawal followed by a stepwise increase in the dose may be attempted. Trientine and zinc have fewer side-effects and are being used increasingly. Zinc inhibits copper absorption in the gut and cannot be used to treat pre-existing copper overload. Although neurological symptoms may not resolve completely, patients with cirrhosis may experience long-term survival if they comply with therapy. Fulminant hepatic failure is not responsive to copper chelation and is universally fatal unless liver transplantation is performed. Transplantation should also be considered in the small fraction of patients with advanced cirrhosis who develop complications of progressive portal hypertension despite therapy.

Hemochromatosis

Incidence and epidemiology

Hemochromatosis is characterized by pathological accumulation of toxic levels of iron in the cells of various organs and tissues, including the liver. Because hepatic inflammation is not a prominent feature of the disease, hemochromatosis technically is not a form of hepatitis but the iron-induced hepatocellular injury leads to clinical and biochemical features similar to chronic hepatitis. Hemochromatosis may be caused by a genetic disorder of iron homeostasis termed hereditary hemochromatosis (HHC), or it may be caused by a secondary disorder, such as transfusional iron overload, sickle cell anemia, or dyserythropoiesis (e.g. thalassemia major). The hepatic manifestations of secondary hemochromatosis are similar to those of HHC but differentiation is usually apparent from the clinical features of the disorders associated with secondary hemochromatosis. Several hepatic disorders including alcoholic liver disease may be associated with uncomplicated iron overload, and differentiation from HHC may be challenging.

Hereditary hemochromatosis is inherited as an autosomal recessive trait, with the responsible gene, designated *HFE*, localized to chromosome 6. It is one of the most common inborn errors of metabolism; the homozygous frequency is 1 in 300 and the heterozygous frequency is 1 in 9. The disease appears to be more common in persons of northern European ancestry but the precise incidence among other racial or ethnic groups is unknown.

Etiology and pathogenesis

The basic pathophysiological mechanism in HHC is increased intestinal absorption of iron in conditions of normal dietary iron intake. A normal adult absorbs 1–2 mg of iron per day, whereas patients with HHC absorb 3–4 mg of iron per day. This increased absorption results in an excess accumulation of 700–1000 mg total body iron per year. The mechanism of enhanced absorption and intestinal cell transport of iron remains poorly defined.

The clinical features of HHC are produced by intracellular accumulation of toxic levels of iron, which causes hepatocellular destruction and fibrosis in the liver. Although the mechanism of iron toxicity remains poorly understood, damage to cellular and organelle membranes by increased lipid peroxidation has been proposed as an important factor. Iron deposition in the heart, pituitary, pancreas, skin, and gonads is responsible for the extrahepatic manifestations of HHC.

Clinical presentation

Liver disease is the most common clinical feature of HHC. Most patients remain asymptomatic until complications of cirrhosis develop but many cases of precirrhotic HHC are diagnosed after detection of asymptomatic hepatomegaly or mild elevations in levels of serum aminotransferases. Advanced liver disease may present with jaundice, weight loss, fatigue, variceal hemorrhage, ascites, and encephalopathy.

The most common extrahepatic manifestation is diabetes mellitus, which occurs in more than 50% of patients with HHC. An additional 50% of patients develop other endocrinopathies, including hypogonadism from pituitary and primary gonadal iron overload. Most patients with advanced disease have bronze or slate gray discolorations of exposed skin from increased melanin production and iron deposition in the basal layers. Degenerative arthropathy with a characteristic predilection for the second and third metacarpophalangeal joints occurs in 25% of patients.

Diagnostic investigation

Serum aminotransferase levels rarely exceed 100 IU/L, and they are normal in many cases. Serum measurements of total body iron levels are almost invariably elevated in HHC. The serum ferritin level is usually higher than 500 ng/mL and is often measured in the thousands. However, the serum ferritin level is elevated in any inflammatory disorder or iron overload condition such as alcoholism. Although a transferrin saturation of more than 55% is more specific for HHC, the predictive accuracy is less than 90% and the sensitivity is less than 80%. Therefore, patients with abnormal iron indexes should have their diagnoses confirmed.

The standard for diagnosing HHC is liver biopsy with hepatic iron quantification and determination of the hepatic iron index. The hepatic iron index (HII) is calculated as micromoles of iron per gram of dry liver divided by the patient's age. A HII higher than 1.9 is diagnostic of hemochromatosis, whereas an index less than 2 essentially excludes HHC. Patients with alcoholic liver disease and those who are heterozygous for HHC often have markedly abnormal serum iron indexes but the HII is always less than 2.0. Histological evaluation with Prussian blue staining usually shows impressive stores of intracellular iron in more than 50% of hepatocytes but this finding may also occur in advanced alcoholic liver disease. Noninvasive magnetic resonance imaging may suggest iron overload but attempts to quantify iron stores with these methods have yet to be validated. Increasingly, diagnosis is made by detecting the C282Y mutation in the *HFE* gene, which detects more than 90% of HHC. A second mutation, H63D, is of less certain clinical import, as is the significance of heterozygotes for C282Y and C282Y/H63D compound heterozygotes.

Management and course

The mainstay of HHC treatment is phlebotomy. The usual regimen removes 1 unit (250 mg of iron) every 1–2 weeks. Patients may require a total of 75–100 sessions over 2–3 years before iron stores return to normal levels. Once the transferrin saturation falls to less than 45% and the serum ferritin level is below 50 ng/mL, patients can be maintained on regimens of phlebotomy every 3–4 months. If diagnosed before the onset of cirrhosis or diabetes, patients with HHC compliant with phlebotomy programs can expect normal survival. Although phlebotomy does not reverse cirrhosis, it improves survival and should be considered at all stages of HHC. In patients with dyserythropoiesis or other causes of anemia intolerant of phlebotomy, chelation therapy with desferoxamine is an alternative. Desferoxamine requires parenteral infusion and removes only 50–75 mg of iron per dose.

In patients with cirrhosis, the 10-year survival rate is 70%. Most deaths caused by HHC are related to complications of liver disease. Up to 30% of patients with HHC develop hepatocellular carcinoma. Screening patients with established cirrhosis by using biannual α-fetoprotein measurement and ultrasound, computed tomography, or magnetic resonance imaging may result in early detection. Patients with advanced cirrhosis should be considered for liver transplantation but the posttransplantation survival of patients with HHC is lower than that of patients with other forms of chronic liver disease, possibly because of a higher incidence of diabetes and cardiac disease.

α_1-Antitrypsin Deficiency

Individuals who have inherited the PiZZ phenotype of α_1-antitrypsin may manifest various liver disorders as a result of the accumulation of mutant Z α_1-antitrypsin in the endoplasmic reticulum of hepatocytes. Patients usually present in infancy with cholestatic hepatitis or cirrhosis but some present in adulthood with chronic hepatitis, cirrhosis, or hepatocellular carcinoma. Only 20% of persons with PiZZ phenotype develop clinical liver disease. The other phenotypes (e.g. PiSS, PiSZ), including those commonly associated with emphysema, are not associated with liver disease. Diagnosis is usually suspected in a patient with liver disease who exhibits decreased levels of the α_1 band in serum protein electrophoresis. Determining the specific phenotype of patients and both parents can provide more direct evidence for the diagnosis. Liver biopsy specimens can confirm the diagnosis by the presence of intracellular periodic acid-Schiff (PAS)-positive globules.

There is no specific treatment for α_1-antitrypsin deficiency, and liver transplantation should be considered in patients with complications of cirrhosis. In addition to treating complications of cirrhosis, transplantation cures the underlying metabolic defect.

Key practice points

- Multiple nonviral etiologies of liver disease exist, and must be considered when evaluating a patient with evidence of liver disease.
- Nonalcoholic fatty liver disease is increasingly prevalent and is the most common etiology of persistent liver test abnormalities in the United States.
- Other less frequent causes of liver test abnormalities include ischemic hepatitis/shock liver, Wilson disease, hemochromatosis and α1-antitrypsin deficiency, in addition to autoimmune and biliary disorders (autoimmune hepatitis, primary biliary cirrhosis, and primary sclerosing cholangitis).

CHAPTER 39
Cholestatic Syndromes

Cholestasis is a defect in bile excretion. It can be classified as intrahepatic or extrahepatic based on the anatomical site of the disturbance. Extrahepatic cholestasis is caused by diseases that structurally impair bile secretion and flow in the large bile ducts. Intrahepatic cholestasis is caused by a functional defect in bile formation and excretion at the level of the hepatocyte and terminal bile ducts. This chapter reviews the common causes of intrahepatic cholestasis (Table 39.1).

Primary Biliary Cirrhosis

Incidence and epidemiology

Primary biliary cirrhosis (PBC) is a chronic, progressive, cholestatic disease that affects mainly middle-aged women. Patients may present as early as age 30 or as late as age 90, with a median age between 40 and 55 at presentation. PBC has been observed in all races but is more common in whites. Some of the highest prevalences have been reported in England and Sweden. Worldwide, PBC accounts for 0.6–2.0% of deaths from cirrhosis. Epidemiological surveys have failed to identify specific environmental risk factors but developed regions have higher incidences than undeveloped regions. It is not known whether this represents a true difference in disease incidence or a detection bias from health screening.

Etiology and pathogenesis

Although several disease associations and well-characterized disturbances in immune regulation suggest that PBC is an immune-mediated disease, the etiology remains unknown. Associated immunological abnormalities include

Yamada's Handbook of Gastroenterology, Third Edition. Edited by Tadataka Yamada and John M. Inadomi.
© 2013 John Wiley & Sons, Ltd. Published 2013 by John Wiley & Sons, Ltd.

Table 39.1 Differential diagnosis of intrahepatic cholestasis

Primary biliary cirrhosis
Sclerosing cholangitis
Hepatocellular disease
    Viral hepatitis
    Alcoholic hepatitis
    Medications
Intrahepatic cholestasis of pregnancy
Systemic infection
Total parenteral nutrition-associated cholestasis
Postoperative cholestasis

antimitochondrial autoantibodies, increased IgM levels, multiple antinuclear antibodies (~30%), circulating immune complexes, and other associated autoimmune phenomena. Autoimmune diseases associated with PBC include Sjögren syndrome, CREST syndrome, autoimmune thyroiditis, and, possibly, rheumatoid arthritis. PBC has also been linked to the HLA-DR8 antigen, which suggests that the disease may have a genetic component.

Liver injury results from the nonsuppurative destruction of small bile ducts in the lobule. Reduced biliary excretion leads to cholestasis and toxic hepatocyte injury from the accumulation of bile acids and copper. The disease evolves through four histologically described stages. In stage I, the portal tracts are expanded by chronic inflammatory cells and noncaseating granulomas adjacent to the damaged bile ducts, including the classic "florid duct lesion." Stage II is characterized by expansion of the inflammatory infiltrate into the hepatic parenchyma and proliferation of the bile ductules. In stage III, interlobular fibrous septa and ductopenia are present. Stage IV represents cirrhosis.

Clinical presentation

Forty percent to 50% of persons with PBC are asymptomatic at presentation. The disease is detected in most of these individuals from elevated serum alkaline phosphatase or γ-glutamyltransferase levels. About 50–60% of patients have presenting symptoms, usually fatigue and pruritus, and in some, upper right quadrant discomfort. Less than 25% present with jaundice. The pruritus may be relentless and profound, prompting the patient to seek advice from a dermatologist before it is recognized as a complication of cholestasis. The skin may become excoriated and hyperpigmented from incessant scratching. Other physical findings include hepatomegaly, splenomegaly, palmar erythema, spider angiomata, xanthomas, and xanthelasma. The last finding correlates with the hypercholesterolemia

Table 39.2 Extrahepatic manifestations of primary biliary cirrhosis

Extrahepatic disease	Prevalence (%)
Sjögren syndrome	30–58
Gallstones	30–50
Decreased pulmonary diffusion capacity	40–50
Renal tubular acidosis	20–33
Osteoporosis	15–40
Bacteriuria	11–35
Arthropathy	4–38
Rheumatoid arthritis	3–26
Hypothyroidism	11–32
Raynaud phenomenon	7–14
CREST* syndrome	3–6
Autoimmune thyroiditis	3–6
Autoimmune anemias	1–2
Psoriasis	1–13
Lichen planus	0.5–6
Ulcerative colitis	0.5–1

*CREST: syndrome of calcinosis, Raynaud phenomenon, esophageal dysmotility, sclerodactyly, and telangiectasias.

(particularly of high-density lipoprotein) which is observed in PBC. The defect in bile acid secretion leads to impaired fat digestion with resultant steatorrhea, weight loss, and fat-soluble vitamin deficiencies. Long-standing cholestasis can also result in bone resorption and osteoporosis, which often lead to vertebral compression fractures and long bone fractures. A rare patient may have hepatic failure or a complication of portal hypertension (e.g. variceal bleeding) as the initial manifestation of PBC.

Most patients with PBC have associated autoimmune diseases. These diseases, of which Sjögren syndrome is by far the most common, usually are mild and survival is dictated by the severity of hepatic dysfunction. Autoimmune thyroiditis with hypothyroidism and CREST syndrome also often occur with PBC and may predate the diagnosis of liver disease. Other diseases associated with PBC include rheumatoid arthritis, gallstones, decreased pulmonary diffusion capacity, psoriasis, Raynaud phenomenon, and distal renal tubular acidosis (Table 39.2).

Diagnostic investigation

Laboratory studies

Patients with PBC typically have elevated serum alkaline phosphatase levels. Similar elevations in levels of 5′-nucleotidase and γ-glutamyltransferase help confirm the hepatic origin of the elevated alkaline phosphatase level. Serum bilirubin levels usually are normal at diagnosis. As the disease progresses, more than 50% of patients develop hyperbilirubinemia, a poor prognostic indicator. As with other cholestatic syndromes, levels of aminotransferases usually are only slightly elevated. Other nonspecific surrogate markers of cholestasis include increased levels of serum bile acids, cholesterol, triglycerides, elevated serum and hepatic copper levels, and decreased levels of fat-soluble vitamins A, D, E, and K.

Serological testing

The immunological abnormalities observed in PBC provide useful diagnostic information. Antimitochondrial antibodies (AMAs) are present in 90–95% of patients with PBC. Although other autoantibodies are present in a large number of cholestatic syndromes, elevated titers of AMAs rarely occur in other diseases and therefore are quite specific for PBC. Similarly, the finding of elevated IgM levels on serum protein electrophoresis, often in the absence of hyperglobulinemia, has high predictive value for PBC. Other serological abnormalities include increased titers of antinuclear antibodies (ANAs) in 25–70% of patients and other autoantibodies but these findings are not specific to PBC and are of limited diagnostic value.

Liver biopsy

Confirmation of PBC requires percutaneous liver biopsy. The pathognomonic lesion is characterized by patchy destruction of interlobular bile ducts with a mononuclear inflammatory infiltrate. Granulomas may be present in some portal tracts but their presence is not required to confirm a diagnosis of PBC. The severity of histological damage can be classified into four distinct stages.

Structural studies

Several imaging procedures may be used to evaluate PBC. These procedures are used primarily to exclude extrahepatic causes of cholestasis. Ultrasound generally demonstrates bile ducts of normal size. Gallstones are revealed in more than 30% of cases. Computed tomographic scanning also helps to exclude bile duct dilation and may demonstrate portosystemic collaterals that suggest portal hypertension. In patients lacking the serological markers of PBC, endoscopic retrograde cholangiopancreatography (ERCP) may be necessary. Although the terminal intrahepatic ducts may be irregular, the larger ducts appear to be normal in size and contour on ERCP.

Management and course

Primary biliary cirrhosis is an invariably progressive disease but the rate of progression varies. About half of the patients with PBC are asymptomatic at presentation but many become symptomatic within 2–4 years. As the disease progresses from the asymptomatic to symptomatic stages, serum alkaline phosphatase and globulin levels often dramatically increase and subsequently reach a plateau. Once symptoms appear, there is an indolent worsening of fatigue and pruritus, usually over the course of years. Patients eventually develop muscle wasting, progressive jaundice, and hepatic dysfunction. Once jaundice develops, life expectancy declines markedly, with mean survival times of 4 years if bilirubin levels are higher than 2 mg/dL and 2 years if higher than 6 mg/dL. The final stage of PBC is marked by complications of portal hypertension, including ascites, variceal hemorrhage, and encephalopathy.

The chronic inflammatory response and immune dysfunction observed in PBC have prompted clinical trials of several immunosuppressive regimens. Corticosteroids fail to alter the biochemical, histological, and clinical progression observed in PBC. Azathioprine, cyclosporine, colchicine, and D-penicillamine may result in biochemical improvements but none of these agents alters disease progression or survival. Some clinical trials of weekly regimens of methotrexate have shown improvement in biochemical and histological abnormalities. Given the potential for toxicity and the lack of clear benefit, the use of methotrexate is not recommended.

The synthetic bile acid ursodeoxycholic acid (ursodiol) is the only approved therapy for PBC. Given at a daily dose of 13–15 mg/kg, ursodiol may stabilize hepatocyte membranes, decrease the rate of biliary epithelial apoptosis, and decrease the production of more toxic bile acids. It also has antioxidant properties, including the ability to inhibit nitric oxide synthase. Several reports describe a decrease in the severity of pruritus in 50% of cases. Most patients experience biochemical improvement but effects on histological improvement have been inconsistent in short-term trials. Long-term studies of ursodiol treatment have shown improved survival and delay in time to transplantation but meta-analysis has not confirmed these results, perhaps due to the short duration of the placebo phase before the cross-over to ursodiol in several large trials.

The control of pruritus is the goal of symptomatic treatment of PBC. Oral antihistamines are occasionally of benefit in cholestasis-associated pruritus. Cholestyramine and colestipol are effective in up to 80% of patients but they often cause profound constipation and bloating. These ionic resins bind intraluminal bile acids and other pruritogens, thus preventing the absorption of these substances. Cholestyramine and other resins also interfere with the absorption of medications such as digoxin, thyroxine, and penicillins. Steatorrhea and fat-soluble vitamin deficiencies can be exacerbated. Patients intolerant of cholestyramine may respond to phenobarbital or rifampin. Refractory pruritus may respond to naloxone or other opioid antagonists, ondansetron, plasmapheresis, or therapy with ultraviolet B light but data are limited.

Survival of patients with PBC depends largely on the clinical and histological stage of disease. The survival times of symptomatic patients are shorter than those of asymptomatic patients. Several models have attempted to predict survival on the basis of clinical variables. The most powerful predictor is the serum bilirubin level. Patients with bilirubin levels higher than 6 mg/dL usually survive less than 2 years. Hypercholesterolemia rarely leads to cardiac disease except in the presence of other cardiac risks or unfavorable lipid profiles. Osteoporosis can be severe so monitoring the vitamin D level and supplementation of calcium and vitamin D as well as estrogen replacement or bisphosphonate therapy are useful in preventing bone loss.

Prediction of survival is critical in enabling the clinician to select optimal candidates for liver transplantation. Transplantation should be considered for patients with complications of portal hypertension, severe symptomatic osteodystrophy, or a predicted survival of less than 2 years. In properly selected candidates, liver transplantation is highly successful in treating PBC; the 2-year survival rate is higher than 80%.

Hepatocellular Diseases

Several liver diseases that characteristically produce hepatocellular injury may demonstrate biochemical and clinical features more consistent with cholestasis. Alcoholic hepatitis may produce profound increases in levels of serum bilirubin and alkaline phosphatase with normal to minimally elevated levels of aminotransferases, a pattern that often correlates with severe hepatocellular injury. Patients with alcoholic hepatitis often have very poor prognoses. Atypical variant forms of acute viral hepatitis A, B, and E include a syndrome of prolonged cholestasis. Although patients with hepatitis C typically manifest acute hepatitis, liver allograft recipients with recurrent infection from hepatitis C virus may rarely develop recurrent cholestatic hepatitis C, which is characterized by pericholangitis and cholestasis with minimal inflammation, rapid graft failure, and poor prognosis.

Intrahepatic Cholestasis of Pregnancy

Pregnancy may be associated with abnormal liver chemistry values attributable to numerous physiological alterations and disease processes. Perhaps the most common finding is a mild increase in the serum alkaline phosphatase level from placental release of this enzyme. Women may also have coincident liver diseases unrelated to their pregnancy, for example, alcohol-, viral-, and immune-mediated liver diseases. The impact of pregnancy on the natural history of these disorders remains unclear. Pregnancy may be complicated by several disorders unique to pregnancy, for example, HELLP syndrome with pre-eclampsia and the rare but devastating syndrome of acute fatty liver of pregnancy. These two disorders present in the third trimester, often with cholestasis and systemic complications such as disseminated intravascular coagulation and renal and hepatic failure. Acute fatty liver and pre-eclampsia-related liver injury require prompt delivery of the fetus. Unless diagnosed early, these disorders have high maternal mortality rates.

The most common liver disease unique to pregnancy is intrahepatic cholestasis of pregnancy. It occurs in less than 1% of all pregnancies in the United States and accounts for 30–50% of all causes of jaundice in pregnancy. It is distinguished from the other disorders by its benign course. The syndrome is similar to the cholestasis associated with estrogen supplements. Moreover, women with a prior history of intrahepatic cholestasis of pregnancy often manifest cholestasis when challenged with oral contraceptives in the nonpregnant state. The etiology remains unknown but familial clustering suggests the presence of a genetically acquired sensitivity to the cholestatic effects of estrogens. Patients usually present with pruritus and mild jaundice in the third trimester. Liver chemistry values demonstrate a cholestatic pattern. A biopsy specimen from the liver reveals bland cholestasis with no inflammatory reaction. A biopsy is occasionally needed to differentiate the syndrome from acute fatty liver of pregnancy or other more morbid disorders. Supportive treatment with ursodiol and cholestyramine may relieve the pruritus; cholestasis and pruritus resolve within 24–48 h of delivery.

Systemic Infection

Systemic Gram-negative bacterial infections are often accompanied by cholestasis. Endotoxemia decreases bile flow and may result in conjugated hyperbilirubinemia, with bilirubin levels in the range of 5–10 mg/dL. Levels of aminotransferases are usually near normal, and the alkaline phosphatase level is variably elevated. Clinical manifestations are dominated by the underlying infection. Cholestasis improves with successful treatment of the responsible micro-organisms.

Cholestasis Associated with Total Parenteral Nutrition

Patients who receive long-term total parenteral nutrition (TPN) may manifest any of several distinct patterns of hepatic dysfunction, including cholestasis. TPN-induced intrahepatic cholestasis is common in premature newborn infants. The mechanism is undefined but probably results from alterations in serum bile acid pools caused by changes in intestinal bacteria. Patients who receive TPN are often subjected to bowel rest; the resulting bile stasis promotes biliary sludge and stone formation. Therefore, extrahepatic cholestasis also should be considered when evaluating patients on long-term TPN.

Postoperative Cholestasis

The postoperative state may be complicated by jaundice caused by cholestasis and impaired bile formation or alterations in the production or excretion of bilirubin. Increased bilirubin production, which may exceed the excretory capacity of the liver, can be caused by several factors in a patient undergoing surgery. Hemolysis caused by systemic infections, transfusion reactions, mechanical trauma caused by artificial valves or a circulatory bypass, or pre-existing red blood cell defects and hemoglobinopathies increase the production of bilirubin. Similarly, massive transfusions and resorption of large hematomas may overwhelm the liver's ability to excrete bilirubin. Increased bilirubin loads lead to predominantly unconjugated hyperbilirubinemia. Patients with Gilbert syndrome, a common autosomal dominant defect of bilirubin conjugation, often develop unconjugated hyperbilirubinemia from physiological stress and fasting in the perioperative period.

Hepatocellular injury also may cause jaundice in postoperative patients. Hypoxia and hypotension in the perioperative period can produce ischemic hepatitis. Drug-induced hepatotoxicity, especially from anesthetic agents, can cause jaundice. Rarely, viral hepatitis acquired from transfusions results in jaundice, weeks after an operation. All of these insults usually produce a marked increase in levels of aminotransferases in addition to hyperbilirubinemia.

Cholestasis in the postoperative state can be extrahepatic or intrahepatic in origin. Patients undergoing biliary surgery are prone to extrahepatic cholestasis if there are retained bile duct stones and bile duct injuries. Systemic infection, medications, and TPN can produce intrahepatic cholestasis. When all other causes of postoperative jaundice and cholestasis have been excluded, the probable diagnosis is benign postoperative intrahepatic cholestasis. This transient syndrome of unknown etiology usually causes conjugated hyperbilirubinemia and elevated serum alkaline phosphatase levels by the third postoperative day. It gradually resolves over 1–2 weeks.

Key practice points

- Cholestasis is a defect in bile excretion. It can be classified as intrahepatic or extrahepatic based on the anatomical site of the disturbance.
- Primary biliary cirrhosis (PBC) results in intrahepatic cholestasis due to destruction of small bile ducts. It is characterized by a positive antimitochondrial antibody and the only recommended treatment is ursodiol.
- PBC, along with other cholestatic liver diseases, can result in jaundice, pruritus, fat-soluble vitamin deficiency, hypercholesterolemia, and reduced bone density.
- Treatment of pruritus in cholestatic liver disease can include antihistamines, cholestyramine, rifampin, naloxone and ultraviolet light therapy.

CHAPTER 40

Alcoholic Liver Disease

Alcohol-related liver diseases are among the most common liver diseases in the United States. It is estimated that 15–20 million people suffer from alcoholism in the United States, and alcohol is considered the third leading cause of preventable mortality. Alcoholism can affect people of all ages but the highest incidence of alcoholism occurs in those between the ages of 45 and 64 years. The male-to-female ratio of alcoholism is approximately 10/1, although the ratio for alcoholic liver disease (ALD) is estimated to be 3/1. This difference likely represents an increased risk of developing cirrhosis in female compared with male alcoholics. Further, there is a more rapid course of liver disease in women who abuse alcohol compared with men. The peak incidence of alcoholic liver disease in men is between ages 40–55 but a decade earlier in women. The amount of alcohol that can be safely consumed is unknown but it is estimated to be 20 g/day (two drinks) for men and 10 g/day (one drink) for women. In men, the risk of alcoholic cirrhosis increases with daily alcohol consumption of 60–80 g/day, with a lesser intake of 20 g/day placing women at risk. Why only a minority of alcoholics develop cirrhosis remains unknown.

Metabolism of ethanol

After ingestion, ethanol undergoes partial first-pass metabolism in the stomach and liver and is subsequently distributed throughout the extracellular and intracellular water space. Most ethanol is metabolized by hepatic alcohol dehydrogenase (ADH) to acetaldehyde, which is subsequently converted by acetaldehyde dehydrogenase (ALDH) to acetate. ADH is the rate-limiting enzyme. Its activity is decreased by fasting, protein malnutrition, and chronic liver disease. ADH is not inducible with chronic ethanol ingestion but several iso-forms with disparate rates of ethanol metabolism have been associated with

---

Yamada's Handbook of Gastroenterology, Third Edition. Edited by Tadataka Yamada and John M. Inadomi.
© 2013 John Wiley & Sons, Ltd. Published 2013 by John Wiley & Sons, Ltd.

differences in the risk of alcoholism and alcohol-related liver disease among different ethnic groups. There are also several ALDH isoforms with differing metabolic rates. Isoforms of ALDH with low activities are common among Asian populations and are associated with lower rates of alcoholism. These persons can experience a flushing syndrome after consuming ethanol. Disulfiram (Antabuse) acts by blocking ALDH. The accumulation of acetaldehyde leads to the clinical syndrome of flushing, nausea, and vomiting. Ultimately, the rate of ethanol metabolism by ADH and ALDH may be crucial in determining the toxicity of alcohol.

A smaller portion of ethanol is oxidized by the cytochrome CYP2E1. This enzyme is inducible by chronic ethanol ingestion and may contribute to the increased rate of ethanol elimination in alcoholics. Because CYP2E1 is responsible for metabolizing other drugs, ethanol can increase or decrease the rate of elimination of some medications

Pathogenesis of alcoholic liver disease

The most common and earliest response of the liver to heavy alcohol use is the development of fatty liver, due to the accumulation of triglyceride droplets in the liver. This phenomenon has in the past been attributed to increasing nicotinamide adenine dinucleotide (NADH) levels generated by ADH and ALDH, resulting in decreased fatty acid oxidation. The resultant increase in fatty acids leads to accelerated triglyceride synthesis. This hypothesis has been challenged recently, and alternative mechanisms may play an equally important pathogenic role.

Chronic alcohol use can induce oxidative stress, resulting in lipid peroxidation which is felt to be a key component in the injury of ALD. Acetaldehyde may alter membrane and cytoskeletal elements and induce the formation of protein adducts that may serve as antigenic stimuli, leading to an inflammatory response. Further, alcohol increases gut-derived lipopolysaccharide (endotoxin) in the portal circulation, which leads to Kupffer cell activation. All of these metabolic alterations interact with cytokines including tumor necrosis factor (TNF)-α and transforming growth factor $\beta 1$ to produce cell necrosis, stellate cell activation, collagen deposition, and fibrosis.

Clinical presentation

The clinical manifestations of alcoholic liver disease can be divided into three disease processes: steatosis, alcoholic hepatitis, and alcoholic cirrhosis. A liver biopsy specimen may show evidence of all three forms of alcoholic liver disease. Steatosis is generally benign, asymptomatic, and reversible with abstinence. Patients with alcohol-related steatosis may be asymptomatic or have mild hepatomegaly.

Laboratory abnormalities in alcoholic fatty liver are typically mild. Bilirubin may be elevated but less than 5 mg/dL. As with all stages of ALD, serum aspartate aminotransferase (AST) and alanine aminotransferase (ALT) levels are usually less than 300 IU/L. The AST is usually higher than the ALT, with AST/ALT ratio ≥2 in the vast majority of cases.

Most morbidity and mortality from alcohol-related liver disease are the result of alcoholic hepatitis and cirrhosis. Although a rare patient may be asymptomatic, patients with alcoholic hepatitis generally experience fever, anorexia, malaise, and abdominal pain. Bilirubin is increased, whereas albumin is decreased and prothrombin time is typically prolonged. Electrolyte abnormalities are common, including hyponatremia, hyperchloremia, hypokalemia, and hypophosphatemia. Most patients with alcoholic hepatitis have physical examination findings of icterus, tender hepatomegaly, tachycardia, and spider angiomata. Severe alcoholic hepatitis manifests portal hypertension, including splenomegaly, enlarged collateral abdominal veins, ascites in 40–70% of cases, encephalopathy in 20%, and upper gastrointestinal bleeding in 30%. Although most patients admitted to hospital with alcoholic hepatitis have simultaneous cirrhosis by biopsy, portal hypertension may be present in the absence of histological evidence of cirrhosis. Mortality rates are high in this population.

Patients may present with alcoholic cirrhosis without progressing through the stages of steatosis or clinically apparent alcoholic hepatitis. At the time of diagnosis, 10–20% of patients with cirrhosis are asymptomatic but most present with nonspecific complaints of weight loss, malaise, failure to thrive, or complications of portal hypertension (e.g. ascites, spontaneous bacterial peritonitis, variceal hemorrhage, and hepatic encephalopathy). Patients with alcoholic cirrhosis often have stigmata of alcoholism on physical examination, including palmar erythema, Dupuytren contracture, testicular atrophy, gynecomastia, and feminization in male patients.

Liver biopsy

The classification of alcoholic liver disease into fatty liver, alcoholic hepatitis, and cirrhosis is based on clinical and pathological correlations; therefore, confirmation of these abnormalities and exclusion of alternative causes of liver disease may require liver biopsy. For patients with coagulopathy, tense ascites, or thrombocytopenia, the risk of biopsy may outweigh the benefit of obtaining pathological confirmation.

Fatty liver or steatosis is characterized histologically by large intracytoplasmic fat droplets often concentrated in the pericentral zone or zone 3. By definition, simple steatosis is not accompanied by significant inflammation or necrosis but pericentral fibrosis, a network of collagen surrounding the central vein, may be present. In addition to alcohol, other causes of fatty liver should

Table 40.1 Potential causes of fatty liver

Macrovesicular fat

Alcoholic steatohepatitis

Nonalcoholic steatohepatitis

Hepatitis C

Toxins and drugs: methotrexate, halogenated hydrocarbons, niacin, HIV protease inhibitors, glucocorticoids, heavy alcohol use

Nutritional disorders: obesity, diabetes, choline deficiency, systemic carnitine deficiency, celiac disease, kwashiorkor, parenteral nutrition

Lipodystrophy

Wilson disease

Aβ-lipoproteinemia

Inflammatory bowel disease

Weber–Christian disease

Q fever

Microvesicular fat*

Reye syndrome

Parenteral alimentation

Yellow fever

Heat stroke

Toxins and drugs: valproic acid, intravenous tetracycline, toxic shock syndromes, salicylate overdosage in children, Jamaican vomiting disease, FIAU, nucleoside reverse transcriptase inhibitors, mycotoxins

Metabolic diseases: cholesterol ester storage disease, galactosemia, Wolman disease, long-chain 3-hydroxyacyl-CoA dehydrogenase deficiency, medium-chain acyl-CoA deficiency

Complications of pregnancy: acute fatty liver of pregnancy, eclampsia, HELLP syndrome

---

*Microvesicular fatty liver is usually the result of mitochondrial damage and defects in lipid oxidation pathways; however, there is significant overlap with many disorders occasionally producing microvesicular fatty liver.

CoA, coenzyme A; FIAU, fialuridine; HELLP, hemolysis, elevated liver enzymes, and low platelet syndrome; HIV, human immunodeficiency virus.

Source: Yamada T et al. (eds) *Textbook of Gastroenterology*, 5th edn. Oxford: Blackwell Publishing Ltd, 2009.

be considered (Table 40.1). In contrast, inflammation and hepatocellular necrosis are hallmarks of alcoholic hepatitis. The inflammatory infiltrate is primarily neutrophilic, and necrosis may range from ballooning degeneration of isolated hepatocytes to confluent centrilobular necrosis. Mallory hyaline and pericellular and perisinusoidal fibrosis, which has a characteristic "chicken wire" appearance, are common. Cirrhosis, the final stage of alcoholic liver disease, requires documenting the presence of bands of fibrosis extending between the portal tracts and the central veins and the presence of regenerative nodules. Alcoholic cirrhosis may be confused with primary hemochromatosis because of the high levels of hepatic iron. These two disorders can be distinguished by calculating the hepatic iron index: the micromoles of iron per gram of dry liver divided by the patient's age. In hemochromatosis, the iron index is higher than 1.9 μmol/g and in alcoholic cirrhosis without hemochromatosis, it is invariably less than 1.9.

There is no pathognomonic histological feature of alcoholic liver disease. Mallory bodies are aggregates of perinuclear eosinophilic material once considered diagnostic of alcohol-induced injury. They are present in at least 30% of patients with alcoholic hepatitis or cirrhosis but they are also present in other liver disorders, including Wilson disease, cholestatic liver disease, nonalcoholic steatohepatitis, drug-induced and total parenteral nutrition-induced liver disease.

Management and prognosis

The prognosis for alcoholic liver disease is determined mainly by the pathological stage at presentation and the patient's ability to abstain from ethanol consumption. The single most important therapeutic intervention is complete avoidance of ethanol consumption. This often requires a multidisciplinary approach, involving social workers, psychiatrists, primary care physicians, hepatologists, and social support groups. No therapy for alcoholic liver disease has any proven benefit if heavy drinking continues.

Alcoholic fatty liver is generally benign and resolves completely after 3–6 weeks of abstinence. The major clinical importance of this condition is its representation of significant alcohol-related end-organ damage, for which patients should be counseled to abstain before more severe or irreversible damage develops.

Alcoholic hepatitis carries a far worse prognosis, with a high associated mortality. Early (2 month) mortality rates range from 19% to 78%. Patients with encephalopathy, renal failure, ascites, and variceal bleeding have higher mortalities. Several methods of predicting disease severity and survival have incorporated clinical and laboratory findings but the most accurate and widely used is the Maddrey discriminant function: serum bilirubin (mg/dL) + [4.6 × (patient's prothrombin time – control prothrombin time)]. A discriminant function of more than 32 identifies patients with severe alcoholic hepatitis who have a 30-day mortality rate higher than 50%.

Corticosteroids have been used to reduce the inflammatory response of alcoholic hepatitis. Several studies have demonstrated improved survival of patients with a discriminant function (DF) of more than 32 or with spontaneous encephalopathy. Studies have used prednisone, prednisolone, or 5-methylprednisolone in doses of 35–80 mg/day for 4–6 weeks. The American College of Gastroenterology has recommended the use of prednisolone 40 mg daily for 4 weeks, followed by a taper, in patients with severe alcoholic hepatitis (DF >32) with hepatic encephalopathy. Treatment should exclude patients with active infection, renal failure, pancreatitis, or gastrointestinal hemorrhage. The mortality rate in this selected group is reduced by 25%.

The possible contribution of protein and calorie malnutrition to alcohol toxicity has led to several trials of enteral and parenteral nutritional supplementation for treating patients with alcoholic hepatitis. These supplements result in accelerated biochemical improvement, and some studies have demonstrated improved survival. Patients with alcoholic hepatitis should have their caloric intake monitored and supplemented if deficient. Aggressive enteral supplementation may be warranted if oral intake is inadequate.

Pentoxifylline, which has anti-TNF-α properties, has been shown to reduce the risk of hepatorenal syndrome in a large study of patients with severe alcoholic hepatitis. Pentoxifylline, given at a dose of 400 mg three times daily, reduced mortality by 40%, due in large part to a reduction in renal failure. Because it has a low side-effect profile, pentoxifylline is being used to treat moderate alcoholic hepatitis and, in conjunction with corticosteroids, to treat severe cases. Numerous additional medications have been studied for the management of alcoholic hepatitis, including anabolic steroids (oxandrolone), propylthiouracil (PTU), infliximab, colchicine and vitamin E, without convincing evidence of benefit and some with potential risk.

As with all forms of alcoholic liver disease, long-term survival of patients with alcoholic cirrhosis is directly related to the stage of the disease and the patient's ability to abstain from ethanol consumption. In cirrhotic patients without jaundice, ascites, or gastrointestinal hemorrhage, 5-year survival rates are 85% with abstinence and 60% with continued heavy drinking. In patients with jaundice or ascites, the 5-year survival rates are 50% with abstinence and 30% with continued drinking. Cirrhotic patients with variceal hemorrhage have the worst prognoses: 5-year survival rates of 35% and 20% for nondrinkers and drinkers, respectively. Much of this survival data predates the use of endoscopic variceal banding and transjugular intrahepatic portosystemic shunts, although these therapies have not shown a survival benefit. Similar to other forms of cirrhosis, treatment is largely supportive.

Liver transplantation should be considered for patients who have abstained for at least 6 months but continue to suffer from complications of portal hypertension and are in Child class B or C. The period of abstinence selects candidates who will probably have low rates of recidivism. Also, it allows for potential improvement in liver function to a condition that may not warrant transplantation. Patients may be referred to a transplant center before completing this prolonged period of abstinence. Although guidelines for pretransplant and posttransplant treatment vary from center to center, survival post transplant has been excellent. With appropriate patient selection, only 10–30% of patients return to drinking. Alcohol-related liver disease accounts for about 25% of adult liver transplants in the United States.

Key practice points

- Alcoholic liver disease is highly prevalent, affecting men more than women (3/1), typically at the ages of 40–55.

- The histological findings in alcoholic fatty liver disease include steatosis in a zone 3 distribution, neutrophilic inflammation, Mallory hyaline and pericentral fibrosis.

- Alcoholic liver disease can be divided into three disease processes: steatosis, alcoholic hepatitis, and alcoholic cirrhosis, and all three can coexist.

- Alcoholic hepatitis carries a poor prognosis. Multiple models exist to measure disease severity, most notably Maddrey's discriminant function.

- Treatment options for severe alcoholic hepatitis (discriminant function >32 +/- encephalopathy) include the use of corticosteroids, nutritional supplementation, and pentoxifylline.

- Ultimately, prognosis of alcoholic liver disease depends on abstinence from alcohol.

CHAPTER 41

Autoimmune Liver Disease

Initially described as a disease of young women, autoimmune hepatitis (AIH) is now known to affect patients of all ages and races. Women are affected four times more often than men. The disease prevalence in the European population is approximately 1.9 per 100,000. Identification of the disease through serological testing and liver biopsy is critical, in order to initiate appropriate treatment and prevent disease progression to cirrhosis and liver failure.

Pathogenesis

The precise etiology of autoimmune hepatitis remains poorly defined but current evidence suggests that a genetic predisposition to aberrant immunological responses is the fundamental pathogenic mechanism. Unaffected relatives of patients with autoimmune hepatitis often have autoantibodies. In addition, associations of the antigens HLA-DRB*301 and DRB*401 with type 1 autoimmune hepatitis and DRB1*07, DRB1*15, and DQB1*06 with type 2 autoimmune hepatitis suggest potential genetic components of autoimmune hepatitis relating to immune dysregulation. It is possible that an environmental agent, such as a hepatotropic virus or a medication, triggers an immune response that remains permanently activated in persons with this putative genetic susceptibility but this hypothesis has not been proven. AIH has been reported to be precipitated by acute viral infection, the use of interferon for hepatitis C treatment, and the use of certain drugs, such as minocycline and nitrofurantoin. The autoantibodies typically associated with AIH, antinuclear antibody (ANA) and anti-smooth muscle antibody (ASMA), are not thought to be pathogenic on their own, and are not infrequently noted in other non-autoimmune liver diseases. Low complement levels are seen in some patients and may portend a worse outcome. Perhaps the most convincing evidence in favor of the role of the immune system in the pathogenesis of autoimmune

Yamada's Handbook of Gastroenterology, Third Edition. Edited by Tadataka Yamada and John M. Inadomi.
© 2013 John Wiley & Sons, Ltd. Published 2013 by John Wiley & Sons, Ltd.

hepatitis is the nearly complete resolution of the inflammatory response with immunosuppressive therapy.

Classification

Autoimmune hepatitis is classified into type 1 (anti-actin) and type 2 (anti-LKM). Type 1 autoimmune hepatitis is the most common form of disease in North America, and occurs in young and older women. It is associated with a high frequency of positive ANA and ASMA. Type 2 is more common in the European population, and typically affects children and adolescents. It is associated with positive anti-liver and kidney microsomal antibodies (LKM), and only rarely with ANA and ASMA. Progression to cirrhosis occurs in 3 years in 82% of patients with type 2 disease, compared to 43% with type 1 disease. Type 1 and type 2 AIH can often be distinguished clinically by the natural history of the disease, the antibody profiles, and the different responses to treatment. Type 3 (anti-SLA) autoimmune hepatitis is rare, and follows a clinical and epidemiological pattern similar to that of type 1, except that serum tests are reliably positive only for anti-soluble liver antigen (SLA). ANAs and SMAs may be negative in this third type.

Clinical presentation

The initial presentation of autoimmune hepatitis can be mild and nonspecific, with fatigue, malaise, and arthralgias. Patients can present with secondary amenorrhea or delayed menarche. Some patients are entirely asymptomatic, and are diagnosed upon further evaluation of abnormal liver tests. That said, the majority of patients will present with markedly abnormal liver tests, and patients may be jaundiced at the time of diagnosis. Occasionally, patients will present with fulminant liver disease and hepatic decompensation. Patients typically report significant fatigue, and can confirm anorexia, pruritus, and right upper quadrant abdominal pain. There may be a personal or family history of other autoimmune diseases. Physical examination can reveal a spectrum of findings, from a normal exam to the presence of jaundice, ascites, and encephalopathy.

Diagnostic investigation

Before treatment begins, patients with autoimmune hepatitis will have elevated serum aminotransferase levels. Typically, aminotransferase levels are threefold to tenfold above normal but occasionally, levels higher than 1000 IU/L are encountered. Patients with advanced disease may present with varying degrees of hyperbilirubinemia or with symptoms of fulminant or subfulminant hepatitis. Similarly, prolongation of prothrombin time, hypoalbuminemia, thrombocytopenia, leukopenia, and anemia may be present in patients with cirrhosis or portal hypertension. Viral testing for hepatitis A, B, and C should be performed to rule out viral infection, and serological testing for alternative causes of liver disease, such as Wilson disease, should be completed.

The key to diagnosing autoimmune hepatitis is documenting the presence of circulating autoantibodies. Testing for ANA, ASMA, anti-LKM, SLA and IgG levels should be performed. Patients with autoimmune hepatitis may have other autoantibodies, including asialoglycoprotein receptor, anti-liver cytosol I, anti-actin, antineutrophil cytoplasmic antibodies, and low titers of antimitochondrial antibodies. Conversely, other chronic liver diseases may have low titers of ANAs and SMAs but titers higher than 1:320 and higher than 1:40, respectively, are unusual. A small group of patients with the typical clinical features of autoimmune hepatitis have no detectable viral serological features or autoantibodies.

Liver histology

The role of liver biopsy is very important in confirming the diagnosis of autoimmune hepatitis, even though histological findings are not entirely specific. Viral hepatitis and drug-induced hepatitis may have indistinguishable histological findings. The typical histological findings in AIH include an interface hepatitis consisting of lymphoplasmacytic chronic inflammatory cells. The intrahepatic bile ducts generally appear normal. Staining for $\alpha 1$-antitrypsin and excess iron should be negative. In patients with a more severe presentation, bridging necrosis may be seen. It is not uncommon to find advanced histological injury, including cirrhosis, at the time of initial diagnosis and biopsy.

Diagnostic scoring systems

Several scoring systems have been proposed to aid the accurate diagnosis of autoimmune hepatitis. The initial scoring system published in 1993 was subsequently modified in 1999, and more recently a simplified version has been proposed. This scoring system uses results of autoantibody and immunoglobulin testing as well as liver histology to allow for a diagnosis of probable or definite AIH (Table 41.1).

Management

Without immunosuppressive therapy, patients with autoimmune hepatitis may progress to liver failure, so AIH patients with elevated aminotransferase levels

Table 41.1 Simplified diagnostic criteria for autoimmune hepatitis

Variable	Cutoff	Points
ANA or SMA	≥1:40	1
ANA or SMA	≥1:80	
or LKM	≥1:40	2*
or SLA	Positive	
IgG	> Upper normal limit	1
	>1.10 times upper normal limit	2
Liver histology (evidence of hepatitis	Compatible with AIH	1
is a necessary condition)	Typical AIH	2
Absence of viral hepatitis	Yes	2
		≥6: probable AIH
		≥7: definite AIH

*Addition of points achieved for all autoantibodies (maximum, 2 points).
AIH, autoimmune hepatitis; ANA, antinuclear antibody; LKM, liver and kidney microsomal antibody; SLA, soluble liver antigen; SMA, smooth muscle antibody.
Source: Hennes EM et al. Simplified criteria for the diagnosis of autoimmune hepatitis. Hepatology 2008; 48(1):169–176.

and inflammation in biopsy specimens should be treated. Fortunately, immuno-suppressive therapy is successful in more than 80% of patients. Therapeutic trials have shown significant survival benefit from the use of corticosteroids, with or without azathioprine. Therapy may be divided into an induction phase and a maintenance or withdrawal phase. Therapy is initiated with prednisone alone or in combination with azathioprine. Both regimens are equally effective in inducing remission. Azathioprine alone is not effective for induction but can be used alone for maintenance. Once remission is achieved, steroids should be tapered and discontinued if possible. Patients who do not tolerate azathioprine can be maintained on prednisone alone or may try an alternative immunosup-pressive agent such as mycophenolate mofetil or a calcineurin inhibitor. There is no consensus on the need to repeat a liver biopsy to establish histological improvement. Patients occasionally can be tapered completely off immunosup-pressants but a significant proportion will relapse in the first few months after stopping therapy. For any patient, the risks of life-long therapy must be weighed against the risk of disease recurrence. A proposed treatment algorithm is outlined in Table 41.2.

Table 41.2 Suggested therapeutic regimen for autoimmune hepatitis

Initial therapy

Prednisone 30–40 mg/day monotherapy or prednisone 30 mg/day and azathioprine 50–100 mg/day combined therapy

Dose reduction

Slowly reduce prednisone (2.5–5 mg every 1–3 months) if ALT in normal range

Maintenance

Minimum-dose prednisone or azathioprine to maintain ALT in normal range

Stop therapy

If ALT and IgG normal for 1–2 years; liver biopsy indicates inactivity

Treatment of relapse

Reintroduce therapy as for initial treatment

Failure to respond

To above, use either high-dose prednisone 40–60 mg/day or another immunosuppressant, or consider liver transplant if appropriate

ALT, alanine aminotransferase.

Source: Yamada T et al. (eds) *Textbook of Gastroenterology*, 5th edn. Oxford: Blackwell Publishing Ltd, 2009.

Key practice points

- The diagnosis of autoimmune hepatitis (AIH) is based on serological and histological findings.
- Type 1 AIH is the most common in the United States, with a high frequency of positive antinuclear and anti-smooth muscle antibodies.
- Type 2 AIH typically affects children and adolescents. It is associated with positive anti-liver and kidney microsomal antibodies (LKM), and only rarely with ANA and ASMA. It is associated with a more aggressive disease course.
- Treatment of AIH is indicated for those with abnormal liver tests and significant inflammation on liver biopsy. Treatment is typically initiated with prednisone and azathioprine. For patients who fail or are intolerant to this regimen, alternative agents such as mycophenolate, cyclosporine or tacrolimus may be used. Most patients require life-long treatment.

CHAPTER 42

End-stage Liver Disease

With progression of liver disease, regardless of etiology, the development of cirrhosis and portal hypertension can occur. Progression to end-stage liver disease can result in multiple potential complications, some of which are life threatening. The identification and management of complications of cirrhosis are the basis of care for the patient with end-stage liver disease, and can significantly affect liver-related morbidity and mortality.

Cirrhosis

Cirrhosis represents the final common pathway of many hepatic disorders characterized by chronic cellular destruction. An intervening stage of increased fibrosis is followed by the formation of parenchymal regenerative nodules. The nodular distortion of the lobules and vascular network defines cirrhosis and ultimately plays a critical role in the development of portal hypertension. The cellular and biochemical events leading to this altered growth response and resulting architectural distortion are not well characterized. Cirrhosis is often classified according to the gross pattern of architectural distortion into micronodular cirrhosis and macronodular cirrhosis. Alcoholic cirrhosis is typically micronodular; uniformly sized parenchymal nodules are separated by thin bands of connective tissue. The cirrhosis that evolves from the bridging necrosis of severe chronic viral hepatitis is often macronodular, characterized by nodules measuring up to several centimeters, separated by thick, asymmetrical bands of connective tissue. This classification has limited clinical use because many disease processes present with either variant. Also, micronodular cirrhosis may transform into macronodular cirrhosis.

A more clinically relevant method of classifying cirrhosis is based on the primary disease processes responsible for hepatocellular injury (Table 42.1). In the United States, most cases of cirrhosis are related to alcoholic liver disease and chronic viral hepatitis. Other common causes of cirrhosis include hereditary

Yamada's Handbook of Gastroenterology, Third Edition. Edited by Tadataka Yamada and John M. Inadomi.

Table 42.1 Causes of cirrhosis

Common	Infrequent	Rare
Chronic hepatitis C	Primary biliary cirrhosis	α1-Antitrypsin deficiency
Chronic hepatitis B	Primary sclerosing cholangitis	Wilson disease
Alcoholic cirrhosis	Autoimmune hepatitis	Sarcoidosis
	Hemochromatosis	Cystic fibrosis
	Nonalcoholic fatty liver disease	Drug-induced (methotrexate,
	Cryptogenic	amiodarone)
	Secondary biliary cirrhosis	Glycogen storage disease

hemochromatosis, primary and secondary biliary cirrhosis, nonalcoholic fatty liver disease (NAFLD), and autoimmune hepatitis. Several rare disorders that frequently are complicated by cirrhosis should always be considered in the differential diagnosis, including Wilson disease and α1-antitrypsin deficiency. Medications such as nitrofurantoin, amiodarone, and methotrexate may produce chronic hepatitis and cirrhosis. Cirrhosis in childhood can be caused by congenital anomalies (e.g. biliary atresia), metabolic conditions (e.g. tyrosinemia, galacto-semia), α1-antitrypsin deficiency, cholestatic liver disease (e.g. total parenteral nutrition, progressive familial intrahepatic cholestasis), Wilson disease, glycogen storage disease, cystic fibrosis, and idiopathic neonatal hepatitis.

When all other causes of cirrhosis are excluded, the diagnosis is idiopathic (cryptogenic) cirrhosis. This disorder may result from an immunological or viral disease process that cannot be detected by serological assays or from "burned-out" NAFLD. Cryptogenic cirrhosis may account for 10–20% of all cases with cirrhosis; it is clinically indistinguishable from other common causes.

Portal hypertension

Pressure gradients in portal circulation follow Ohm's law, which states that the pressure gradient is equal to the product of flow and resistance. Portal hyper-tension occurs if there is increased splanchnic flow or increased resistance in the hepatic vasculature. In cirrhosis, both mechanisms contribute to the development of portal hypertension. Nodular regeneration and fibrosis in the space of Disse increase postsinusoidal and sinusoidal resistance, respectively. Cirrhosis is also accompanied by increased splanchnic flow from decreased tone in the splanchnic arterioles. The mechanisms responsible for splanchnic arteriolar vasodilation are poorly understood but may involve nitric oxide. In extrahepatic causes of portal hypertension, such as portal vein thrombosis or massive splenomegaly, either increased resistance or increased flow is the principal mechanism of increased portal pressure. The anatomical site of increased flow or resistance has been used to

Table 42.2 Classification and differential diagnosis of portal hypertension

Prehepatic causes
Portal vein thrombosis
Splenic vein thrombosis
Arterioportal fistula
Splenomegaly

Intrahepatic causes
Cirrhosis
Fulminant hepatitis
Veno-occlusive disease
Budd–Chiari syndrome
Schistosomiasis
Metastatic malignancy

Posthepatic causes
Right ventricular failure
Constrictive pericarditis
Inferior vena cava web

classify portal hypertension into prehepatic, intrahepatic, and posthepatic portal hypertension (Table 42.2). Intrahepatic causes are often further subdivided into presinusoidal, sinusoidal, and postsinusoidal according to the site of increased resistance. This subclassification has limited value because many forms of cirrhosis may involve more than one site of vascular distortion in relationship to the sinusoids.

Clinical presentation

Although patients with early cirrhosis may be asymptomatic, cirrhosis is typified by a general decline in health with nonspecific complaints of anorexia, weight loss, malaise, fatigue, and weakness. More advanced disease may present with one of the complications of portal hypertension.

Endocrine manifestations

Patients with cirrhosis may manifest several endocrine disturbances. The prevalence of diabetes mellitus increases in all forms of cirrhosis but particularly in patients with hemochromatosis, alcoholic liver disease, or hepatitis C. Hypogonadism in males and females is also common in hemochromatosis and alcoholic liver disease, primarily because of the direct gonadal toxicities of iron and alcohol, respectively. In addition, androgenic steroids may bypass metabolism in the liver and subsequently undergo conversion in adipose tissue to the estrogenic steroid estrone. Increased plasma estrogen levels may lead to gynecomastia, telangiectasia, and palmar erythema.

Pulmonary manifestations

End-stage liver disease is often accompanied by pulmonary disorders. Chronic hyperventilation is probably caused by the same central nervous system alterations responsible for hepatic encephalopathy. Patients may have hypoxemia because of mismatches of ventilation and perfusion induced by ascites, which restrict the ventilation of dependent lung spaces. The hepatopulmonary syndrome, a distinct form of right-to-left shunting with impaired gas exchange caused by intrapulmonary vascular dilation, is increasingly recognized. This condition is potentially reversible by transplantation. Portopulmonary hypertension, in contrast, is caused by pulmonary vasoconstriction, which produces markedly elevated pulmonary pressure and is a relative contraindication to liver transplantation. Patients with or without ascites may develop a transudative pleural effusion, termed hepatic hydrothorax, which may impair respiratory function. Hydrothorax probably develops from ascites traversing pores in the diaphragm. The onset of hepatic hydrothorax often signals rapid clinical deterioration.

Renal manifestations

Numerous disturbances of sodium and water homeostasis are observed In cirrhosis but the most devastating complication is renal failure caused by the hepatorenal syndrome. In its most severe form, hepatorenal syndrome type I progresses to oliguric renal failure and prerenal physiology despite adequate filling pressure. It is associated with extreme intrarenal vasoconstriction that leads to sodium retention. Potential precipitants include intravascular volume depletion from hemorrhage, diuretics, or paracentesis. Alternative causes of renal failure include acute tubular necrosis caused by hypovolemia, nephrotoxic drugs, nonsteroidal anti-inflammatory agents, and radiocontrast agents. These disorders can often be distinguished from hepatorenal syndrome on the basis of a normal or elevated urine sodium concentration. Pulmonary artery catheter placement or central venous pressure monitoring should be considered because they facilitate optimal management of volume status. Hepatorenal syndrome type 1 usually is irreversible without transplantation. A milder form, hepatorenal syndrome type 2, affects many cirrhotics and is characterized by a mildly depressed glomerular filtration rate and marked sodium and water retention refractory to diuretics.

Diagnostic investigation

Laboratory results

Liver chemistry values are obtained in essentially all patients with suspected liver disease or portal hypertension but the patterns and degrees of abnormality are variable and are determined by the primary disorder. Notably, patients with pathological evidence of cirrhosis may have normal biochemical profiles.

Coagulation profiles, complete blood counts, electrolytes, and albumin should all be obtained. Patients with advanced cirrhosis will have a prolonged prothrombin time and a decrease in serum albumin levels because of impaired hepatic synthetic function. Protein malnutrition and vitamin K deficiency, which are particularly common in alcoholics, may also produce these abnormalities. Patients with portal hypertension may have thrombocytopenia, anemia, or leukopenia on the basis of congestive hypersplenism. Thrombocytopenia from splenic sequestration rarely is less than 30,000 per μl; lower levels suggest an alternative diagnosis, such as drug-induced, immune-mediated, or disseminated intravascular coagulation-associated thrombocytopenia. In addition to splenic sequestration, anemia may result from gastrointestinal hemorrhage, nutritional deficiencies (e.g. folate, iron, or vitamin B_{12}), or hemolysis. Hyponatremia, hypokalemia, and renal insufficiency are common complications of the altered renal hemodynamics and sodium and water homeostasis observed in cirrhosis.

An accurate determination of the cause of cirrhosis requires a serological evaluation, whose extent is largely dictated by the clinical setting. The initial screen should include serum assays for antibody to hepatitis C, antibodies to hepatitis B core antigen and surface antigen, hepatitis B surface antigen, antimitochondrial antibodies, antinuclear antibodies, anti-smooth muscle antibodies, ferritin, transferrin, total iron-binding capacity, and serum protein electrophoresis to measure the α1 band and γ-globulins. Patients younger than age 50 should be screened for Wilson disease with an assay of serum ceruloplasmin. In the second stage, selected patients may require specialized studies based on the preliminary results above, for example, hepatitis C viral RNA, hepatitis B DNA.

Imaging and endoscopic studies

Imaging procedures are often helpful in providing evidence of cirrhosis or portal hypertension. Ultrasound, computed tomographic (CT), and magnetic resonance imaging (MRI) studies may demonstrate lobular, heterogeneous, hepatic parenchyma or findings attributable to portal hypertension, including ascites, splenomegaly, and portosystemic collaterals. Standard ultrasound and CT scanning are insensitive methods for detecting varices but Doppler ultrasound may demonstrate portal vein thrombosis or hepatofugal flow. Upper gastrointestinal endoscopy permits detection of varices or portal hypertensive gastropathy but does not allow differentiation of cirrhosis from other causes of portal hypertension. MRI and CT with contrast may help exclude primary vascular causes of portal hypertension, including the hepatic vein thrombosis of Budd–Chiari syndrome and portal vein thrombosis. Patients with suspected secondary biliary cirrhosis caused by primary sclerosing cholangitis should undergo magnetic resonance cholangiopancreatography (MRCP) or endoscopic retrograde cholangiopancreatography (ERCP).

Liver biopsy

Liver biopsy is the only definitive means of diagnosing cirrhosis and often provides clues to the underlying cause. Liver biopsy also can be used to quantify iron and copper if hemochromatosis or Wilson disease is in the differential diagnosis. In the setting of coagulopathy, the risk of biopsy-associated hemorrhage often outweighs the benefit of obtaining information from the biopsy specimen. A transjugular biopsy may be performed if histological confirmation is deemed critical.

Portal venous pressure measurement

Although not frequently needed in clinical practice, direct and indirect measurements of portal pressure are the definitive means of diagnosing portal hypertension. The more commonly used indirect method involves angiographic positioning of a balloon occlusion catheter in the hepatic vein and, with the balloon inflated, measuring the hepatic vein wedge pressure. Analogous to pulmonary capillary wedge pressure, the hepatic vein wedge pressure measures sinusoidal pressure and is an estimate of portal pressure. It is inaccurate if the causes of portal hypertension are presinusoidal or prehepatic because the major pressure gradient is upstream from the sinusoids. The difference between the hepatic vein wedge pressure and free hepatic vein pressure provides an estimate of the portosystemic gradient, or the pressure drop across the resistance bed of the liver. This is termed the hepatic venous pressure gradient, or HVPG. A portosystemic gradient higher than 5 mmHg is consistent with portal hypertension, whereas a gradient higher than 12 mmHg identifies patients at risk for variceal hemorrhage. The pressure in the portal circulation can be measured directly by a pressure transducer placed in the portal vein. This can be done through the parenchyma from the hepatic vein, similar to transjugular intrahepatic portosystemic shunt (TIPS) or transhepatic placement. The risk of bleeding from the transhepatic approach prohibits the routine use of this procedure.

Management

Clinical management of patients with cirrhosis is focused on control of ascites, varices and hepatic encephalopathy, and screening of hepatocellular carcinoma. The management of ascites is reviewed separately in Chapter 14, and hepatocellular carcinoma is reviewed in Chapter 43.

Management of variceal hemorrhage

Any form of portal hypertension can lead to the formation of portosystemic collaterals. The major sites of collateral formation are through the umbilical vein, producing abdominal wall collaterals (the caput medusae); through the superior rectal vein to the middle and inferior rectal vein, producing rectal varices; and through the coronary and left gastric veins to the azygos vein, producing gastroesophageal varices. Collaterals may form in numerous other sites within the abdomen but hemorrhage from gastroesophageal varices is the primary cause of morbidity from portosystemic collaterals.

The formation of varices is closely related to portal pressure. Varices are not encountered below a threshold portosystemic gradient of 12 mmHg but for unclear reasons, many patients with pressures above this level never develop significant varices. Bleeding occurs in 25–30% of patients with varices but variables for identifying patients at high risk are less than perfect. Absolute portal pressures above the threshold of 12 mmHg do not correlate well with the risk of bleeding but the endoscopic size of varices does seem to indicate the patients at highest risk. Variceal hemorrhage is historically associated with a 50% mortality rate, and without subsequent preventive treatment, the risk of rebleeding is nearly 70%. These high morbidity and rebleeding rates have led to several interventions for treating acute bleeding as well as preventing initial or recurrent variceal hemorrhage. In-hospital mortality rates of patients with cirrhosis and variceal bleeding decreased by two-thirds between 1985 and 2000 (42.6% to 14.5%), although the rate remains as high as 32–36% in class C patients. Despite improving therapeutic options for patients, the long-term survival has not significantly changed.

Primary prevention of acute variceal hemorrhage includes nonselective β-adrenergic antagonists (e.g. propranolol, nadolol and carvedilol). β-Blocker therapy in multiple studies reduced the rate of first bleeds as well as rebleeding. These medications should be dose titrated to a 25% decrease in resting heart rate. Contraindications include bradycardia, hypotension, congestive heart failure, reactive airway disease, and peripheral vascular disease. For large varices, endoscopic band ligation can be used for primary prophylaxis and reduces the rate of initial variceal bleeding. Still, β-adrenergic antagonists are the most widely used therapy for the primary prevention of variceal bleeding.

Acute variceal hemorrhage from esophageal or gastric varices is a medical emergency. Patients should be managed in intensive care; volume resuscitation and optimizing the hemodynamic status are the first priorities. Nonvariceal hemorrhage may account for up to 50% of gastrointestinal bleeding in patients with known cirrhosis. Therefore, early upper gastrointestinal endoscopy is needed to confirm the source of bleeding. Endoscopic band ligation has replaced sclerotherapy as the first-line treatment for endoscopic management of gastroesophageal varices. Band ligation has superior efficacy with fewer side-effects. Injection sclerotherapy of varices is occasionally used for acute variceal bleeding that is difficult to control, particularly if extensive bleeding impairs visualization and makes banding difficult. Complications of sclerotherapy include esophageal ulceration, pneumonia, and bacteremia. Combination therapy with banding and sclerotherapy does not have higher rates of efficacy than either technique alone and has more complications. Thus, combination treatment should not be used routinely.

Continuous infusion of the somatostatin analog octreotide (25–50 µg/h for 24–48 h) reduces splanchnic blood flow by inhibiting the vasodilating hormones (e.g. glucagon) and lowers portal pressure. It does not cause systemic vasoconstriction and thus is safer than vasopressin. If portal hypertensive bleeding is suspected, therapy should be started immediately and continued for 72 h. In some studies, octreotide was as effective as endoscopic therapy in controlling acute hemorrhage but most centers use octreotide and endoscopic therapy together. Continuous infusion of vasopressin (0.1–0.4 U/min) may also control acute hemorrhage but 50% of patients fail to respond and side-effects of systemic vasoconstriction, including myocardial and cerebral ischemia, are common. Vasopressin therapy should be limited to less than 24–48 h.

If bleeding persists despite the above measures, balloon tamponade is sometimes required. Balloon tamponade is 90% effective in stopping variceal hemorrhage but it is only a temporizing measure, usually while awaiting TIPS. Adverse effects are common and include esophageal rupture and aspiration. Tamponade should never be continued for longer than 24–36 h and should be limited to inflating the gastric balloon whenever possible. Endotracheal intubation should be performed before balloon insertion to prevent airway compromise. In refractory or recurrent variceal hemorrhage, portosystemic shunting should be considered by using TIPS or a surgically created shunt. Although both procedures are highly effective in controlling hemorrhage, encephalopathy results in 10–20% of patients. The lower morbidity and less invasive nature of TIPS make it the logical choice in this setting.

After acute variceal bleeding has been stopped, secondary prophylactic interventions lower the risk of rebleeding. The preferred therapy is endoscopic band ligation. Complete obliteration of varices is the goal, and several sessions separated by approximately 2 weeks are often required. Once the varices are obliterated, endoscopic surveillance to detect recurrence is usual, annually or biannually.

Pharmacotherapy with the nonselective β-adrenergic antagonists also reduces the rate of rebleeding but does not improve survival. Combination therapy with long-acting nitrates may be as effective as endoscopic therapy. Many clinicians use propranolol as an adjuvant means of preventing rebleeding.

Transjugular intrahepatic portosystemic shunt has added a new dimension to therapies for secondary prophylaxis of variceal bleeding. Although TIPS clearly has a role in patients with hemorrhage refractory to endoscopic therapy, its role in secondary prophylaxis remains to be established. Reports suggest that TIPS improves rebleeding rates compared with endoscopic therapy but risks of encephalopathy have generally limited the applicability of TIPS to failure of endoscopic therapy with rebleeding.

Management of hepatic encephalopathy

The mechanism for developing hepatic encephalopathy (HE) in severe liver disease remains ill defined. Possible explanations include decreased clearance of gut-derived neurotoxins, including ammonia; disturbances of central

Table 42.3 West Haven criteria for clinical grading of hepatic encephalopathy

Stage 0	No abnormality detected
Stage I	Trivial lack of awareness, euphoria, or anxiety
	Shortened attention span
	Impairment of addition or subtraction
Stage II	Lethargy
	Disorientation for time
	Obvious personality change
	Inappropriate behavior
Stage III	Somnolence to semi-stupor but responsive to stimuli
	Confusion
	Gross disorientation
	Bizarre behavior
Stage IV	Coma
	Tests of mental state not possible

Source: Yamada T et al. (eds) *Principles of Clinical Gastroenterology*. Oxford: Blackwell Publishing Ltd, 2008.

neurotransmission resulting from an accumulation of false neurotransmitters that activate γ-aminobutyric acid receptors or catecholamines; and accumulation of glutamate in astrocytes. None of these explanations is satisfactory. Although serum ammonia is often elevated in hepatic encephalopathy, some patients have normal ammonia levels.

Hepatic encephalopathy is often graded according to the patient's level of consciousness, using the West Haven criteria (Table 42.3). Other indexes exist, including the Glasgow Coma Scale for patients in stage III–IV and the portosystemic encephalopathy (PSE) index. Minimal hepatic encephalopathy, previously called subclinical, can be measured by Reitan trail testing, other neuropsychiatric testing, electroencephalography, or evoked potentials. Imaging of the brain has little diagnostic yield but may be more important to exclude other causes, such as intracranial hemorrhage in an alcoholic patient with coagulopathy.

New-onset HE or acute decompensation of chronic HE should always prompt a search for precipitating causes. Common causes include gastrointestinal hemorrhage, psychotropic medications (in particular benzodiazepines), electrolyte and fluid disturbances, infection, new-onset renal insufficiency, constipation, and medical or dietary noncompliance. In addition to providing specific therapy for HE, the clinician should always attempt to correct the precipitating factors.

Because many of the responsible neurotoxins appear to be produced by intestinal flora, therapy is directed at altering the colonic microenvironment.

Table 42.4 Child–Turcotte–Pugh classification system

Prothrombin time	Bilirubin	Albumin	Ascites	Encephalopathy	Score
0–4 sec above control	0–2.0 mg/dL	>3.5 mg/dL	Absent	Absent	1
4–6 sec above control	2.0–3.0 mg/dL	2.8–3.5 mg/dL	Nontense	Grade I–II	2
>6 sec above control	>3.0 mg/dL	0–2.8 mg/dL	Tense	Grade III–IV	3

Class A = 5–6 points; class B = 7–9 points; class C = 10–15 points.

Lactulose, titrated to produce 2–3 soft stools per day, is the first-line therapy. It promotes catharsis and lowers intraluminal pH to decrease ammonia absorption. It can cause flatulence and bloating; higher doses cause diarrhea, with possible fluid and electrolyte disturbances. Rifaximin is a minimally absorbed enteric antibiotic which is now approved by the Food and Drug Administration for treatment of HE. It has been shown in studies to reduce the risk of overt HE recurrence and may reduce HE-related hospitalizations. The antibiotics metronidazole or neomycin also may be added to treat refractory HE but generally are second-line agents because of side-effects, including nephrotoxicity with neomycin and neuropathy with metronidazole. Other agents being studied include benzoate, L-ornithine-L-aspartate, branched-chain amino acids, levodopa, and bromocriptine.

Severe restriction of dietary protein is no longer recommended as a means of preventing encephalopathy in cirrhotic patients, as long-term nitrogen restriction is potentially harmful. Protein intake of 1–2 g/kg/day is generally recommended.

Orthotopic liver transplantation

The decision to perform orthotopic liver transplantation depends mostly on the expected surival of the patient with end-stage liver disease. Several prognostic indicators have been developed, including the Child–Turcotte–Pugh classification (Table 42.4) and the Model for End-Stage Liver Disease (MELD). MELD is a mathematical model based on log-transformed serum bilirubin, serum creatinine, and the international normalized ratio (INR) for prothrombin time. It predicts 3-month mortality more accurately than a Child–Turcotte–Pugh score and is now used to prioritize candidates for transplantation. The 3-year survival rate for patients with Child–Turcotte–Pugh class C disease is 30%, whereas the corresponding survival rate for patients in Child–Turcotte–Pugh class A may exceed 90%. Three-year survival rates for class B patients are intermediate and average 50–60%. Because orthotopic liver transplantation has a 1-year mortality rate of approximately 10%, patients at Child–Turcotte–Pugh stage A are better served with medical therapy. Conversely, the posttransplant 3-year survival rate is higher than 70–80% in most centers. Patients in Child–Turcotte–Pugh class B or C clearly benefit from transplantation. The benefit of orthotopic liver transplantation for any person must also account for the individual's clinical complications such as spontaneous bacterial peritonitis, intractable ascites, refractory encephalopathy, recurrent variceal bleeding, or debilitating fatigue.

Pretransplant evaluation should include an assessment for contraindications and an evaluation of factors that may complicate the posttransplant period. Absolute contraindications include active ethanol or substance abuse, extrahepatic or metastatic malignancy, untreated sepsis, and severe cardiopulmonary disease. Relative contraindications include human immunodeficiency virus infection, previous malignancy, and poor social support. Chronological age is not a contraindication but patients significantly older than 70 are acceptable candidates for orthotopic liver transplantation only if there are no other comorbidities. The evaluation usually includes ultrasound with Doppler examination, cardiac stress testing, contrast-enhanced (bubble) echocardiography, serological testing for herpes viruses (e.g. cytomegalovirus, herpes simplex virus, and varicella zoster virus), serum α-fetoprotein, and tuberculosis skin testing. Women require a Papanicolaou smear. Women older than 40 years should undergo mammography, and all patients older than 50 should have screening colonoscopies.

Investigation of a patient's social support system is critical and requires the input of a trained social worker. Psychiatric consultation should be sought for all patients with prior substance or alcohol abuse. Dental evaluation may be necessary. The complex decision to approve a patient for orthotopic liver transplantation requires the input of several disciplines. This multidisciplinary approach should consider the medical and social implications of transplantation as well as the limited availability of donor organs and the long pretransplant waiting period.

Key practice points

- Cirrhosis is the common endpoint of multiple liver diseases, and is the result of progressive fibrosis leading to nodular distortion of the liver.

- Portal hypertension results from increased splanchnic flow and increased resistance to flow (at the level of the sinusoid and/or pre- or postsinusoidal).

- Numerous complications can develop in patients with cirrhosis and portal hypertension, including variceal bleeding, hepatic encephalopathy, ascites, and hepatocellular carcinoma. More rare complications include hepatic hydrothorax, hepatopulmonary syndrome and portopulmonary hypertension.

- Liver transplant should be considered for patients with poor expected survival and no significant contraindications based on multidisciplinary evaluation.

CHAPTER 43

Hepatocellular Carcinoma

Hepatocellular carcinoma (HCC) is the fifth most common cancer and the third leading cause of cancer deaths worldwide. While all forms of cirrhosis are associated with an increased risk of hepatocellular carcinoma, the risk is particularly high in patients with cirrhosis secondary to chronic viral infection, and in hepatitis B-infected patients even in the absence of cirrhosis. Due to regional variations in the prevalence of chronic hepatitis B and C infections, there is signficant geographic variation in the incidence of HCC. The highest regional incidence is in eastern Asia, followed by sub-Saharan Africa, South East Asia, and southern Europe. In the United States, there has been a well-documented rise in the number of HCC cases over the past decade. This recent increase in incidence has been attributed to chronic hepatitis C infection.

Risk factors

Ninety percent of patients with hepatocellular carcinoma have coexisting cirrhosis. Certain causes of cirrhosis are more highly associated with HCC than others. Chronic viral hepatitis, hemochromatosis, and alcoholic cirrhosis carry a higher risk of HCC, while cirrhosis secondary to autoimmune hepatitis and Wilson disease carries a lower risk. Hepatitis B infection can result in HCC in the absence of cirrhosis, and the risk is highest in those with high serum HBV DNA levels. Regardless of underlying liver disease, men are more likely than women to develop HCC, with a male-to-female ratio of almost 3/1. A family history of HCC is a signficant risk factor for liver cancer development. The risk of developing HCC increases with advancing age, although a significant proprtion of HCC occurs in young and middle-aged individuals. The use of tobacco and alcohol, dietary exposure to aflatoxin, and oral contraceptive use have also been identified as additional factors that increase HCC risk.

Yamada's Handbook of Gastroenterology, Third Edition. Edited by Tadataka Yamada and John M. Inadomi.

There are emerging data suggesting that diabetes and obesity are risk factors for hepatocellular carcinoma, which will likely have a significant impact on the epidemiology of the disease in future decades. Recent epidemiological studies have identified factors which potentially decrease the risk for HCC, including high serum retinol levels and high coffee consumption. Alcohol cessation, clearance of HCV virus with treatment, and iron depletion of hemochromatosis patients all reduce, although do not eliminate, the risk of HCC in cirrhotic patients.

Pathogenesis

Although the precise molecular mechanisms of hepatocellular carcinogenesis are not fully understood, hepatocellular carcinoma probably results from activation of proto-oncogenes, deactivation of tumor suppressor genes (e.g. *p53* and *pRb*), changes in growth factors or growth factor signaling processes (e.g. insulin-like growth factor [IGF] or transforming growth factors [TGF]), changes in telomeric length and activity, or microsatellite instability. Genetic injury may result from a variety of sources. Perhaps the best described is random integration of the hepatitis B virus (HBV) genome into the host genome, as well as transactivating features of the hepatitis B x protein that can activate proto-oncogenes such as c-*myc* and c-*fos*. Although hepatitis C virus (HCV) is an RNA virus and does not have the same direct mutagenic capacity as HBV, any chronic inflammatory state can generate free radicals capable of inducing genetic injury. In addition, the HCV core protein appears to be a cell signaling activator. Similarly, the regenerative response in cirrhosis may lead to chromosomal rearrangements that foster unrestrained proliferation (Figure 43.1).

Multiple genetic abnormalities have been identified in hepatocellular carcinoma and in dysplastic nodules. However, it is likely that the process is multifactorial and further genetic studies are needed. For reasons that remain poorly defined, some forms of cirrhosis have exceptionally high incidences of hepatocellular carcinoma, whereas other diseases have a low incidence. Further characterization of the cellular and genetic events that lead to hepatocellular carcinoma may clarify these discrepancies.

Clinical presentation

Ninety percent of patients with hepatocellular carcinoma have superimposed cirrhosis, and many of the presenting signs and symptoms are often mistakenly attributed to coexisting cirrhosis. Nonspecific symptoms of fatigue, anorexia, weight loss, and jaundice are common. Patients may complain of right upper quadrant pain or increasing abdominal girth. Hepatocellular carcinoma may cause well-compensated cirrhosis to become decompensated, with progressive ascites, encephalopathy, jaundice, or hemorrhage. Invasion of the portal and, less

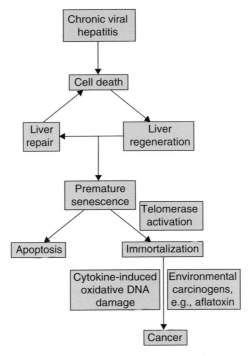

Figure 43.1 The role of chronic hepatitis with recurrent liver injury, regeneration, and repair in the development of hepatocellular carcinoma. Premature senescence of liver cells occurs by apoptosis. Cells undergoing telomerase activation escape apoptosis. The resulting immortalized cells are susceptible to the influence of oxidative and environmental carcinogen-induced DNA damage, leading to the eventual development of transformed neoplastic hepatocytes. (Source: Yamada T et al. (eds) *Textbook of Clinical Gastroenterology*, 5th edn. Oxford: Blackwell Publishing Ltd, 2009.)

commonly, hepatic veins can greatly worsen portal hypertension that leads to refractory ascites or variceal bleeding. Hepatocellular carcinoma should be suspected in all new cases of portal vein thrombosis. Patients can occasionally exhibit paraneoplastic phenomena, such as fever and hypercalcemia. Rarely, patients will present with hemoperitoneum due to tumor rupture, which requires urgent angiography for embolization. On physical examination, an abdominal mass may be palpable, and a bruit related to arterioportal shunting may be heard.

Diagnostic investigation

Laboratory studies

Aminotransferase levels are often mildly elevated but can be normal. Alkaline phosphatase may be elevated in infiltrative tumor of if there is biliary obstruction due to malignancy. In advanced tumors, serum bilirubin may be markedly elevated. Paraneoplastic hypercalcemia and erythrocytosis have been observed. The tumor marker most often associated with hepatocellular carcinoma is

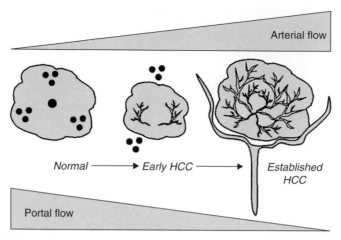

Figure 43.2 Schematic representation of arterialization during hepatocellular carcinoma (HCC) development. (Source: Yamada T et al. (eds) *Textbook of Clinical Gastroenterology*, 5th edn. Oxford: Blackwell Publishing Ltd, 2009.)

α-fetoprotein (AFP), which is a glycosylated protein expressed in proliferating hepatocytes. Although chronic hepatitis and cirrhosis may be associated with levels in the hundreds, levels higher than 400 ng/mL are likely to be caused by hepatocellular carcinoma. An AFP level higher than 1000 ng/mL associated with a liver mass is diagnostic of hepatocellular carcinoma. Unfortunately, AFP is elevated in only 60–70% of patients with hepatocellular carcinoma and may be only mildly elevated in certain tumors, which compromises the ability of AFP to serve as a screening test for early hepatocellular carcinoma.

Imaging studies

The difficulty in imaging the cirrhotic liver is to distinguish macroregenerative nodules, also known as dysplastic nodules, from hepatocellular carcinoma. The distinguishing feature of HCC is increased arterial vascularity, which results in enhancement on the arterial phase compared with the surrounding normal liver, and "washout" of contrast from the lesion on the portal venous and delayed phases, unlike the surrounding liver tissue (Figure 43.2). For lesions >2 cm in size, this enhancement pattern is associated with a 98% specificity for the diagnosis of HCC, and liver biopsy is not required (Figure 43.3).

Management

The safety, tolerability, and outcome of hepatocellular carcinoma treatment is dependent on the severity of the underlying liver disease, tumor characteristics such as size and vascular invasion, the patient's performance status, and the efficacy of the treatment intervention.

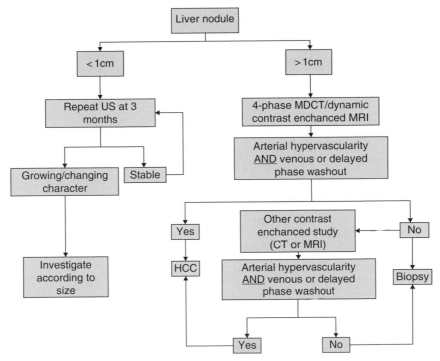

Figure 43.3 Diagnostic algorithm for suspected HCC. CT, computed tomography; MDCT, multidetector CT; MRI, magnetic resonance imaging; US, ultrasound. (Source: Bruix J, Sherman M. Management of hepatocellular carcinoma: an update. Hepatology 2011;53:1020–1022. Copyright © 2011 American Association for the Study of Liver Diseases.)

Surgical resection

Resection of HCC is limited to patients with Child A cirrhosis with localized disease. Patients with signficant liver dysfunction and/or portal hypertension (hepatic venous pressure gradient >10 mmHg) are unlikely to tolerate a liver resection. Patients with extrahepatic tumor spread or diffuse liver involvement by HCC are unlikely to benefit from resection. Resectability rates, therefore, are typically very low, ranging from 5% to 20%. The typical 5-year recurrence rates after resection are around 50%, due to new or recurrent tumors.

Liver transplant

Orthotopic liver transplantation (OLT) for patients with hepatocellular carcinoma offers significant advantages over partial hepatectomy. It can be used for patients with advanced liver disease, and it removes the existing cancer and the diseased liver with its underlying neoplastic potential. Numerous studies have shown excellent results of liver transplantation for patients with single lesions smaller than 5 cm or up to three lesions, each 3 cm or smaller (stage I–II disease). Patients who meet these "Milan" criteria are now given additional priority for OLT. Other studies have suggested that larger tumors can also be transplanted, such as the University of California, San Francisco (UCSF) criteria that extend to 8 cm hepatocellular carcinoma, suggesting that the current algorithm may be too restrictive.

Despite the additional priority given to hepatocellular carcinoma, with the potential for tumor growth and spread while on the waiting list, many centers treat the lesions prior to OLT with locoregional therapies. None of these therapies has been subjected to randomized controlled trials in combination with OLT and, therefore, the optimal approach remains to be defined. Living donor liver transplantation has also been used to shorten waiting time and may be an optimal use of the reduced-sized graft because of the usually reasonably preserved hepatic function in patients with hepatocellular carcinoma. The impact of regeneration on the risk of HCC recurrence after living donor liver transplantation remains controversial.

Locoregional therapy
Percutaneous ethanol injection
Percutaneous ethanol injection (PEI) is widely accepted as a form of therapy for small (<3 cm), discrete HCC lesions. The advantage of PEI is its relatively simple technique and low cost. PEI can be performed even for patients with advanced liver disease. Larger lesions may require several rounds of therapy, and the extent of necrosis achieved is dependent on the tumor size. Survival data have been reported but there have been no prospective, randomized controlled trials comparing PEI to other therapies.

Radiofrequency ablation
Radiofrequency ablation (RFA) is emerging as a preferred therapeutic option in the management of HCC. RFA destroys tissue by thermal energy. It is typically performed via the percutaneous approach with ultrasound guidance. RFA can be done via a laparoscopic approach if necessary, due to tumor location or proximity to structures such as diaphragm or colon. Large blood vessels act as a heat sink and thereby reduce the effectiveness of RFA for tumors adjacent to large veins. The accumulating data regarding RFA suggest that it may be equivalent to surgical resection for small tumors.

Transarterial chemoembolization
Transarterial chemoembolization (TACE) is a technique that uses angiography to selectively embolize the arterial supply of an HCC. A cytotoxic agent, such as doxorubicin, is injected into the feeding artery of the tumor, either as a suspension or adhered to drug-eluting beads. This results in both selective ischemic and chemotherapeutic effects on the HCC. The value of TACE as a palliative measure has been established in recent trials demonstrating survival benefit over untreated controls. The risks of TACE include arterial pseudoaneurysm formation, worsening liver function tests, hepatic abscess, and ischemic cholangiopathy/cholecystitis. The technique cannot be used if there is significant portal venous thrombosis.

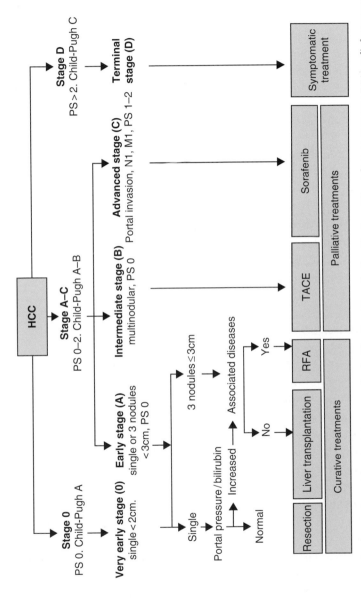

Figure 43.4 The BCLC staging system for HCC. M, metastasis classification; N, node classification; PS, performance status; RFA, radiofrequency ablation; TACE, transarterial chemoembolization. (Source: Bruix J, Sherman M. Management of hepatocellular carcinoma: an update. Hepatology 2011;53:1020–1022. Copyright © 2011 American Association for the Study of Liver Diseases.)

Transaterial radioembolization

Transaterial radioembolization (TARE) is similar to TACE, with radiolabeled particles infused via the hepatic artery into the HCC. The embolic load of radioembolization microspheres is small, and therefore does not occlude the vasculature as in TACE. TARE can therefore be administered to patients with portal venous thrombosis. There are risks of radiation injury to the lungs or gastrointestinal tract, therefore a planning angiogram is necessary during which any hepatic artery branches that supply the stomach and duodenum are occluded, and the degree of shunt to the lungs is measured. TARE may provide superiority in downstaging patients to resection, RFA, or transplantation.

Systemic therapy

Hepatocellular carcinoma is typically refractory to currently available cytotoxic therapies, with overall response rates <20%. Further, systemic chemotherapy is often poorly tolerated in patients with advanced liver disease. Recent advances in understanding of the molecular pathogenesis of HCC have led to potential treatment targets, including tyrosine kinase signaling pathways and their downstream proangiogenic pathways mediated by vascular endothelial growth factor (VEGF). The tyrosine kinase inhibitor sorafenib has shown modest survival benefit in patients with advanced HCC. Large studies have been completed in patients with Child–Turcott–Pugh Class A disease, and the safety and tolerability of the drug are being evaluated for those with more advanced liver disease. It is part of the BCLC staging and treatment system which has become widely accepted into clinic practice (Figure 43.4).

Surveillance

The key to improved outcomes for hepatocellular carcinoma is early detection via a surveillance program. Screening of patients with cirrhosis or with HBV without cirrhosis by ultrasound every 6 months is recommended. Consideration should be given to measuring AFP levels at the same interval, which may increase sensitivity for tumor detection. Multiphase computed tomography or magnetic resonance imaging should be used for inadequate ultrasound imaging, to further evaluate any unclear lesions or unexplained elevation in AFP.

Key practice points

- Hepatocellular carcinoma is a leading cause of cancer deaths worldwide.
- Primary risk factors are cirrhosis of any cause and hepatitis B even in the absence of cirrhosis.
- The diagnosis depends largely on imaging characteristics which reflect the increased arterial vascularity of the tumor. Liver biopsy is often not required for diagnosis.
- Treatment modalities include surgical resection, transplantation, various locoregional therapies (transarterial chemoembolization, transarterial radioembolization, radiofrequency ablation, percutaneous ethanol injection) and chemotherapy.

CHAPTER 44

Infections of the Gastrointestinal Tract

Bacterial and viral infections of the large and small intestine cause disease by direct destruction of intestinal epithelial cells or mediated by toxin production. Ingestion of food or water contaminated with pathogens accounts for most cases. An estimated 76 million cases of food-borne disease occur per year in the United States, accounting for 325,000 hospitalizations and 5000 deaths. The most common bacterial and viral pathogens of the gastrointestinal tract are reviewed below.

BACTERIAL INFECTIONS OF THE GASTROINTESTINAL TRACT

Infection with *Campylobacter* Species

Incidence and epidemiology

Campylobacter species (*Campylobacter jejuni* and *Campylobacter coli*) are the most common cause of bacterial diarrhea in the United States. The Centers for Disease Control and Prevention estimate that *Campylobacter* is responsible for 2 million illnesses per year. Seasonal variation of infection exists and the peak incidence is during the summer. The organism is transmitted by ingesting contaminated poultry, unpasteurized milk, or contaminated water, or by exposure to infected pets. Children younger than 5 years are most susceptible to infections caused by *Campylobacter*.

Clinical presentation

The incubation period of *Campylobacter* is 18 hours to 8 days. A prodrome of fever, headache, malaise, and myalgia may precede symptoms of watery and bloody

Yamada's Handbook of Gastroenterology, Third Edition. Edited by Tadataka Yamada and John M. Inadomi.

diarrhea with abdominal pain. Other reported symptoms include nausea, vomiting, and weight loss. Although the disease usually resolves within 1 week, some patients experience a relapsing course similar to ulcerative colitis. Physical examination may reveal localized tenderness suggestive of appendicitis. Complications of infections with *Campylobacter* species include bacteremia, hemorrhage, toxic megacolon, Reiter syndrome, erythema nodosum, urticaria, cholecystitis, pancreatitis, abortion, Guillain–Barré syndrome, and hemolytic uremic syndrome.

Diagnostic investigation

Laboratory studies may show evidence of volume depletion and peripheral leukocytosis. Stool examination usually reveals leukocytes and erythrocytes. The diagnosis is confirmed by positive stool cultures. Rapid detection methods that use DNA probes and polymerase chain reaction (PCR) have been developed although are not widely available.

Management

The mainstay of therapy for infections with *Campylobacter* species is fluid and electrolyte replacement. By the time a diagnosis is confirmed, most patients will have experienced a decrease in their symptoms, obviating the need for treatment. For severe dysentery, relapsing symptoms, systemic infection, or immunosuppression, antibiotic therapy can effectively eradicate the organism. Erythromycin (500 mg, twice daily, or 250 mg, four times daily, for 5 days) is efficacious but there is no evidence that the antibiotics reduce the duration or severity of symptoms. Ciprofloxacin is an alternative choice but quinolone-resistant strains are frequent. Azithromycin (500 mg daily for 3 days) is effective in areas of quinolone resistance. Adding an aminoglycoside is recommended for cases of systemic infection.

Infection with *Shigella* Species

Incidence and epidemiology

About 15,000 cases of shigellosis occur annually in the United States. Most infections (69%) occur in children younger than 5 years. The organism is transmitted by the fecal–oral route, via infected food or water, or in chronic care facilities, day-care centers, and nursing homes. Shigellosis is highly contagious, requiring only small inoculums (180 organisms) to establish infection. Ninety percent of infections occur from *Shigella sonnei* or *Shigella flexneri*, although *Shigella dysenteriae* has been associated with pandemic disease.

Clinical presentation

Shigella infection is characterized by the acute onset of bloody diarrhea with mucus, accompanied by fever and abdominal pain. After a 1–3-day incubation period, symptomatic disease generally persists for 5–7 days in adults and 2–3 days in children. The illness may have two phases: an initial small bowel phase of severe watery diarrhea, followed by a dysenteric phase with smaller volumes of blood-tinged mucus or blood clots. Symptoms may be severe in malnourished children or debilitated adults, whereas some healthy individuals may note only mild diarrhea. Physical examination may reveal lower abdominal tenderness with normal or increased bowel sounds. Dehydration may occur in some cases but peritoneal findings are rare and should suggest other diagnoses. The infection most severely affects the rectosigmoid colon but 15% of cases exhibit pancolitis.

Complications of *Shigella* infection include bacteremia, Reiter syndrome, and the hemolytic uremic syndrome. Bacteremia has a 20% mortality rate as a result of renal failure, hemolysis, thrombocytopenia, gastrointestinal hemorrhage, and shock. Reiter syndrome, a triad of arthritis, urethritis, and conjunctivitis, occurs most commonly in men between ages 20 and 40 and presents 2–4 weeks after infection with *Shigella* species (or certain strains of *Salmonella*, *Yersinia*, or *Campylobacter*). Eighty percent of patients who develop Reiter syndrome are HLA-B27 positive. The arthritic manifestations, which are distributed asymmetrically, often are chronic and relapsing and require management with nonsteroidal anti-inflammatory drugs (NSAIDs). Although hemolytic uremic syndrome is most often associated with enterohemorrhagic *Escherichia coli* infection, it may complicate infections with *Shigella*. The syndrome is characterized by microangiopathic hemolytic anemia, thrombocytopenia, and renal failure. It has been postulated that hemolytic uremic syndrome results from the systemic effects of Shiga toxin. The syndrome has a mortality rate of less than 10%.

Diagnostic investigation

Examination of stool will identify leukocytes and erythrocytes. The laboratory diagnosis of infection with *Shigella* species is made by identification in stool culture.

Management

Antibiotics reduce the duration and severity of symptoms in shigellosis, shorten the period of fecal excretion of the organism, and are recommended for all patients with diarrhea, except those with mild symptoms. Ciprofloxacin is the drug of choice, or azithromycin in cases of fluoroquinolone resistance. As for other diarrheal illness, oral or intravenous rehydration should be administered. Antidiarrheal agents are contraindicated because they may prolong symptoms and delay clearance of the organism. Oral vaccines against infection with *Shigella* are being developed.

Infection with *Escherichia Coli*

Most strains of *E. coli* do not produce gastrointestinal disease. However, four clinically and epidemiologically distinct syndromes are associated with *E. coli*: enterotoxigenic, enteropathogenic, enteroinvasive, and enterohemorrhagic infections. Enterotoxigenic and enteropathogenic *E. coli* infections affect the small intestine, while enteroinvasive and enterohemorrhagic infections primarily affect the colon.

Enterotoxigenic *Escherichia coli*

Enterotoxigenic *E. coli* (ETEC) causes disease by producing a heat-labile toxin and two heat-stable toxins. The heat-labile toxin increases cAMP levels, leading to chloride secretion and secretory diarrhea. One of the heat-stable toxins activates guanylate cyclase. Disease occurs in the absence of invasion or damage to intestinal epithelial cells. ETEC is a major cause of diarrhea in children in developing countries and accounts for most cases of traveler's diarrhea resulting from ingesting food contaminated by human waste.

Patients with ETEC present with watery diarrhea, abdominal cramping or pain, headache, arthralgias, myalgias, vomiting, and low-grade fever. The period of illness is generally 2–5 days. Less than 10% of patients complain of symptoms for more than 1 week. Dehydration is severe only in the very young or very old. Fluid and electrolyte replacement are emphasized. Therapy includes trimethoprim-sulfamethoxazole (double strength [DS] twice daily for 3 days), fluoroquinolone twice daily for 3 days (ciprofloxacin 500 mg, norfloxacin 400 mg, ofloxacin 300 mg), or ciprofloxacin (one 750 mg dose). Prophylaxis with bismuth subsalicylate, two 262 mg tablets four times daily, is more than 60% effective in preventing illness. Probiotic prophylaxis using *Lactobacillus* species also may be efficacious. Vaccine trials have met with variable success.

Enteropathogenic *Escherichia coli*

Enteropathogenic *E. coli* (EPEC) produces disease as a result of its ability to adhere to the epithelial cell and destroy microvilli. It is an endemic pathogen with fecal–oral transmission and affects primarily infants and children younger than 2 years. Older children and adults may serve as reservoirs for this illness. Patients with EPEC present with profuse watery diarrhea and associated symptoms of vomiting, fever, failure to thrive, metabolic acidosis, and possibly life-threatening dehydration. The diagnosis is by stool culture with serotyping, documentation of tissue culture adherence, or detecting the adherence factor by DNA probe techniques. Therapy relies on fluid and electrolyte replacement, as the illness is usually self-limited.

Enteroinvasive *Escherichia coli*

Enteroinvasive *Escherichia coli* (EIEC) is a rare cause of traveler's diarrhea. The pathogenesis initiates with attachment and invasion of colonocytes by the organism, which proliferates within cells and finally destroys the host cell. EIEC possesses a virulence plasmid identical to that possessed by *Shigella*. The clinical presentation of EIEC includes fever, malaise, anorexia, abdominal cramps, and watery diarrhea, followed by passage of blood-tinged stool or mucus. Fecal blood and leukocytes are present in many but not all patients. Laboratory confirmation of EIEC in clinical practice requires serotyping *E. coli* O and H antigens. The disease usually is self-limited and uncomplicated.

Treatment should concentrate on fluid and electrolyte replacement. The role of antibiotic therapy in EIEC infection is undefined but it is reasonable to give patients with dysentery a 5-day course of either trimethoprim-sulfamethoxazole (160 mg/800 mg, twice daily), ampicillin (500 mg, four times per day), or ciprofloxacin (500 mg, twice daily).

Enterohemorrhagic *Escherichia coli*

Infection with enterohemorrhagic *Escherichia coli* (EHEC) is caused by the O157:H7 strain, which is transmitted to humans in poorly cooked ground beef, unpasteurized dairy products or fruit juices, and fecally contaminated water. The highest incidence of infection occurs in children younger than 5 years, although elderly patients are also affected. Outbreaks are clustered in schools, day-care centers, and nursing homes. Factors that enhance EHEC virulence include adhesins that provide attachment to host cells, plasmid-encoded hemolysin, and two Shiga-like toxins that cause damage through thrombus formation and vasculitis leading to ischemia and hemorrhage. After an incubation of 3–9 days, EHEC-associated hemorrhagic colitis manifests watery diarrhea and abdominal cramping pain, followed by bloody diarrhea 2–5 days later. The severity of blood loss ranges from blood-tinged mucus to passage of large clots. Vomiting is present in three-quarters of patients, whereas fever is generally absent.

Complications of infection with EHEC include hemolytic uremic syndrome and intestinal hematoma causing intestinal obstruction, rhabdomyolysis, and pancreatic necrosis with subsequent development of diabetes mellitus. Fecal leukocytes are typically not present. *E. coli* O157:H7 can be identified by culturing on sorbitol-MacConkey medium and agglutination with O157 and H7 antiserum.

The most important goal of treatment is replacement of fluid and electrolytes. Recovery without sequelae is the usual outcome, although patients with hemolytic uremic syndrome may have long-term renal failure or neurological deficits. Antibiotics are not recommended for this infection because they do not diminish the duration of symptoms or prevent complications and may increase the risk of developing hemolytic uremic syndrome. Novel therapies for treating *E. coli* O157:H7 include reagents that bind the Shiga-like toxins to prevent interaction with host cell receptors.

Infection with *Salmonella* Species

Etiology and pathogenesis

Although all *Salmonella* are grouped into a single species, *Salmonella choleraesuis*, there are seven species subgroups, of which subgroup I contains almost all the serotypes that cause human disease. Nontyphoidal *Salmonella* species account for 1.5 million cases of food-borne enteric illness in the United States annually. *Salmonella* may be acquired from infected eggs, poultry, beef, dairy products, pet turtles, carmine red dye, aerosols, marijuana, thermometers, endoscopes, and platelet transfusions. Outbreaks of infection tend to occur during the summer and autumn, likely from picnics and barbecues during which food is not cooked at temperatures necessary to kill the organism (>150°F for 12 min). Person-to-person transfer is important only in institutional settings where fecal contamination is prevalent. Other persons at risk include patients with malignancy, immunosuppression, alcoholism, hypochlorhydria, sickle cell anemia, cardiovascular disease, hemolytic anemia, or schistosomiasis, and those who have recently undergone surgery.

The development of symptomatic infection depends on the volume of organisms ingested and various host factors. Diarrhea develops only if the mucosa of the small intestine is invaded. The pathogenicity is poorly understood but is thought to involve regulatory proteins that control the synthesis of proteins at the level of transcription. Unlike *Shigella* infection, *Salmonella* only rarely causes ulceration, hemorrhage, and microabscesses. Invasion of the bloodstream by nontyphoidal *Salmonella* species is infrequently beyond the mesenteric lymph nodes, and blood cultures are positive in less than 10% of cases.

Clinical presentation, diagnosis, and management

Nontyphoidal *Salmonella* species are associated with a spectrum of disease severity ranging from infrequent loose stools to a cholera-like diarrhea with dehydration. Associated symptoms include fever, abdominal pain, nausea, and vomiting. Symptoms manifest within 48 h of exposure and persist for 3–7 days. Complications include osteomyelitis, focal abscesses, bacteremia, sepsis, and infection of aortic or iliac aneurysms. Diagnosis is by stool culture and the mainstay of treatment is supportive care.

Antimicrobials are not recommended for mild-to-moderate disease because they may prolong intestinal carriage of the organism and increase the risk of relapse. Antimicrobials do not shorten symptom duration. Indications for antibiotics include extremes of age, immunodeficiency, sepsis, abscess, osteomyelitis, and chronic typhoid carrier states. Multidrug resistance is emerging in the United States, mediated by large complex plasmids. In seriously ill patients, administration of two antimicrobial agents of different classes for 10–14 days orally or parenterally is indicated. Antibiotics with proven efficacy include ampicillin, amoxicillin, trimethoprim-sulfamethoxazole, chloramphenicol, cefotaxime, ceftriaxone, and quinolones. To eradicate the chronic carrier state, 6-week regimens of amoxicillin and trimethoprim-sulfamethoxazole and norfloxacin or ciprofloxacin for 3 weeks have known efficacy.

Salmonella Typhi

Etiology and pathogenesis

The pathogenesis of *Salmonella typhi* resides with the Vi antigen, which prevents antibody binding and subsequent phagocytosis by the host. The organism is transmitted by the fecal–oral route and humans are the only known reservoir. Initially, transient bacteremia results from organism release from dying macrophages in Peyer patches. Persistence of *Salmonella typhi* in the circulating macrophages leads to seeding of distant sites and a second phase of bacteremia that coincides with enteric fever.

Clinical presentation, diagnsosis, and management

After an incubation period of about 1 week (range 3–60 days), enteric fever (temperature of 39–40°C) develops and persists for 2–3 weeks. Associated symptoms include headache, malaise, mental confusion, anorexia, abdominal discomfort, bloating, and upper respiratory symptoms. Initially, diarrhea may be short-lived and resolves prior to the onset of fever, only to recur in the late phase of illness. The liver and spleen may be enlarged, and abdominal tenderness may mimic appendicitis. Rose spots – a faint salmon-colored maculopapular rash on the anterior trunk – develop in 30% of patients but last only 3–4 days. Relative bradycardia (pulse slow for degree of fever) may be seen. Hematological abnormalities include leukopenia and anemia. Complications include hemorrhage, intestinal perforation, pericarditis, orchitis, and splenic or liver abscess.

A combination of cultures from blood, bone marrow, and intestinal secretions will provide the diagnosis in more than 90% of patients, although the sensitivity of blood culture alone is 50–70%. Third-generation cephalosporins and fluoroquinolones are effective in treating typhoid fever and have replaced chloramphenicol as the treatment of choice. Symptom relapse occurs in 3–13% of cases. Oral (live attenuated virus) and parenteral (whole-cell and purified capsular polysaccharide) vaccines are effective in preventing illness.

Infection with *Yersinia* Species

Etiology and pathogenesis

Yersinia species are Gram-negative, nonlactose-fermenting coccobacilli that cause gastrointestinal illness primarily in children. *Yersinia enterocolitica* causes 0.1% of reported food-borne illness in the United States. The organism is transmitted by the fecal–oral route, by animals (e.g. dogs), and by contaminated milk, ice cream, tofu, and water.

Clinical presentation, diagnosis, and management

Yersinia enterocolitica manifests clinically as a self-limited, febrile, diarrheal illness. Abdominal pain often occurs in the right lower quadrant and may mimic appendicitis. Other symptoms include vomiting, dysentery, arthritis, and pharyngitis. Most cases resolve over 2–3 days, although diarrhea can persist for months, especially in children. Rare complications of appendicitis, intestinal perforation, ileocolic intussusception, peritonitis, toxic megacolon, or cholangitis have been reported. Sepsis is uncommon but is associated with iron overload states (e.g. hemochromatosis, cirrhosis, and hemolysis). Focal *Yersinia* infections may involve the meninges, joints, bone, sinuses, and pleural spaces. Thyroiditis or glomerulopathy have developed in the postinfectious state. Moreover, patients who are HLA-B27 positive are susceptible to postinfectious Reiter syndrome, carditis, arthritis, rashes, erythema nodosum, ankylosing spondylitis, and inflammatory bowel disease.

Yersinia is diagnosed by stool examination that shows leukocytes and erythrocytes and by stool cultures using special techniques specific for *Yersinia* species. There is no evidence supporting the general use of antimicrobial therapy because the disease is usually self-limited and antibiotics do not decrease the risk of postinfectious complications. If septicemia occurs, however, therapy may consist of aminoglycosides, tetracycline, chloramphenicol, trimethoprim-sulfamethoxazole, piperacillin, or third-generation cephalosporins.

Infection with *Vibrio Cholerae*

Etiology and pathogenesis

Cholera causes an estimated 100,000 deaths worldwide each year out of 5.5 million total cases annually. Cholera is caused by *Vibrio cholerae*, a motile, monoflagellated, Gram-negative, curved rod that classically causes voluminous watery diarrhea by elaborating an enterotoxin. The disease is endemic in southern Asia, Africa, and Latin America. Cholera is transmitted mainly via seafood or fecally contaminated water, and the disease primarily affects children (age 2–9) and women of child-bearing age who live in crowded conditions with poor water and waste sanitation. Other persons at increased risk of infection include those with hypochlorhydria or impaired immune function. Person-to-person transmission is not considered important.

There are seven *Vibrio* species that are known to cause gastroenteritis. Although the risk of cholera in the United States is small, cases involving serogroups O1 and O139 have been reported. Cholera toxin consists of an "A" subunit, which is internalized and irreversibly activates mucosal adenylate cyclase, thus producing massive electrolyte and fluid secretion, and a "B" subunit, which binds to specific surface receptors and enables the A subunit to enter into the cell. The inoculum required to produce illness is larger than 10^6 organisms.

Clinical presentation, diagnosis, and management

The clinical presentation of cholera is highly variable, ranging from subclinical gastroenteritis to severe cholera (cholera gravis) that may lead to hypovolemic shock within 1 h. After an incubation period of a few hours to 7 days, cholera manifests with diarrhea, which is described as having the consistency of rice water. Associated symptoms include vomiting, metabolic acidosis, hyponatremia, hypokalemia, hypoglycemia, lethargy, altered sensorium, and seizures. Paralytic ileus, muscle cramps, weakness, and cardiac arrhythmias may result secondary to electrolyte abnormalities. The diagnosis is based on the characteristic clinical presentation, direct stool examination identifying the "shooting star" motility under dark-field or phase microscopy or stool culturing of *V. cholerae* O1 or *V. cholerae* O139 Bengal.

The mainstay of therapy is prompt initiation of oral rehydration with glucose and electrolyte solutions endorsed by the World Health Organization. Intravenous lactated Ringer solution may be required to treat severe dehydration or concomitant vomiting. Antibiotics reduce the volume and duration of diarrhea and shorten the period of excretion of *V. cholerae*. Tetracycline (250–500 mg, four times daily for 3 days) and doxycycline are effective, as are streptomycin, chloramphenicol, trimethoprim-sulfamethoxazole, nalidixic acid, ampicillin, and furazolidone. Eradication with a single 1 g dose of ciprofloxacin has been effective. Primary infection with *V. cholerae* confers immunity to subsequent infection for at least 3 years. Parenteral and oral vaccines have been formulated but they confer only about 50% protection.

Other *Vibrio* Species

Etiology and pathogenesis

Vibrio parahaemolyticus is found in salt water or in its inhabitants and frequently causes food-borne illness in the United States. Reported cases generally involve ingestion of raw or incorrectly stored seafood or contamination of food with seawater. It elaborates an enterotoxin and produces inflammation in the small intestine. In addition to *V. parahaemolyticus*, a group of vibrios termed non-O1 cholera vibrios (they do not agglutinate in antiserum against O-group 1 antigen) can cause gastroenteritis. Infection may result from ingesting oysters, eggs, and potatoes or from exposure to dogs. Other vibrios (e.g. *fluvialis*, *furnissii*, *hollisae*, and *mimicus*) may also cause diarrheal illness.

Clinical presentation, diagnosis, and management

Vibrio parahaemolyticus produces a range of illness from mild diarrhea to dysentery after an incubation of longer than 24 h, with associated nausea, vomiting, headache, and fever. Non-O1 cholera vibrio illness presents with diarrhea, which lasts 1–6 days and is associated with abdominal cramping, fever, nausea, and vomiting. Most cases of gastroenteritis caused by *V. parahaemolyticus* and non-O1 cholera vibrios are self-limited, and antibiotics do not shorten the duration of symptoms. Severe illness, however, may be effectively treated with tetracycline.

Additional Food-borne Bacterial Pathogens

Staphylococcus aureus

Staphylococcus aureus is a Gram-positive coccus that accounts for 1–2% of recognized food-borne illness in the United States. Epidemics often occur during warm weather, reflecting the association of *Staph. aureus* outbreaks with large gatherings (e.g. picnics). The high sugar or salt content of certain foods (e.g. salads, pastries, and meats) allows selective growth of the organism. The organism produces at least seven enterotoxins and a δ-toxin that can evoke fluid secretion in the intestine. The clinical features of food poisoning with *Staph. aureus* include nausea, vomiting, and diarrhea. These symptoms occur with an attack rate of 80–100% within 8h after ingesting preformed enterotoxin. Full recovery usually occurs within 48h. The diagnosis is clinical but may be confirmed by culturing the organism from the food or food handler.

Bacillus cereus

Bacillus cereus is an aerobic, motile, spore-forming Gram-positive rod. It accounts for less than 1% of food-borne disease in the United States. The organism produces two types of toxins, depending on the media upon which it grows. Two distinct clinical syndromes are associated with food-borne illness caused by *B. cereus*. Patients with the emetic illness present with vomiting and cramping. Symptoms appear 1–6h after ingestion and persist for 2–10h. Patients with the diarrheal illness have profuse watery diarrhea, abdominal cramping, and occasional vomiting. The illness has an incubation period of 6–24h and lasts for 16–48h. The diagnosis is based primarily on clinical information. Both syndromes are self-limited. Prevention of *B. cereus* infection requires proper food handling and storage.

Clostridium botulinum

Clostridium botulinum is a ubiquitous, anaerobic, spore-forming, Gram-positive bacterium that produces a neurotoxin capable of blocking acetylcholine release at the neuromuscular junction. Incorrectly canned food is the usual source of infection. Mild nausea, vomiting, abdominal pain, and diarrhea occur within 12–36h after ingestion. Associated neurological symptoms may also be present, including diplopia, ophthalmoplegia, dysarthria, dysphagia, dysphonia, descending weakness, paralysis, postural hypotension, and respiratory muscle paralysis. The latter is the major cause of mortality and occurs in 15% of patients; otherwise, full recovery may take months. The diagnosis is confirmed by detecting botulinum toxin in the stool and vomitus of infected patients or in the contaminated food. Electromyography can be used to differentiate this illness from Guillain–Barré syndrome. Treatment is supportive in addition to administering the antitoxin early in the course of disease.

Clostridium perfringens

Clostridium perfringens is a nonmotile, obligate anaerobe that is responsible for approximately 2% of all food-borne cases reported to the Centers for Disease Control and Prevention (CDC). Spores are heat resistant and grow in temperatures that vary from 15° to 50°C. The organism produces a heat-labile enterotoxin that binds to mucosal cell surfaces, causing structural damage and leading to loss of electrolytes, fluids, and proteins. Most outbreaks occur in the autumn and winter and result from ingesting incorrectly stored beef, fish, poultry, pasta salads, and dairy products. *C. perfringens* causes watery diarrhea and cramping abdominal pain 8–24 h after ingestion of contaminated food. The disease is self-limited and full recovery is expected within 24 h, although dehydration may cause death of elderly patients. *C. perfringens* has also been implicated in antibiotic-associated diarrhea. Other toxins (e.g. α-toxin and β-toxin) can produce necrotizing enterocolitis, ileus, and pneumatosis intestinalis. Definitive diagnosis is made by demonstrating more than 10^5 organisms per gram in contaminated food or more than 10^6 spores per gram in stools of affected individuals, or by detecting *C. perfringens* enterotoxin in assays.

Therapy for infection with *C. perfringens* is supportive, although oral metronidazole (400 mg, three times per day for 7–10 days) may facilitate eradication of the infection.

Listeria monocytogenes

Listeria monocytogenes is a nonspore-forming, Gram-positive bacillus that is notorious for causing gastrointestinal illness from ingesting unpasteurized milk products, although an association with ingesting contaminated meats, fruits, vegetables, and seafood is also known. It is uncommon and is reported to the CDC in only 0.1% of food-borne outbreaks. Populations at risk include pregnant women, infants, immunosuppressed individuals, the elderly, veterinarians, and laboratory workers. The varied clinical presentation of *Listeria* ranges from mild febrile illness to an overt episode of bacteremia, meningitis, and sepsis. Complications include perinatal listeria septicemia (granulomas and abscesses in multiple organs), cervical adenitis, endocarditis, arthritis, osteomyelitis, brain abscess, peritonitis, and cholecystitis. It is diagnosed by isolating the organism with "tumbling motility." Early treatment with ampicillin and an aminoglycoside is indicated because of the seriousness of the illness. Trimethoprim-sulfamethoxazole, macrolides, and tetracycline have also been advocated; cephalosporins are not effective. The duration of therapy has not been well studied but at least 2 weeks, and up to 6 weeks, is recommended.

Aeromonas, Plesiomonas, and Edwardsiella

Aeromonas species, *Plesiomonas shigelloides*, and *Edwardsiella tarda* are pathogens responsible for gastroenteritis (including traveler's diarrhea), wound infection, and meningitis. All are water-borne: *Aeromonas* species are commonly identified and isolated from freshwater fish and shrimp, *P. shigelloides* is present in contaminated oysters and seafood, and *E. tarda* is found primarily in water and aquatic animals. All produce illness by elaborating an enterotoxin and by cytotoxic activity.

Enterocolitis Induced by *Clostridium Difficile*

Incidence and epidemiology

Clostridium difficile is the most common cause of nosocomial diarrhea. The inpatient incidence is 20–60 cases per 100,000 patient-days; however, the incidence among outpatients is only 22 cases per 100,000 person-years. *C. difficile* may be isolated from the stool of only 3% of healthy individuals, whereas the prevalence among hospitalized patients is 20%. The major risk factors for symptomatic *C. difficile* infection are exposure to antimicrobials, hospitalization, and host susceptibility. The antibiotics most commonly used for treatment include clindamycin, ampicillin, and cephalosporins. *C. difficile* is prevalent in chronic care facilities, nursing homes, newborn nurseries, and neonatal intensive care units. To reduce transmission of *C. difficile*, hospital personnel should wear disposable gloves when handling stool or linen, and they should wash their hands after patient contact. Incontinent patients with diarrhea caused by *C. difficile* should be placed in isolation. Bleach solutions may be effective against environmental contamination.

Pathogenesis

Clostridium difficile is a Gram-positive, obligate anaerobic rod. Colonic damage is mediated by the release of two potent toxins, A and B. These toxins inactivate Rho proteins, leading to collapse of the cell cytoskeleton, increased tight junction permeability, and fluid secretion. An intense inflammatory response is initiated by the toxins and mediated by nuclear factor-κB (NF-κB), which in turn increases production of interleukin-8 (IL-8), tumor necrosis factor-α (TNF-α), prostaglandin E$_2$, and leukotriene B$_4$.

Clinical presentation

Clostridium difficile is associated with a wide spectrum of disease ranging from, in order of decreasing severity, pseudomembranous colitis, antibiotic-associated colitis without pseudomembranes, to antibiotic-associated diarrhea. Pseudomembranous colitis presents with diarrhea and cramps generally within the first week of antibiotic therapy, although delays in symptom onset of up to 6 weeks have been reported. Associated symptoms include fever, nausea, vomiting, tenesmus, and dehydration. Physical findings may include abdominal distension and diffuse tenderness. Peripheral leukocytosis usually is present. Occult fecal blood loss is common but hematochezia is rare. Complications of pseudomembranous colitis include toxic megacolon, perforation, and peritonitis. Findings that suggest a fulminant course include fever, tachycardia, localized abdominal tenderness with guarding, ascites, decreased bowel sounds, and signs of toxemia. In these cases of toxic megacolon, striking leukocytosis (white blood cell count of up to 40,000–80,000 cells/µL), and hypoalbuminemia, caused by protein-losing enteropathy, may be present.

Antibiotic-associated colitis without pseudomembranes follows a more benign course, with insidious development of fecal urgency, cramps, watery diarrhea, malaise, fever, and abdominal tenderness. Antibiotic-associated diarrhea without colitis is characterized by the absence of systemic findings and by diarrhea that resolves when antibiotics are stopped. Infection with *C. difficile* can also complicate the course of inflammatory bowel disease. A stool toxin assay is recommended for patients with Crohn's disease or ulcerative colitis who have unexplained relapses, especially after recent exposure to antibiotics.

Diagnostic investigation

Stool examination reveals leukocytes in 50% of patients with pseudomembranous colitis but fecal leukocytes are less common with milder infections caused by *C. difficile*. The gold standard for diagnosing *C. difficile* intestinal infection is a tissue culture assay. If a stool specimen submitted for testing contains toxin, cellular rounding or detachment of cultured human fibroblasts is observed after an incubation of 24–48 h. The cytotoxin assay is positive in 95–100% of patients with pseudomembranous colitis and in 60–75% of patients with colitis without pseudomembranes. Enzyme-linked immunosorbent assays that detect *C. difficile* toxins are also widely available and used. Although less sensitive than the cell culture assay, results are available the same day and are highly specific for infection. *C. difficile* stool cultures do not differentiate asymptomatic carriers from patients with colitis and thus are of limited clinical use.

Sigmoidoscopy is not necessary to diagnose infection with *C. difficile*; however, endoscopic evaluation may be considered for very ill, hospitalized patients for whom reliance on stool toxin assays may delay initiation of appropriate therapy. Endoscopic diagnosis hinges on the presence of pseudomembranes, which appear as yellow-white raised plaques 2–5 mm in diameter. Histological examination of the pseudomembrane reveals a summit lesion, which is composed of fibrin, mucus, and inflammatory cells erupting from an epithelial microulceration.

Management

The initial step in management should be to discontinue the inciting antimicrobial, which effectively resolves symptoms in 15–23% of patients. In patients who do not respond, metronidazole and vancomycin have proven efficacy in eradicating infection. Oral metronidazole (250 mg four times daily, or 500 mg three times daily, for 10 days) is the recommended initial course for treating pseudomembranous colitis. In patients with ileus, intravenous metronidazole (500 mg every 6 h) is an alternative therapy. Oral vancomycin (125 mg, four times daily for 10 days) can effectively eradicate *C. difficile* after 1 week. Opiate antidiarrheals (e.g. loperamide, diphenoxylate with atropine) are not recommended for treating severe colitis but may be useful in mild cases.

Fifteen percent to 20% of patients with pseudomembranous colitis relapse after successful antibiotic treatment, usually 1–2 weeks after completing therapy. Possible etiologies for relapse include persistence of spores or vegetative forms of the organism or reinfection from environmental sources. A repeated course of the initial antibiotic regimen is recommended. Various strategies are available for multiple relapses (Table 44.1). Prolonged courses of antibiotics with a tapering dose have had therapeutic success, as have regimens combining oral vancomycin and rifampicin or vancomycin and an anion exchange resin (e.g. cholestyramine, colestipol) that binds the *C. difficile* toxins. Because resins also bind the antibiotics used for therapy, they should be administered at least 1 h before or after the antibiotic. More novel eradication strategies include oral administration of nonpathogenic organisms (e.g. *Saccharomyces boulardii*) that inhibit the growth of *C. difficile*, rectal infusions of feces or stool transplantation, and intravenous infusions of immunoglobulin.

VIRAL INFECTIONS OF THE GASTROINTESTINAL TRACT

Infection with Rotavirus

Epidemiology and pathogenesis

Rotavirus is a nonenveloped, spherical, segmented, double-stranded RNA virus that is the single most important cause of severe diarrhea in young children worldwide. It is estimated that rotavirus infects 1 million people annually in the United States, mainly children from age 3 months to 36 months, although it also causes symptomatic infection in elderly or immunocompromised adults. In the United States, rotavirus infections usually occur in the fall, although infection occurs year round in tropical regions. Transmission is by fecal–oral transfer, most likely person to person, and children and asymptomatic adults are the major reservoirs. Recurrent infections with differing serotypes are not uncommon. Infection with rotavirus causes loss of mature villus absorptive cells and loss of brush border hydrolases, resulting in fluid loss and osmotic diarrhea. In addition, a nonstructural protein of the virus appears to have enterotoxin-like activity and may augment diarrhea.

Table 44.1 Treatment recommendations for first-occurrence C. difficile-associated diarrhea and recurrences

	Agent	Adult dose*	Duration	Side-effects
First-line treatment, first occurrence	Metronidazole	250 mg tid	10 days	Disulfiram-like reaction, nausea, vomiting, metallic taste in mouth, peripheral neuropathy (rare during short-course therapy). Should not be used during pregnancy
	Vancomycin	125 mg po qid	10 days	None
First recurrence (confirm diagnosis with antigen test for all recurrences; consider withholding treatment if symptoms are not severe)	Metronidazole	250 mg tid	14 days	Disulfiram-like reaction, nausea, vomiting, metallic taste in mouth, peripheral neuropathy (rare during short-course therapy). Should not be used during pregnancy
	Vancomycin	250 mg po tid	14 days	None
7-week taper	Tapering course of vancomycin	125 mg po qid	1 week	
		125 mg po tid	1 week	
		150 mg qd	1 week	
		125 mg qod	2 weeks	
		125 mg q3days	2 weeks	

Third and subsequent recurrences	Tapering vancomycin as above, plus:		
	Saccharamyces boulardii	500 mg po bid	30 days started during the last week of the taper	None
	or			
	Cholestyramine	4 g po per day	Starting during the last week of the taper	Bloating, constipation, medication interactions

* Dosage recommendations are for adults and might need adjustment based on body habitus and other factors.

bid, twice a day; po, orally; qd, once a day; qid, four times a day; q3days, every 3 days; qod, every other day; tid, three times a day.

Source: Yamada T et al. (eds) *Textbook of Gastroenterology*, 5th edn. Oxford: Blackwell Publishing Ltd, 2009.

Clinical presentation, diagnosis, and management

Most rotavirus infections are not associated with symptomatic disease. Clinical cases present after an incubation period of 1–3 days with a rapid onset of fever, malaise, vomiting, and watery diarrhea. The illness typically lasts 3–8 days. A mild elevation of blood urea nitrogen and metabolic acidosis are common. Stools are watery but devoid of red or white blood cells. A number of diagnostic assays have been developed to detect rotavirus infection. Solid-phase immunoassays have sensitivities and specificities higher than 90%. Nucleic acid hybridization assays are also available, as are reverse transcriptase–polymerase chain reaction (PCR) assays; however, both are generally more expensive than solid-phase immunoassays. Electrophoretic analysis of stool RNA is both sensitive and inexpensive. Culture of the virus from fecal specimens is also feasible.

Therapy for rotaviral diarrhea is supportive. Oral rehydration therapy is the cornerstone of treatment; no effective antiviral medication is available. Several live, attenuated, rotavirus vaccines are being tested.

Infection with Norwalk Virus

Epidemiology and pathogenesis

Norwalk virus is a nonenveloped, round, viral particle that causes epidemic diarrhea in both developed and underdeveloped countries. The virus, named after the 1968 outbreak of gastroenteritis that affected half of the teachers and students of an elementary school in Norwalk, Ohio, was the first evidence of a viral etiology for diarrhea. The settings of Norwalk virus outbreaks include homes, schools, cruise ships, swimming pools, and military facilities. Transmission is primarily through the fecal–oral route, although person-to-person, air-borne, and fomite transmissions have also been implicated. Primary and secondary attack rates higher than 50% and higher than 30%, respectively, have been reported. Biopsy specimens of the small intestine show broad and blunted villi, crypt cell hyperplasia, cytoplasmic vacuoles, and infiltration of the lamina propria with polymorphonuclear and mononuclear cells. Brush border enzymes are reduced and gastric emptying may be delayed.

Clinical presentation, diagnosis, and management

The incubation period is 10–50h. The most frequently reported symptoms are nausea, abdominal cramps, headache, diarrhea and fever, which last 12–72h. There are no commercially available diagnostic tests for Norwalk virus infection. Research centers have diagnosed infection through detection of viral antigen by enzyme-linked immunosorbent assay (ELISA), the presence of viral RNA by reverse transcriptase–PCR, or the serological response to infection. Therapy centers on fluid and electrolyte replacement and symptomatic treatment of diarrhea. Prevention should be directed toward hand washing and hygienic food preparation.

Infection with Astrovirus

Epidemiology and pathogenesis

Astrovirus infection mainly affects children but it also occurs in institutionalized elderly patients. Other groups at risk of infection are bone marrow transplant recipients and patients infected with human immunodeficiency virus. Viral aggregates are seen in enterocytes, which appear to cause villus atrophy and crypt cell hyperplasia.

Clinical presentation, diagnosis, and management

After an incubation period of 1–4 days, symptoms that consist of watery diarrhea with vomiting, fever, and abdominal pain ensue for about 2–3 days. An ELISA based on monoclonal antibodies to all eight types of human astroviruses is commercially available. Supportive therapy is advocated. Immunoglobulin administered intravenously, orally, or by a combination of routes has been reportedly efficacious, although not yet studied in controlled clinical trials.

Infection with Enteric Adenovirus

Epidemiology and pathogenesis

Adenoviruses are DNA viruses, of which serotypes 40 and 41 in particular are known to cause gastroenteritis. The infection affects mainly children younger than age 2. Viral infection appears to vary geographically but does not exhibit seasonal variation. Infection is transmitted from person to person.

Clinical presentation, diagnosis, and management

The presentation of adenovirus is similar to that of other viral agents. The incubation period is about 7 days. Symptoms include watery diarrhea and vomiting, in addition to respiratory complaints and fever. An ELISA kit is available for diagnosis. Viral particles can be evaluated directly by electron microscopy and by PCR. The goal of therapy is rehydration and adequate nutritional intake.

Key practice points

- Bacterial infections of the gastrointestinal tract are common, and can lead to significant disease. The most common pathogens include *Campylobacter*, *Shigella*, *Salmonella*, *Yersinia*, *E. coli*, and *Vibrio* species.

- *Clostridium difficile* is an increasingly common infection. Retreatment for relapse or reinfection may be necessary.

- Viral infections of the gastrointestinal tract are most commonly due to rotavirus, norovirus (including Norwalk virus), adenovirus, and astrovirus infections.

- Treatment is usually supportive for both bacterial and viral infections of the gastrointestinal tract, although there is a role for antibiotic use for certain infections.

CHAPTER 45

Vascular Lesions: Ectasias, Tumors, and Malformations

A variety of vascular lesions manifests in the gastrointestinal tract. They can be broadly categorized as ectasia, vascular neoplasia, and other vascular lesions (Table 45.1).

Dieulafoy Lesion

The Dieulafoy lesion is an arterial malformation associated with massive gastrointestinal hemorrhage; it accounts for 1.5% of acute upper gastrointestinal bleeding episodes. In addition to lesions in the stomach and duodenum, Dieulafoy lesions have also been reported in the jejunum, ileum, colon, and rectum.

Clinical presentation

Upper gastrointestinal Dieulafoy lesions usually present with massive upper gastrointestinal bleeding and an absence of associated gastrointestinal symptoms. Hypotension, orthostasis, tachycardia, and prerenal azotemia are common. Lower gastrointestinal lesions manifest as hematochezia with hemodynamic instability.

Diagnostic investigation

Upper gastrointestinal endoscopy is the principal means of diagnosing an upper tract Dieulafoy lesion. There may be a pigmented protuberance, identifying the vessel stump, and an adherent clot with little surrounding edema. No ulceration is present; if one is seen, the visualized lesion is a visible vessel in an ulcer, not a Dieulafoy lesion. Lesions of the colon are similar in appearance to upper tract

Yamada's Handbook of Gastroenterology, Third Edition. Edited by Tadataka Yamada and John M. Inadomi.
© 2013 John Wiley & Sons, Ltd. Published 2013 by John Wiley & Sons, Ltd.

Table 45.1 Vascular lesions of the gastrointestinal tract

Vascular ectasia disorders
Angiodysplasia
Gastric antral vascular ectasia ("watermelon stomach")
Telangiectasia associated with multisystem disease (e.g. hereditary hemorrhagic telangiectasia, CREST
syndrome, Turner syndrome)

Vascular tumors
Hemangiomas
Multiple hemangioma syndromes (e.g. intestinal hemangiomatosis, universal hemangiomatosis, blue
rubber bleb nevus syndrome, Klippel–Trénaunay–Weber syndrome)
Malignant vascular tumors (e.g. angiosarcoma, hemangiopericytoma, Kaposi sarcoma)

Other vascular lesions
Dieulafoy lesion
Miscellaneous (e.g. multiple phlebectasia, pseudoxanthoma elasticum, Ehlers–Danlos syndrome)

CREST, syndrome of calcinosis, Raynaud phenomenon, esophageal dysmotility, sclerodactyly,
and telangiectasia.

lesions. Active bleeding may obscure endoscopic visualization, in which case
angiography may be used to identify the bleeding vessel.

Management and course

Initial management consists of fluid resuscitation and replacement of blood loss.
Acid suppression is of no benefit. Endoscopic therapy is used to treat the
Dieulafoy lesion: injection therapy with epinephrine or polidocanol, bipolar
electrocoagulation, thermal coagulation, laser photocoagulation, band ligation,
and hemoclips. Up to 85% of patients achieve long-term hemostasis with this
approach. Angiography with selective left gastric artery embolization has been
used with limited success to treat gastric Dieulafoy lesions. If nonsurgical
attempts to control bleeding fail, surgical vessel ligation, wedge resection, or
proximal partial gastrectomy may be necessary. Colonic lesions unresponsive to
endoscopic therapy should be managed surgically. Mortality averaged 25% in
the past but diagnostic and therapeutic advances have dramatically improved
the survival of patients with this condition.

Key practice points: Dieulafoy lesions
- A Dieulafoy lesion is identified endoscopically as a pigmented protuberance, possibly an
  adherent clot with little surrounding edema or ulceration.
- Endoscopic management includes clipping, banding, electrocautery, or injection therapy.

Angio-ectasia

Angio-ectasias consist of dilated, tortuous, thin-walled blood vessels lined by endothelium with little or no smooth muscle. Vascular ectasias that occur in association with lesions of the skin or other organs are termed telangiectasias.

Clinical presentation

Angio-ectasia clinically manifests with painless gastrointestinal hemorrhage. Most colonic lesions are located in the right colon and are associated with low-grade chronic bleeding or iron deficiency anemia but 10–15% of patients present with acute massive hemorrhage. Up to 60% of patients have multiple angio-ectasias within the same portion of the intestinal tract. Although the percentage of angio-ectatic lesions that bleed is unknown, autopsy series suggest that most do not produce clinically evident bleeding.

Diagnostic investigation

Endoscopy is the procedure of choice for diagnosing angio-ectasia. Upper gastrointestinal endoscopy, small bowel enteroscopy, capsule endoscopy, and colonoscopy are the primary methods for identifying angio-ectasia in the gastrointestinal tract. The lesions range in diameter from 0.2 to 1.0 cm and typically are discrete and bright red, composed of a dense reticular network of vessels. Angiography may identify colonic angio-ectasia overlooked on colonoscopy or angio-ectasia lesions in the small intestine not visualized by enteroscopy plus capsule endoscopy. The characteristic angiographic findings include a vascular tuft during the arterial phase of the study, rapid filling of the dilated vein, and slowly emptying veins. Because angio-ectasias bleed only intermittently, angiography demonstrates active bleeding in only 10–20% of patients. ^{99m}Tc-labeled erythrocyte scintigraphy is more sensitive in detecting acute hemorrhage but it can identify only the general region of bleeding. Patients with acute lower tract bleeding should undergo emergency colonoscopy or erythrocyte scintigraphy as the initial imaging procedure. Positive erythrocyte scans should be followed by angiography or colonoscopy.

Management and course

Many angio-ectasias are asymptomatic and are incidentally noted by endoscopy for nonbleeding indications. About one-quarter of patients who bleed from angio-ectasias experience recurrent hemorrhage within 1 year, and one half rebleed over a 3-year period. Any therapeutic intervention for these patients must consider this natural history of angio-ectasia. Patients with mild, chronic blood loss who do not require transfusion are best managed conservatively with oral iron supplements. Several reports have suggested a benefit from estrogen alone or in combination with progesterone, especially for patients with renal failure or hereditary hemorrhagic telangiectasia. Other series have failed to demonstrate decreased transfusion requirements.

Although the efficacy of hormonal therapy for sporadic angio-ectasias remains in question, an empirical trial of oral contraceptives containing low-dose estrogen is often worthwhile for selected patients. Gynecomastia in males and recurrent menstruation in postmenopausal females may limit compliance. Hormonal therapy should be avoided for patients with histories of thromboembolism, atherosclerotic disease, or hormone-sensitive neoplasms.

Patients with acute bleeding or chronic bleeding who require transfusion should undergo more invasive therapy. Successful outcomes have been reported using multiple endoscopic methods, including heater probe thermocoagulation, electrocoagulation with multipolar or argon plasma coagulation, photocoagulation using Nd:YAG lasers, and injection therapy with alcohol or epinephrine. Local expertise and availability dictate the preference for instruments to control hemorrhage. In all series evaluating endoscopic therapy, multiple sessions are often necessary, and 50% of patients experience persistent or recurrent bleeding (presumably from angio-ectasias at other sites).

Angiography may be used to provide selective intra-arterial infusion of vasopressin to control acute bleeding, which is successful in 50–90% of cases. One-third of patients rebleed after infusion; thus angiographic embolization is often required to prevent recurrent hemorrhage. Complications of embolization include abdominal pain, fever, and occasionally bowel infarction, which necessitates emergency colectomy.

If medical and endoscopic therapies fail to control bleeding, surgical resection should be considered. Preoperative angiography can often define the extent of angio-ectasia in the small intestine and the colon. Recurrent hemorrhage after surgery occurs in one-quarter to one-third of patients and is generally from unresected lesions in the remaining intestine.

Key practice points: angio-ectasia

- Up to 60% of patients have multiple angio-ectasias within the same portion of the intestinal tract.
- Recurrent bleeding from angio-ectasias is common.
- Endoscopic therapy with a noncontact method of electrocautery (argon plasma coagulation [APC]) or laser can be effective but multiple sessions are often required.
- If medical and endoscopic therapies fail then surgical resection should be considered.

Gastric Antral Vascular Ectasia

Gastric antral vascular ectasia (GAVE), also known as "watermelon stomach," is a distinctive syndrome of vascular ectasias localized in the gastric antrum. The mean age at presentation is 70 (range: 50–90), with a female-to-male ratio of 5/1. Although endoscopic surveys have been limited, the disorder is rare and is observed in less than 0.03% of upper endoscopic examinations.

Clinical presentation, diagnosis, and management

Gastric antral vascular ectasia generally presents with iron deficiency anemia from chronic occult gastrointestinal bleeding. Acute upper gastrointestinal hemorrhage is uncommon, and the lesion is painless.

Upper gastrointestinal endoscopy is the only definitive means of diagnosing GAVE. There is a characteristic appearance of erythematous longitudinal antral folds that converge toward the pylorus in a pattern reminiscent of a watermelon. Distinguishing GAVE from other gastropathies is based on the endoscopic pattern of dilated vessels or by demonstrating that the lesions blanch when compressed with biopsy forceps. Biopsy specimens reveal hypertrophied mucosa, dilated and tortuous mucosal capillaries occluded by fibrin thrombi, and dilated or tortuous submucosal veins. Angiography and barium radiography are generally of limited diagnostic value for this condition.

Management and course

Patients may require iron supplementation and blood transfusion. Endoscopic therapy with multipolar or argon plasma electrocoagulation, heater probe coagulation, or laser therapy successfully controls bleeding but multiple sessions may be required. Endoscopic therapy is generally well tolerated but is associated with complications, including perforation, stenosis, ulceration, and recurrent hemorrhage. Estrogen-progesterone therapy and other medical therapies have been largely anecdotal and are of uncertain clinical benefit. A transjugular intra-hepatic portosystemic shunt (TIPS) is not effective in controlling hemorrhage. If patients do not respond to endoscopic therapy, antrectomy is essentially curative.

Systemic Telangiectasia Syndromes

When vascular ectasias occur in conjunction with vascular lesions of the skin or other organs, they are termed telangiectasias. Hereditary hemorrhagic telangiectasia, also known as Osler–Weber–Rendu syndrome, is an autosomal dominant disorder associated with vascular ectasia of the skin, mucous membranes, and internal organs. The disease prevalence is about 10 per 100,000 population, with equal gender distribution.

Clinical presentation, diagnosis, and management

Patients usually present in childhood with recurrent and severe epistaxis. Gastrointestinal hemorrhage occurs in 25% of cases. Bleeding from a source in the upper intestinal tract, characterized by melena and hematemesis, is more common than lower tract bleeding. Bleeding from a posterior nasal or pharyngeal source presents similarly and should be considered in the differential diagnosis. The diagnosis of hereditary hemorrhagic telangiectasia should be considered in individuals with telangiectasia, recurrent epistaxis, and compatible family histories. Gastrointestinal lesions are identified by endoscopic examination, and most are located in the stomach and duodenum. Endoscopic thermocoagulation, electrocoagulation, and photocoagulation are effective in controlling bleeding. Estrogen-progesterone therapy improves epistaxis and may reduce the rate of gastrointestinal bleeding. The role of surgery is limited because of the diffuse nature of the disorder.

Bleeding gastrointestinal telangiectasias also occur in the CREST (calcinosis, Raynaud phenomenon, esophageal dysmotility, sclerodactyly, and telangiectasia) variant of progressive systemic sclerosis. These patients have vascular lesions on the hands, lips, face, and tongue, as well as other signs of systemic sclerosis. Gastrointestinal hemorrhage is not a dominant feature of this disorder but has been reported from telangiectasias in the colon, stomach, and small intestine. The therapeutic approach is similar to that for sporadic angiodysplasia.

Hemangiomas

Hemangiomas are benign vascular growths that usually are detectable at or shortly after birth but often do not produce symptoms until young adulthood (often in the third decade of life). They are a rare etiology of gastrointestinal hemorrhage, although the precise incidence is unknown.

Clinical presentation

Many hemangiomas are asymptomatic but the most common clinical presentation is gastrointestinal hemorrhage. Capillary hemangiomas tend to cause low-grade chronic bleeding with iron deficiency anemia but cavernous lesions may produce massive bleeding. Most cavernous lesions are located in the rectosigmoid region, so painless hematochezia is a common presenting symptom. Polypoid and expansive lesions may cause nausea, vomiting, and abdominal pain as a result of obstruction or intussusception. Multiple hemangiomas throughout the digestive tract, a condition termed intestinal hemangiomatosis, affect 10% of patients. In the rare neonatal syndrome of universal hemangiomatosis, cavernous lesions are disseminated to other organs, including the brain and skin.

Two other rare disorders associated with diffuse cutaneous and gastrointestinal hemangiomas are the blue rubber bleb nevus syndrome and Klippel–Trénaunay–Weber syndrome. In the former, cutaneous lesions affect the limbs, trunk, and face. Their blue color and rubbery consistency are the source of the syndrome's descriptive name. Lesions also occur throughout the gastrointestinal tract and may produce occult bleeding. In the latter syndrome, patients have distinctive soft tissue and bony hypertrophy of one limb. Gastrointestinal lesions are cavernous and are usually located in the rectum.

Diagnostic investigation

Upper and lower gastrointestinal endoscopy can diagnose hemangiomas in the stomach, proximal duodenum, and colon. Capillary lesions appear as punctate red nodules, whereas cavernous lesions are violet-blue, sessile, polypoid lesions. The color, submucosal location, and compressibility distinguish the latter from colonic adenomas. On barium radiography, larger lesions can be mistaken for adenomatous polyps or carcinoma. Angiography and capsule endoscopy are useful for detecting hemangiomas in the small intestine. The characteristic pooling of contrast in the venous phase is a typical finding in angiographic images of large cavernous lesions but may be absent in images of small lesions.

Management and course

Small capillary hemangiomas may be amenable to endoscopic obliteration by coagulation, band ligation, or polypectomy but large cavernous lesions have high rates of massive hemorrhage or perforation using this therapy. Symptomatic sporadic hemangiomas are best managed by surgical resection. In disorders with multiple gastrointestinal hemangiomas, conservative therapy with iron supplementation is recommended initially. Persistent hemorrhage or obstruction at a defined site requires surgical resection.

Key practice points: hemangiomas

- Small capillary hemangiomas may be treated endoscopically with electrocautery such as APC.
- Large cavernous venous lesions have high rates of hemorrhage or perforation with endoscopic therapy.

Miscellaneous Vascular Lesions

Angiosarcomas, epithelioid hemangioendotheliomas, and hemangiopericytomas are malignant neoplasms that originate from the cellular components of blood vessels. All may be complicated by gastrointestinal hemorrhage or obstruction. Kaposi sarcoma is another vascular neoplasm that frequently disseminates to the gastrointestinal tract. This represents one of the most common causes of gastrointestinal bleeding in patients with acquired immunodeficiency syndrome. Gastrointestinal bleeding also occurs in patients with pseudoxanthoma elasticum, as a result of an abnormal vascular structure. This disorder of elastin synthesis typically presents with bleeding from arterioles in the gastric fundus. Gastrectomy is the definitive therapy.

Ehlers–Danlos syndrome is a heterogeneous group of genetic disorders of collagen metabolism. Patients characteristically have skin hyperextensibility, bruise easily, and have hypermobile joints. Diagnosis is by clinical presentation, family pedigree analysis, and identifying genetic or biochemical defects. Patients with type IV Ehlers–Danlos syndrome can present with gastrointestinal hemorrhage from spontaneous arterial rupture due to vascular and perivascular connective tissue fragility. There is an increased risk of intramural intestinal hematomas, colonic diverticular hemorrhage, and intestinal perforation.

CHAPTER 46
Multiple Choice Questions

Questions

Chapter 1

1.1 What is the best initial test in a patient with complete esophageal obstruction?
 a. Barium esophagram
 b. Video esophagram
 c. Upper endoscopy
 d. Chest CT
 e. Esophageal manometry

1.2 What is the manometric characteristic of achalasia?
 a. Aperistalsis of the esophageal body
 b. Diminished amplitude of esophageal body contractions
 c. Absence of esophageal body contractile activity
 d. Esophageal contractile pressure >240 mmHg

1.3 What is the most common etiology of odynophagia in an immunocompromised patient?
 a. Foreign body ingestion
 b. Bacterial infection
 c. Nonbacterial infection
 d. Pill-associated ulceration

Chapter 2

2.1 True or false: Esophageal manometry is abnormal in the majority of patients with noncardiac chest pain?
 a. True
 b. False

Yamada's Handbook of Gastroenterology, Third Edition. Edited by Tadataka Yamada and John M. Inadomi.
© 2013 John Wiley & Sons, Ltd. Published 2013 by John Wiley & Sons, Ltd.

2.2 Ergonovine is used to:
  a. Treat nutcracker esophagus
  b. Test for esophageal sensitivity to acid
  c. Test for esophageal spasm
  d. Test for coronary artery spasm
  e. Treat noncardiac chest pain due to costchondritis

2.3 All the following are consistent with an esophageal source of chest pain *except*:
  a. Symptoms exacerbated by ingesting cold or hot liquids
  b. Symptoms awaken the patient from sleep
  c. Symptoms brought on by exertion
  d. Symptom relief with antacids
  e. Pain radiating to the neck

Chapter 3

3.1 Endoscopic electrocautery therapy is indicated for which one of the following findings?
  a. Gastric ulcer with a flat, red spot
  b. Duodenal ulcer with a clean base
  c. Gastric ulcer with a visible vessel
  d. Colonic ulcer with a flat, red spot
  e. Mallory–Weiss tear with a clean base

3.2 Intravenous antibiotics are recommended for which of the following groups?
  a. Alcoholics with Mallory–Weiss tears
  b. Patients with hepatitis C and peptic ulcer bleeding
  c. Patients with *Helicobacter pylori*-associated peptic ulcer bleeding
  d. Patients with cirrhosis and GI bleeding of any cause
  e. Patients with diverticular hemorrhage

3.3 Which of the following is not recommended for the treatment of esophageal variceal hemorrhage?
  a. Endoscopic sclerotherapy
  b. Endoscopic variceal band ligation
  c. Transjugular intrahepatic portosystemic shunt
  d. Sengstaken–Blakemore tube placement
  e. Argon plasma coagulation

Chapter 4

4.1 Pharyngitis, gingival erosions, parotid swelling and scarred knuckles are consistent with which of the following causes of weight loss?
  a. Anorexia nervosa
  b. Bulimia nervosa

    c. Alzheimer's disease

    d. Adult rumination syndrome

    e. Chronic pancreatitis

4.2 Merycism is characterized by which of the following?

    a. Repetitively regurgitating food from the stomach, rechewing it, and then reswallowing it

    b. Repetitive binges of overeating followed by acts to avert weight gain

    c. Pancreatic calcifications with pancreatic insufficiency

    d. Mood changes, sleep disruption, anhedonia, and low self-esteem

    e. Distortion of body image, inability to interpret hunger and satiety, with a preoccupation with eating and a sense of ineffectiveness

4.3 In severe malnutrition due to anorexia nervosa, refeeding should be established:

    a. At 90% of goal caloric intake and increase by 5% every week until goal is achieved

    b. At 110% of goal caloric intake until goal is achieved

    c. At 125% of goal caloric intake until goal is achieved

    d. At 200 calories above baseline intake and increase by 250 calories every 5 days for a goal of 1.5 kg weight gain per week as an inpatient or 0.75 kg per week as an outpatient

    e. At 500 calories above baseline intake and increase by 400 calories every 5 days for a goal of 2.5 kg weight gain per week as an inpatient or 2.0 kg per week as an outpatient

Chapter 5

5.1 Which of the following is most appropriate for a 17-year-old man with no significant past medical history, on no medications, who calls the nurse helpline reporting a 1-day history of vomiting with myalgias and diarrhea?

    a. Stool studies for ova and parasites

    b. Colonoscopy

    c. Barium upper GI study

    d. No work-up at this time

    e. Gastric emptying study

5.2 Which of the following conditions would be most likely to have an associated succussion splash?

    a. A pyloric channel ulcer

    b. Viral gastroenteritis

    c. Psychogenic vomiting

    d. Erythromycin-associated vomiting

    e. Intracranial hemorrhage

5.3 Which of the following would be most consistent with psychogenic vomiting?

a. Small bowel lumenal dilation on barium radiography
b. Stable weight
c. Feculent emesis
d. Delayed gastric emptying on scintigraphy
e. Tachygastria on electrogastrography

Chapter 6

6.1 In a patient with a suspected perforation, what test should be performed as quickly as possible?

a. Abdominal ultrasound
b. Abdominal series radiography (supine and upright or decubitus)
c. Upper endoscopy
d. Upper GI with barium

6.2 A patient presents with abdominal pain and has a positive Carnett sign on physical examination. What is the likely etiology of the patient's pain?

a. Irritable bowel syndrome
b. Cholecystitis
c. Rectus sheath hematoma
d. Appendicitis

6.3 A patient is evaluated in the emergency department for worsening RUQ abdominal pain. The patient has a positive Murphy sign on physical exam and has a fever to 39°C. Labs demonstrate a leukocytosis but no LFT abnormalities. What is the next appropriate step in management?

a. Surgery
b. Request interventional radiology to place a percutaneous cholecystostomy tube
c. ERCP
d. IV hydration, pain management, and IV antibiotics

Chapter 7

7.1 You diagnose irritable bowel syndrome in a 26-year-old woman based on classic symptoms and normal laboratory tests including hemoglobin/iron, albumin and B_{12}/folate. She complains of increased gas and flatulence and would like your advice about further testing to evaluate her symptoms. The best next step in management is:

a. Glucose hydrogen breath testing
b. SmartPill pH, temperature and pressure measurements
c. Antibody to tissue transglutaminase
d. Reassurance

7.2 Which of the following sources of complex carbohydrate is completely absorbed in healthy individuals?

a. Oat

b. Potato

c. Corn

d. Rice

Chapter 8

8.1 What is the best management of a patient who presents with acute small intestinal obstruction?

a. Neostigmine intravenously

b. Water-soluble contrast enema

c. Colonic decompression by colonoscopy

d. Surgery

8.2 What is the optimal initial management for a patient with acute colonic pseudo-obstruction?

a. Surgery

b. Interventional radiology placement of a cecostomy tube

c. Nasogastric tube suctioning, discontinuation of narcotics and other potential exacerbating drugs and correction of potential electrolyte disturbances

d. Neostigmine

8.3 A patient with acute colonic pseudo-obstruction and a cecal diameter of 10 cm is initially treated with nasogastric tube insertion with suctioning, intravenous hydration, frequent position changes and correction of electrolyte disturbances. The next day repeated plain abdominal radiographs reveal a cecum diameter of 12 cm. What is the best management option?

a. Surgery

b. Decompression of colon by colonoscopy

c. Neostigmine

d. Cecostomy tube placement by interventional radiology.

Chapter 9

9.1 In a 23-year-old woman with long-standing constipation in the absence of abdominal pain, with normal physical examination and basic laboratory tests, what is the next best step in management?

a. Colonoscopy

b. Flexible sigmoidoscopy

c. CT abdomen and pelvis

d. Empirical trial of polyethylene glycol

9.2 A patient with chronic constipation describes an increase in bowel movements to once every third day with use of polyethylene glycol, but remains concerned about symptoms that include a sensation of "incomplete evacuation" with each movement. What is the next best test to identify the cause of symptoms?
   a. Colonic transit test
   b. Colonoscopy with biopsies
   c. Anorectal manometry
   d. CT abdomen and pelvis

9.3 What is the best initial therapy for dyssynergic defecation?
   a. Sphincter myotomy
   b. Botulinum toxin sphincter injection
   c. Biofeedback
   d. Nitroglycerin topical ointment

Chapter 10

10.1 A 34-year-old woman presents with watery diarrhea. Her stool tests include the absence of red or white cells, negative bacterial culture and *C. difficile*, and concentrations of sodium of 65 and potassium 15. What is the most likely cause of her diarrhea?
   a. Magnesium-containing laxative
   b. Irritable bowel syndrome
   c. VIP-secreting tumor
   d. Senna-containing laxative

10.2 A 19-year-old college student complains of nausea, vomiting and diarrhea since yesterday evening. She and several friends ate at an Asian restaurant in the afternoon and within 6 h, two of the five diners had acute onset of nausea and vomiting, followed by watery diarrhea. Minor abdominal cramping is also noted, but no blood is seen in stool. No travel history is noted. What is the most likely cause of symptoms?
   a. Enterotoxigenic *E. coli*
   b. *Bacillus cereus*
   c. *Campylobacter jejuni*
   d. *Shigella*

Chapter 11

11.1 On CT scan, a 45-year-old man was incidentally found to have a well-circumscribed, round, 3 cm mass that appeared to arise from the wall of the stomach. What is the next appropriate step in evaluation?
   a. Esophagogastroduodenoscopy
   b. Upper GI series with barium

    c. Follow-up CT scan in 6 months to assess for interval growth

    d. EUS FNA

11.2 A 64-year-old woman presents to her physician with complaints of new-onset jaundice and a 15 lb unintentional weight loss over the past 3 months. LFTs demonstrate elevated bilirubin, alkaline phosphatase, AST, and ALT. CA 19-9 is also elevated. True or false: given the elevated CA 19-9, a diagnosis of pancreatic cancer can be made.

    a. True

    b. False

Chapter 12

12.1 A patient with prolonged jaundice due to primary biliary cirrhosis would be expected to have all of the following except:

    a. Vitamin D deficiency

    b. Diminished bone density

    c. Low cholesterol levels

    d. Severe pruritus

12.2 Jaundice in the newborn is often due to physiological neonatal jaundice, breast milk jaundice, or Lucey–Driscoll syndrome. The pathophysiology of these conditions relates to:

    a. Impaired hepatocyte secretion of bilirubin

    b. Reduced activity of uridine diphosphate glucuronosyltransferase (UGT)

    c. Increased destruction of red blood cells

    d. Inadequate caloric intake

12.3 A patient has been hospitalized in the intensive care unit for postoperative sepsis, and has been critically ill. Fortunately, he is responding to antibiotics and clinically improving. Of the following, the least likely etiology for persistent hyperbilirubinemia is:

    a. Renal failure

    b. Covalent binding of bilirubin to albumin

    c. Development of gallstones

    d. Ongoing use of total parenteral nutrition (TPN)

Chapter 13

13.1 Which of the following is true?

    a. Antimitochondrial antibody is positive in approximately 50% of patients with PBC

    b. Anti-liver kidney microsomal (LKM) antibody is associated with older patients with autoimmune hepatitis

    c. Anti-LKM antibodies are associated with a more benign course of autoimmune hepatitis

    d. Anti-smooth muscle antibodies may be present in up to 50% of PBC patients

13.2 Which of the following is false regarding the diagnosis of Wilson disease?
    a. Ceruloplasmin is a copper storage protein
    b. Free serum copper is low in Wilson disease
    c. Urinary copper can be markedly elevated in chronic cholestatic liver disease
    d. Ceruloplasmin can be low in advanced liver disease of any etiology

13.3 Which of the following diseases is characterized by a low serum alkaline phosphatase level?
    a. Primary biliary cirrhosis (PBC)
    b. Primary sclerosing cholangitis (PSC)
    c. Wilson disease
    d. Cholangiocarcinoma

Chapter 14

14.1 Routine analysis of ascites fluid should include:
    a. Total protein
    b. White blood cell count with differential
    c. Albumin
    d. Glucose

14.2 All the following are associated with high serum-ascites albumin gradient (SAAG), low protein ascites, except:
    a. Alcoholic hepatitis
    b. Hepatitis C cirrhosis
    c. Congestive heart failure
    d. Nodular regenerative hyperplasia

14.3 In a patient with tense ascites who develops hepatorenal syndrome (HRS), all the following should be part of management, except:
    a. Intravenous fluids and/or albumin
    b. Discontinue nephrotoxic medications
    c. Increase diuretic doses
    d. Consider use of octreotide and midodrine

Chapter 15

15.1 Which of the following findings is not typically seen with hypocalcemia?
    a. Trousseau sign
    b. Hyporeflexia

   c. Heart block

   d. Seizures

   e. Paresthesias

15.2 What is the daily caloric requirement of a 70 kg person who is postoperative?

   a. 1400–1750 kcal

   b. 1750–2100 kcal

   c. 2100–2800 kcal

   d. 3000–4000 kcal

15.3 In a patient with an active Crohn's flare who is unable to tolerate any oral intake, how soon should TPN be initiated?

   a. In 14–21 days

   b. In 10–14 days

   c. In 1–7 days

   d. TPN is contraindicated during a Crohn's flare

Chapter 16

16.1 Which of the following is not an accepted indication for performing endoscopy?

   a. Surveillance of Barrett esophagus

   b. Evaluation of suspected upper GI bleeding

   c. Evaluation of suspected perforated duodenal ulcer

   d. Evaluation of dysphagia

16.2 A 67-year-old man is scheduled for upper endoscopy for evaluation and management of solid food dysphagia. He is on coumadin for a mechanical heart valve in the mitral position. What is the appropriate management of his anticoagulation therapy?

   a. Coumadin should be held for 2 days and low molecular weight heparin should be administered until the night before the scheduled procedure

   b. Coumadin should be held for 5–7 days prior to the procedure and low molecular weight heparin should be administered until the night before the scheduled procedure

   c. Coumadin should be held for 5–7 days. No bridge therapy is needed

   d. Coumadin should not be held for the procedure

Chapter 17

17.1 What is the most common cause of noncardiac chest pain?

   a. High-amplitude contractions of the esophageal body

   b. Simultaneous contractions of the esophageal body

   c. Gastroesophageal acid reflux

   d. Hypertensive LES

17.2 Which is the defining characteristic of achalasia?
   a. Nonrelaxation of the lower esophageal sphincter
   b. Aperistalsis of the esophageal body
   c. Absence of esophageal body contractions

17.3 What is the most common cause of oropharyngeal dysphagia?
   a. Cerebrovascular accident
   b. Parkinson disease
   c. Myasthenia gravis
   d. Polymyositis

Chapter 18

18.1 Which of the following is best able to detect the presence of gastroesophageal reflux?
   a. Upper gastrointestinal endoscopy
   b. Esophageal impedance
   c. Esophageal manometry
   d. Ambulatory esophageal pH monitoring
   e. Barium esophagram

18.2 What is the most common adverse event associated with PPIs?
   a. *C. difficile*-associated diarrhea
   b. Nosocomial pneumonia
   c. Bone fracture
   d. Myocardial infarction
   e. Increased heartburn upon discontinuation of drug

18.3 What is the recommended management of Barrett esophagus with high-grade dysplasia?
   a. Esophagectomy
   b. Endoscopic surveillance every 3 months
   c. Endoscopic therapy
   d. Chemoprevention with selective COX-2 inhibitors

18.4 What is the most common cause of heartburn symptoms that persist despite PPI therapy?
   a. Excessive gastric acid production
   b. Functional heartburn
   c. Nonacid reflux
   d. Alkaline reflux

18.5 What is the most common endoscopic finding in patients with documented GERD?
   a. Normal
   b. Barrett esophagus

    c. Erosive esophagitis

    d. Esophageal stricture

Chapter 19

19.1 Which of the following is a strong risk factor for esophageal adenocarcinoma?

    a. Alcohol

    b. Smoking

    c. African-American race

    d. Intestinal metaplasia

19.2 Current guidelines recommend which of the following for patients with confirmed Barrett esophagus with high-grade dysplasia?

    a. Esophagectomy

    b. Intensive endoscopic surveillance

    c. Endoscopic therapy

    d. Repeated endoscopy with four-quadrant biopsies every 0.5 cm

19.3 Which of the following is associated with esophageal squamous cell carcinoma (ESCC)?

    a. White race

    b. Heartburn

    c. Alcohol

    d. Intestinal metaplasia

Chapter 20

20.1 For patients with established diabetic gastroparesis, which therapy should be pursued if medical therapy fails to alleviate symptoms?

    a. Gastric pacing

    b. Venting gastrostomy and feeding jejunostomy

    c. Total parenteral nutrition

    d. Total gastrectomy

20.2 In patients with early dumping syndrome, what is the best therapy in addition to dietary modifications?

    a. Omeprazole 40 mg daily

    b. Metoclopramide 10 mg three times daily

    c. Octreotide 50 µg three times daily

    d. Insulin, regularly titrated to maintain glucose below 130

20.3 Which of the following scintigraphic-based gastric emptying protocols is most accurate for diagnosing gastroparesis?

    a. 2-h liquid

    b. 2-h solid

    c. 4-h liquid

    d. 4-h solid

Chapter 21

21.1 What is the most common cause of hypergastrinemia in a 24-year-old patient presenting with recurrent duodenal ulcer disease?
   a. Gastrinoma (Zollinger–Ellison syndrome)
   b. Acid suppression therapy
   c. Pernicious anemia
   d. Laboratory error

21.2 What is the most clinically expeditious method to differentiate hypergastrinemia due to gastrinoma from gastrin elevation due to PPI therapy?
   a. Basal and maximal acid output
   b. Secretin stimulation
   c. Gastric pH
   d. Serum chromogranin A

21.3 In addition to a PPI, what is the best retreatment regimen for patients who have persistent *H. pylori* despite being adherent to a 14-day course of clarithromycin, amoxicillin, and PPI?
   a. Clarithromycin and metronidazole
   b. Bismuth, metronidazole, and amoxicillin
   c. Amoxicillin for 5 days followed by clarithromycin and tinidazole for 5 days

21.4 A 58-year-old man comes to the emergency department with symptoms of melena and epigastric pain for 2 days. His exam is notable for orthostatic hypotension, reduced bowel sounds, and epigastric tenderness with guarding. His rectal examination reveals melena but his nasogastric lavage consists of bile-stained nonbloody fluid. His laboratory tests are notable for a Hb of 7.5 mg/dL, a HCT of 22 and a white blood count of 18.3. He is resuscitated with crystalloid and colloid and an intravenous PPI infusion is initiated. He is no longer orthostatic and repeated Hb is 9.7 mg/dL. What is the next best step in management?
   a. Upper gastrointestinal endoscopy
   b. Interventional radiology embolization
   c. CT scan of the abdomen
   d. *H. pylori* serology

Chapter 22

22.1 A 28-year-old woman is referred to your office for symptoms of epigastric discomfort, nausea, and bloating. The symptoms do not wake her from sleep, are not associated with weight loss, and have been constant for the past several months. She takes oral contraceptives but no other prescription or over-the-counter medication. Her examination is normal and her laboratory tests reveal a normal complete blood count and liver tests. What is the next best step in management?

a. Proton pump inhibitor
b. *H. pylori* eradication
c. Upper endoscopy
d. CT scan of the abdomen

22.2 The patient in question 22.1 responds initially to a 4-week trial of PPI but her symptoms recur while still taking the medication. *H. pylori* stool antigen testing is negative. Upper endoscopy is performed. What is the most likely finding?

a. Gastric ulcer
b. Duodenal ulcer
c. Erosive esophagitis
d. Normal

22.3 The patient in questions 22.1 and 22.2 remains symptomatic on PPI therapy. What is the next best step in management?

a. Abdominal CT scan
b. Gallbladder scintigraphy with ejection fraction
c. Magnetic resonance angiography
d. Reassurance

22.4 The patient remains symptomatic. What is the next best therapeutic option?

a. Sequential therapy for *H. pylori* eradication
b. High-dose proton pump inhibitor
c. Metoclopramide
d. Tricyclic antidepressant (TCA)

Chapter 23

23.1 Which of the following is not a high-risk feature in evaluation of a gastrointestinal stromal tumor?

a. >10 mitosis/50 HPF
b. Tumor diameter >10 cm
c. Tumor with mucosal ulceration and GI bleeding
d. Tumor diameter >5 cm with >5 mitosis/50 HPF

23.2 A patient underwent EGD to evaluate epigastric pain and was found to have evidence of a 3 cm malignant-appearing ulcer with biopsies demonstrating intestinal-type gastric adenocarcinoma. Which is the next most appropriate test?

a. EUS
b. PET

    c. CT

    d. Upper GI series

Chapter 24

24.1 Which of the following grains is tolerated by most patients with celiac disease?

    a. Wheat

    b. Barley

    c. Oats

    d. Rye

    e. Malt

24.2 Which of the following tests is no longer recommended as part of the diagnostic evaluation of suspected celiac disease?

    a. Anti-tTG IgA

    b. Antiendomysial antibody

    c. Total IgA

    d. Antigliadin antibodies

    e. Small intestinal biopsy

24.3 All the following are true statements about celiac disease *except*:

    a. Celiac disease is more common in Caucasians than in Asians or people of African descent

    b. Celiac disease is associated with dermatitis herpetiformis

    c. A gluten-free diet will result in recovery of normal intestinal histology within 48 h

    d. A gluten-free diet is considered to be protective against the development of lymphoma

    e. Histological findings on small bowel biopsy may be milder than expected due to gluten restriction in the diet or use of immunosuppressant medications

Chapter 25

25.1 What is the most likely composition of nephrolithiasis in a patient with short bowel syndrome?

    a. Calcium oxalate

    b. Calcium phosphate

    c. Sodium hydroxyapatite

    d. Calcium urate

25.2 A patient with short bowel syndrome suddenly becomes obtunded after eating a pizza. A significant metabolic acidosis with respiratory alkalosis is revealed. What is the most likely etiology of this presentation?

    a. New-onset diabetic ketoacidosis

    b. Alcoholic ketoacidosis

    c. Salicylate overdose

    d. D-lactic acidemia

25.3 How should the patient in question 25.2 be treated?

    a. Intravenous insulin and fluids

    b. N-acetylcysteine

    c. Antibiotics

    d. Bicarbonate infusion

25.4 What type of fat source is best absorbed in a patient with short bowel syndrome?

    a. Short-chain triglycerides

    b. Medium-chain triglycerides

    c. Long-chain triglycerides

Chapter 26

26.1 Patients with familial adenomatous polyposis (FAP) syndrome should have which of the following performed every 1–2 years for surveillance purposes?

    a. Double balloon enteroscopy

    b. CT scan

    c. Side-viewing upper endoscopy

    d. Standard upper endoscopy

26.2 Which lab test should be orderd if carcinoid syndrome is suspected?

    a. CA 19-9

    b. CEA

    c. Urinary 5-HIAA

    d. Liver function panel

Chapter 27

27.1 Which of the following statements about diverticular disease is *true*?

    a. Approximately half of diverticular hemorrhage emanates from the right colon

    b. Diverticulosis is more common in the proximal colon (i.e. cecum, ascending and transverse colon) than in the sigmoid colon

    c. Diverticulitis is precipitated by seeds, corn or nuts

    d. Most patients with diverticulosis will develop complications (i.e. diverticulitis or bleeding) at some point in their lifetime

    e. Barium enema is recommended during an acute attack of diverticulitis to delineate the severity of strictures and determine if fistulization is present

27.2 Which of the following is *not* an indication for surgery for acute diverticulitis?

    a. Peritonitis

    b. Abscess formation

    c. Intractable symptoms

    d. Fistula formation

    e. Recurrent diverticulitis with first episode at age 45

27.3 True or false: Diverticulosis commonly causes symptoms?

    a. True

    b. False

Chapter 28

28.1 Which of the following is effective for treating functional constipation?

    a. Lubiprostone

    b. Dicyclomine

    c. Alosetron

    d. Tricyclic antidepressants

    e. Atropine with diphenoxylate

28.2 Why is alosetron not approved for men and available only through a restricted prescription program?

    a. High potential for abuse by patients

    b. Risk of new-onset ulcerative colitis

    c. Risk of prostate cancer

    d. Association with ischemic colitis

    e. Teratogenicity

28.3 Which of the following is an appropriate therapy for a patient with diarrhea-predominant IBS?

    a. Polyethylene glycol solution

    b. Tegaserod

    c. Lubiprostone

    d. Tricyclic antidepressant

Chapter 29

29.1 A 34-year-old patient with ulcerative proctitis presents with worsened diarrhea, abdominal pain, and tenesmus. What is the best initial evaluation?

    a. CT scan of the abdomen

    b. Colonoscopy

    c. Stool examination for *C. difficile* toxin

    d. Stool electrolytes

29.2 A 24-year-old woman with pan-ulcerative colitis presents with abdominal pain, distension, and diarrhea. On examination, she is febrile and her abdomen is notable for absent bowel sounds, distension, tenderness with rebound, and guarding. Her WBC is 21,000 and her albumin is 2.8 mg/dL.

CT scan of the abdomen reveals dilation of the cecum to 10 cm with bowel wall edema but no free peritoneal air. What is the best step in management?

a. Intravenous steroids

b. Infliximab IV

c. Cyclosporine IV

d. Surgical intervention

29.3 A 29-year-old woman with ileal Crohn's disease presents with renal colic. What is the most likely composition of her stones?

a. Calcium phosphate

b. Calcium urate

c. Sodium hydroxyapatite

d. Calcium oxalate

Chapter 30

30.1 A 57-year-old patient presents with 10 lb weight loss and occasional bright red blood per rectum. Laboratory studies reveal iron deficiency anemia. What is the best initial evaluation?

a. Barium enema

b. CT scan of the abdomen and pelvis

c. EGD

d. Fecal occult blood test

e. Colonoscopy

30.2 A 42-year-old man presents for his annual check-up. His review of systems is completely negative. His family history is notable for colon cancer in his brother at age 48 and his father at age 62. His maternal aunt was diagnosed with breast cancer in her 50s and his paternal uncle had ureteral cancer age 67. What do you recommend?

a. Annual FOBT beginning at age 50

b. Colonoscopy every 10 years beginning at age 50

c. CT colonography every 5 years

d. Colonoscopy now, in addition to referral for genetics counseling

e. Colonoscopy every 10 years beginning now

30.3 A 77-year-old woman with a history of a negative colonoscopy 10 years ago, diabetes mellitus, and COPD requiring home oxygen asks what colorectal cancer screening she should undergo. What do you recommend?

a. Annual FIT screening

b. Double contrast barium enema

c. Flexible sigmoidoscopy with FOBT

d. Colonoscopy

e. None of the above

Chapter 31

31.1 Which of the following statements about hemorrhoids is *not* true?
  a. Hemorrhoids occur in up to 50% of adults in the United States
  b. Second-degree hemorrhoids prolapse and require digital reduction
  c. Surgical hemorrhoidectomy is the treatment of choice for most third-degree hemorrhoids
  d. Most first-degree hemorrhoids can be managed with high-fiber diet, adequate fluid intake, sitz baths and good anal hygiene
  e. Thrombosis of an external hemorrhoid can produce severe pain and bleeding

31.2 Severe anal pain with scant red bleeding is a classic presentation of:
  a. Solitary rectal ulcer
  b. Anal fistula
  c. Pruritus ani
  d. Anal fissure
  e. Rectal prolapse

31.3 Botulinum toxin injection is used to treat which of the following?
  a. Anal fistula
  b. Anal fissure
  c. Anal carcinoma
  d. Solitary rectal ulcer
  e. Fecal incontinence

Chapter 32

32.1 Which of the following is true regarding pancreatic enzymes therapy?
  a. Immediate-release enzymes (nonenteric coated) have been shown to be effective in the treatment of chronic pancreatitis pain in a randomized controlled trial
  b. Delayed-release enzymes (enteric coated) have been shown to be effective in the treatment of chronic pancreatitis pain in a randomized controlled trial
  c. The mechanism of action of pancreatic enzyme replacement therapy is to increase pancreatic exocrine output in response to a meal
  d. They are inexpensive

32.2 When should enteral nutrition with nasojejunal feeding be started in a patient diagnosed with severe acute pancreatitis?
  a. On the 7th hospital day
  b. Once the prediction of severe acute pancreatitis is made
  c. Enteral nutrition should be avoided since it may exacerbate the patient's pancreatitis. Instead start TPN
  d. Once the lipase is below five times the upper limit of normal

32.3 What is the theoretical advantage of placing a feeding tube past the ligament of Treitz?
- **a.** Less likely that the tube will be displaced
- **b.** Avoids the risk of tube tip trauma to the major papilla
- **c.** Higher concentration of CCK and secretin-secreting cells in the duodenum
- **d.** Lower concentration of CCK and secretin-secreting cells in the duodenum

32.4 In the setting of acute biliary pancreatitis, when should cholecystectomy be performed?
- **a.** Always shortly after presentation
- **b.** Shortly after presentation for mild acute pancreatitis, delayed days to weeks after presentation for severe acute pancreatitis
- **c.** Shortly after presentation for severe acute pancreatitis, delayed days to weeks after presentation for mild acute pancreatitis
- **d.** Always delayed days to weeks after presentation
- **e.** Cholecystectomy is not necessary after acute biliary pancreatitis

32.5 Which of the following is not an indication for pseudocyst drainage?
- **a.** Pseudocyst size greater than 6 cm
- **b.** Vomiting due to gastric outlet obstruction
- **c.** Infection of the pseudocyst
- **d.** Obstructive jaundice with pruritus
- **e.** Abdominal pain with anorexia and weight loss

Chapter 33

33.1 What is the best method for establishing the diagnosis of pancreatic cancer?
- **a.** CA 19-9
- **b.** CEA
- **c.** CT scan
- **d.** EUS FNA
- **e.** PET/CT

33.2 What is the approximate risk of malignancy in a patient with main duct IPMN?
- **a.** <20%
- **b.** 25%
- **c.** 50%
- **d.** 70%

33.3 An EUS FNA is performed to evaluate a 2 cm pancreatic cyst in the body of the pancreas. There are no pancreatic duct abnormalities identified and no masses are appreciated. Cyst fluid aspiration is performed and

demonstrate a CEA of 560 ng/dL and and amylase of 30 U/L. What is the most likely diagnosis?
a. Serous cystadenoma
b. Mucinous cystadenoma
c. Side branch IPMN
d. Main duct IPMN

Chapter 34

34.1 A cholangiocarcinoma involving the hilum and left and right hepatic ducts is called a:
a. bismuth tumor
b. Klatskin tumor
c. Krukenberg tumor
d. Caroli tumor

34.2 Which of the diseases listed below is *not* associated with primary sclerosing cholangitis?
a. Ulcerative colitis
b. Recurrent pancreatitis
c. Sjögren syndrome
d. Celiac sprue

34.3 Which type of biliary cyst is characterized by one or more cystic dilations of the intrahepatic ducts without extrahepatic duct disease?
a. Type I
b. Type II
c. Type III
d. Type IV
e. Type V

Chapter 35

35.1 Which of the following symptoms is not part of the Charcot triad?
a. RUQ abdominal pain
b. Fever
c. Hypotension
d. Jaundice

35.2 A patient who is post cholecystectomy presents with recurrent episodes of severe biliary-type pain. Evaluation of the patient during episodes of pain shows no laboratory or imaging abnormalities. If the patient has SOD, which type would it be most consistent with?
a. Type I
b. Type II

c. Type III
d. Type IV

Chapter 36

36.1 A 67-year-old man with Crohn's ileitis presents with fever, anorexia, abdominal pain, hypotension, and leukocytosis. What is the best initial evaluation?
   a. Colonoscopy
   b. Abdominal ultrasound
   c. Plain abdominal x-ray (3 views)
   d. CT scan of the abdomen and pelvis
   e. Barium enema

36.2 A 24-year-old man with Crohn's ileitis who has been treated with azathioprine for over 2 years presents with new-onset drainage from an erythematous lesion on his abdomen. A CT scan demonstrates an ileocutaneous fistula. What is the best next step in management?
   a. Cyclosporine IV
   b. Intravenous steroids
   c. Infliximab IV
   d. Surgical intervention

36.3 An infant presents with respiratory distress, nausea, and vomiting. Chest radiography reveals a posterolateral diaphragmatic hernia with a left thoracic air–fluid level and mediastinal displacement. This finding fits which of the following types of hernias?
   a. Hernia of Morgagni
   b. Hernia of Bochdalek
   c. Spigelian hernia
   d. Omphalocele
   e. Internal hernia

Chapter 37

37.1 True or false: A vigorous immune response to acute hepatitis B infection leads to greater clinical illness and a greater chance of chronic infection.

37.2 Hepatitis B is considered chronic if:
   a. HBcAb IgG is present beyond 6 months
   b. HBcAb IgM is present beyond 3 months
   c. HBsAg is present beyond 6 months

37.3 Which of the following viruses is associated with fulminant liver failure in pregnant women?
  a. HAV
  b. HBV
  c. HCV
  d. HEV

Chapter 38

38.1 Which of the following is true?
  a. It is estimated that 50% of NASH patients will progress to cirrhosis
  b. A hepatic iron index (HII) of 2.5 is consistent with hemochromatosis
  c. The peak time of onset of Wilson disease is the fourth decade of life
  d. Kayser–Fleischer rings are always present in patients with Wilson disease

38.2 Each of the following can be used in the pharmacotherapy of Wilson disease, except:
  a. Penicillamine
  b. Trientine
  c. Zinc
  d. Ursodiol

38.3 Each of the following is a typical histological feature of nonalcoholic steatohepatitis, except:
  a. Hepatocyte ballooning
  b. Steatosis
  c. Pericellular fibrosis
  d. Bile ductular proliferation

Chapter 39

39.1 Which of the following are potential causes of alkaline phosphatase elevation during the third trimester of pregnancy?
  a. Placental release of alkaline phosphatase
  b. HELLP syndrome
  c. Cholestasis of pregnancy
  d. All of the above

39.2 Typical diagnostic findings in primary biliary cirrhosis include all of the following except:
  a. Positive antimitochondrial antibody (AMA)
  b. Elevated serum IgM level
  c. Dilated bile ducts on ultrasound
  d. Granulomas on liver biopsy

39.3 Appropriate medications to prescribe for a patient with PBC include all the following except:

   a. Ursodiol 15 mg/kg

   b. Ursodiol 5 mg/kg

   c. Calcium supplementation

   d. Vitamin D supplementation

Chapter 40

40.1 Which of the following statements about alcoholic hepatitis is *false*?

   a. Portal hypertension can exist without cirrhosis

   b. Most patients admitted to hospital with alcoholic hepatitis have cirrhosis

   c. Alcoholic hepatitis typically results in AST >300 IU/L

   d. Continued use of alcohol is associated with a high mortality rate

40.2 Which of the following is *not* typical of liver biopsy findings in alcoholic hepatitis?

   a. Pericentral steatosis

   b. Lymphocytic inflammation

   c. Pericellular fibrosis

   d. Mallory hyaline

40.3 Alcoholic hepatitis patients with a Maddrey discriminant function >32:

   a. Have a 30-day mortality >50%

   b. Will likely derive survival benefit from a course of corticosteroids

   c. Are too ill to benefit from alcohol abstinence

   d. Benefit from nutritional supplementation

Chapter 41

41.1 Which of the following is false?

   a. Liver biopsy does not play a significant role in the diagnosis of autoimmune hepatitis (AIH)

   b. AIH patients with a positive anti-LKM antibody (type 2) only rarely have a positive ANA

   c. The diagnostic scoring systems for AIH take into account the results of viral serologies

   d. High levels of serum IgG support the diagnosis of AIH

41.2 Which of the following is false regarding liver biopsy findings in AIH?

   a. Viral hepatitis and drug-induced hepatitis may have similar histological findings to AIH

   b. Bridging necrosis can be seen on biopsies of patients with a severe presentation

   c. Moderate (2–3+) iron staining is commonly seen on liver biopsy in AIH patients

   d. The inflammation seen in AIH typically consists of lymphoplasmacytic inflammatory cells

Chapter 42

42.1 Which of the following is *true*?

   a. A patient with a hepatic venous pressure gradient (HVPG) of 15 is more likely to experience variceal bleeding than a patient with an HVPG of 12

   b. Hepatopulmonary syndrome is due to pulmonary vascular vasoconstriction

   c. Type 1 hepatorenal syndrome (HRS) is more severe than type 2 HRS

   d. Type 1 HRS is associated with severe intrarenal vasodilation

42.2 Which of the following is not an appropriate choice for the purposes of variceal prophylaxis?

   a. Propranolol

   b. Carvedilol

   c. Atenolol

   d. Nadolol

Chapter 43

43.1 Which of the following statements about hepatocellular carcinoma is *false*?

   a. 90% of patients with HCC have underlying cirrhosis

   b. HCC affects men and women equally

   c. HCC is the third leading cause of cancer deaths worldwide

   d. HCC can occur in hepatitis B patients who do not have cirrhosis

43.2 Radiographic features of HCC include all of the following *except*:

   a. HCCs typically have arterial enhancement

   b. HCCs remain enhancing in portal and delayed phases of multiphase CT or MRI

   c. CT and MRI can assess for portal venous invasion

   d. Liver masses that meet radiographic criteria for HCC do not require biopsy for diagnosis confirmation

43.3 Which of the following statements about HCC treatment is *true*?

   a. The majority of tumors are resectable

   b. The recurrence rates after resection are approximately 5% at 5 years

   c. A patient with a 3 cm HCC can receive priority for liver transplantation

   d. Transarterial chemoembolization (TACE) can be used safely in patients with bilirubin >5

Chapter 44

44.1 All the following are helpful in making the diagnosis of *C. difficile* colitis, except:
   a. Tissue culture assay
   b. Stool culture
   c. Enzyme-linked immunosorbent assay for toxins A and B
   d. Colonoscopic findings

44.2 Which of the following is *false* regarding enterohemorrhagic *E. coli* (EHEC) infection?
   a. The disease is caused by the O157:H7 strain
   b. It is most prevalent in children <5 years of age
   c. EHEC is associated with the development of hemolytic uremic syndrome
   d. Treatment includes hydration and antibiotics

44.3 Which of the following is *false* regarding *Campylobacter jejuni* infection?
   a. *C. jejuni* is the most common cause of bacterial enterocolitis in the United States
   b. *C. jejuni* cannot be isolated from stool culture
   c. Infected individuals may present with right lower quadrant abdominal pain and bloody diarrhea
   d. Infection is associated with the development of Reiter syndrome and Guillain–Barré syndrome

Chapter 45

45.1 Which of the following is not consistent with the diagnosis of a Dieulafoy lesion?
   a. Ulcerated lesion with a pigmented protuberance
   b. Pigmented protuberance without an associated ulcer
   c. Adherent clot without an associate ulcer
   d. Large clot in the stomach without any obvious mucosal abnormality

45.2 Which of the following is not appropriate in the management of GAVE?
   a. Argon plasma coagulation
   b. Bipolar electrocautery
   c. Transjugular intrahepatic portosystemic shunt (TIPS)
   d. Nd:YAG laser therapy

Answers

Chapter 1

1.1 (c) Upper endoscopy. In the case of complete obstruction contrast studies of the esophagus are contraindicated due to the risk of pulmonary aspiration. Upper endoscopy is useful for diagnosis and treatment, since acute obstruction can often be relieved endoscopically.

1.2 (a) Aperistalsis of the esophageal body. Achalasia is diagnosed by the presence of aperistalsis of the nonstriated muscle portion of the esophageal body. Absent relaxation of the lower esophageal sphincter is also common but incomplete relaxation may also be found. It is important to note that aperistalsis does not mean the absence of contractions but rather that the observed contractions along the length of the esophagus are simultaneous.

1.3 (c) Nonbacterial infection. The most common causes of odynophagia in immunocompromised individuals are fungal infection (*Candida* esophagitis) and viral infections (HSV and CMV).

Chapter 2

2.1 (b) False: manometry detects potentially pathogenic motor abnormalities in only a minority of patients with noncardiac chest pain.

2.2 (d) Test for coronary artery spasm. Ergonovine can be given during cardiac catheterization to test for epicardial coronary vasospasm.

2.3 (c) Noncardiac chest pain from esophageal sources is often indistinguishable from angina, including radiation in a pattern similar to angina. However, esophageal pain is rarely brought on by exertion.

Chapter 3

3.1 (c) Gastric ulcer with a visible vessel. Electrocautery therapy is appropriate for actively bleeding ulcers or ulcers with a visible vessel. If an adherent clot is present, some advocate removing the clot (e.g. with a snare) and then treating the underlying lesion.

3.2 (d) Patients with cirrhosis and GI bleeding of any cause. Meta-analysis of randomized, controlled trials have demonstrated improvement in morbidity and mortality among patients with cirrhosis admitted with GI bleeding of any cause. While patients with *Helicobacter pylori*-associated peptic ulcer disease should receive appropriate antibiotic therapy, intravenous antibiotics are not generally indicated. Of note, in the setting of complicated peptic ulcer bleeding, documentation of eradication of *Helicobacter pylori* is recommended.

3.3 (e) Argon plasma coagulation. Endoscopic therapy for variceal hemorrhage includes sclerotherapy or band ligation. Transjugular intrahepatic portosystemic shunt (TIPS) and surgical portocaval shunts can reduce the pressure gradient within the liver to reduce the risk of variceal hemorrhage. In the setting of massive variceal hemorrhage, especially after failed endoscopic therapy, a Sengstaken–Blakemore tube can be placed to help stabilize the patient (e.g. while getting the patient ready for TIPS placement). There is no role for endoscopic argon plasma coagulation in the treatment of variceal hemorrhage.

Chapter 4

4.1 (b) Bulimia nervosa. These physical exam findings all result from self-induced vomiting. While adult rumination syndrome may produce the oral findings, the scarring of the knuckles results from scraping of the knuckles on the teeth.

4.2 (a) Repetitively regurgitating food from the stomach, rechewing it, and then reswallowing it is characteristic of Merycism, also known as adult rumination syndrome. Choice (b) is characteristic of bulimia nervosa, while choices (c), (d) and (e) are characteristic of chronic pancreatitis, depression, and anorexia nervosa, respectively. About half of all cases of unexplained weight loss are attributable to organic disease, whereas psychiatric conditions, especially in the elderly, comprise the majority of the remaining cases. Parkinson disease and Alzheimer disease are common neurological etiologies of weight loss.

4.3 (d) In severe malnutrition, rapid refeeding should be avoided because of potential gastroduodenal dilation and refeeding pancreatitis or diarrhea. For anorexia nervosa, feedings are re-established at 200–250 calories above the intake at time of presentation and are increased by 250–300 calories every 5 days to ensure a weekly weight gain of 1.5 kg as an inpatient and 0.75–1.0 kg as an outpatient. The goal for refeeding is to achieve 90–100% of ideal body weight.

Chapter 5

5.1 (d) No work-up at this time. Acute onset of vomiting in association with myalgias and diarrhea suggests an infectious etiology. Diagnostic evaluation is reserved for patients with chronic symptoms or in the setting of comorbidity, such as in a person with diabetes in whom diabetic ketoacidosis must be excluded.

5.2 (a) A pyloric channel ulcer can cause gastric outlet obstruction either through acute inflammation and edema at the pylorus (where the stomach connects to the duodenal bulb) or through chronic inflammation and scarring. A succussion splash, heard through a stethoscope placed on the abdomen during side-to-side movement of the abdomen, is classically found in gastric obstruction and gastroparesis.

5.3 (b) Stable weight. Psychogenic vomiting will typically be associated with a stable weight. However, small bowel luminal dilation suggests a dysmotility or obstruction. A scintigraphic gastric emptying study can also assess for dysmotility and a delay suggesting gastroparesis, as does tachygastria on electrogastrography. Feculent emesis suggests a distal bowel obstruction, gastrocolic fistulae, or bacterial overgrowth.

Chapter 6

6.1 (b) Abdominal series radiography (supine and upright or decubitus). Rapid diagnosis of a perforated viscus is essential as these patients typically require surgical management. Abdominal radiography will demonstrate evidence of free air within the abdomen, rapidly confirming the diagnosis of a perforated viscus.

6.2 (c) Rectus sheath hematoma. The Carnett test can distinguish intra-abdominal discomfort from abdominal wall pain. Increased tenderness upon raising the head and tensing the abdomen suggests a superficial abdominal wall source.

6.3 (d) IV hydration, pain management, and IV antibiotics. This patient has evidence of acute cholecystitis. Initial management involves supportive care with IV hydration, pain management, and IV antibiotics. The patient should have a surgical consult; however, the timing of surgery will depend on the severity of symptoms and the patient's overall risk of undergoing surgery.

Chapter 7

7.1 (d) reassurance. Carbohydrate absorption is not a feature of IBS. Anti-TTG may detect celiac disease but this is unlikely with normal iron absorption and absence of malabsorption. The SmartPill is used to quantify transit through the stomach, small and large intestine using temperature and pH changes; however, her symptoms do not suggest a motility disorder. Reassurance is the best initial course of management.

7.2 (d) Rice. Only rice and gluten-free wheat are 100% absorbed in healthy individuals.

Chapter 8

8.1 (d) Surgery. Complete small intestinal obstruction should be treated surgically. Water-soluble contrast enemas are useful to rule out distal colonic obstruction and may be able to induce catharsis in patients with pseudo-obstruction but are not useful for small intestinal obstructive disease. Colonic decompression will not alleviate acute obstruction and neostigmine is contraindicated under these circumstances.

8.2 (c) Initial management should be conservative and consist of NG tube insertion, frequent position changes, correction of electrolyte abnormalities, nothing by mouth. Neostigmine has been illustrated in controlled clinical trials to relieve symptoms and reduce colonic distension but should be reserved for patients in whom conservative measures have failed to improve symptoms.

8.3 (c) While colonoscopic decompression is a viable alternative, the use of neostigmine in a patient without cardiovascular or other contraindications is less invasive and has proven benefit in reducing distension and other symptoms.

Chapter 9

9.1 (d) In the absence of warning symptoms or signs, structural evaluation is not necessary in patients less than 40 years of age. An empirical trial of fiber or osmotic laxative is advocated prior to more invasive testing.

9.2 (c) Anorectal manometry. Colonic transit tests may be abnormal in defecatory disorders in addition to colonic inertia. For this reason, assessment of colonic transit is recommended only after excluding a defecatory disorder. In this age group malignancy and other structural lesions are unlikely; therefore, CT scans are rarely useful. Colonoscopy is likewise unlikely to identify the source of constipation and biopsies would need to be full thickness in order to rule out Hirshsprung disease.

9.3 (c) Biofeedback has been illustrated to reduce symptoms and improve physiology of patients with dyssynergic defecation. The principal focus is improved relaxation of the anal sphincter during defecation and improved pushing forces. Neither myotomy or botulinum injections to the sphincter lead to improvement in the majority of patients.

Chapter 10

10.1 (a) Magnesium-containing laxatives. The stool electrolytes indicate the presence of unmeasured osmotically active molecules. 290 mOsm (plasma) − 2 × ([Na] + [K]) = 130 mOsm. VIP-secreting tumors cause secretory diarrhea, as does senna ingestion. Irritable bowel syndrome does not cause osmotic diarrhea.

10.2 (b) *Bacillus cereus*. *Campylobacter* and *Shigella* would not present within hours of ingestion of the infected food. Enterotoxigenic *E. coli* is typically found in undercooked meat, while *B. cereus* most often occurs in the setting of cooked rice that is reheated (as is commonly used for fried rice).

Chapter 11

11.1 (d) EUS FNA. The mass described in the CT scan is likely to represent a subepithelial mass that will require EUS to image and also to perform EUS-guided FNA of the lesion for a tissue diagnosis. EGD and upper GI series are unlikely to provide any additional information and endoscopic imaging of the lesion can be performed at the time of EUS.

11.2 (b) False. Although the clinical presentation is consistent with pancreatic cancer, an elevated CA 19-9 can be seen in benign lesions in the presence of biliary obstruction as well as cholangiocarcinoma, which can present similarly. Furthermore, CA 19-9 should not be used to establish the diagnosis of pancreatic cancer; however, it can be a useful marker to monitor patients following surgery or response to chemotherapy. The baseline CA 19-9 should be established after the biliary system has been decompressed.

Chapter 12

12.1 (c) Patients with prolonged cholestasis typically develop hypercholester-olemia, in addition to fat-soluble vitamin deficiency, bone density loss, and pruritus.

12.2 (b) UGT is the hepatic enzyme responsible for bilirubin conjugation. Breast milk jaundice is due to the presence of a UGT inhibitor in breast milk. Lucey–Driscoll syndrome is due to a UGT inhibitor in the mother's blood. Physiological neonatal jaundice reflects inadequate UGT activity in many newborns, which typically improves by day 14 of life.

12.3 (c) In the critically ill patient with jaundice, hyperbilirubinemia can persist despite improvement of the underlying illness. With prolonged jaundice, circulating bilirubin may bind covalently to albumin, which prevents its elimination until the albumin is degraded. Conjugated bilirubin is cleared by renal glomeruli and bilirubin levels may increase in renal failure. Total parenteral nutrition causes hyperbilirubinemia as a result of intrahepatic cholestasis. While gallstones are a common cause of extrahepatic jaundice in the United States, and can be caused by TPN use, they are less likely to be a cause of persistent jaundice in an ICU patient.

Chapter 13

13.1 (d) ASMA is positive in >90% of patients with PBC. Anti-LKM antibodies are associated with aggressive autoimmune hepatitis in young women. It is true that ASMA may be present in 30–50% of patients with PBC.

13.2 (b) Free serum copper is typically high in Wilson disease.

13.3 (c) PBC is a cholestatic liver disorder, with impaired bilirubin excretion and associated alkaline phosphatase elevation. PSC and cholangiocarcinoma can result in bile duct obstruction, with resultant alkaline phosphatase elevation. Wilson disease is notable for a typically low alkaline phosphatase, and an elevated bilirubin to alkaline phosphatase ratio.

Chapter 14

14.1 (d) Routine analysis of ascites fluid should include total protein, albumin, cell counts, and culture. Glucose is not routinely checked, although it may be used when evaluating for secondary peritonitis.

14.2 (c) Congestive heart failure is typically associated with high SAAG, high protein ascites.

14.3 (c) The development of HRS is a severe complication that can develop in patients with ascites. Management includes holding diuretics, providing intravenous fluids and albumin, potential use of octreotide and midodrine, and consideration of TIPS and/or liver transplantation.

Chapter 15

15.1 (b) Hyporeflexia. Hyperreflexia, as opposed to hyporeflexia, is typically seen in patients with hypocalcemia.

15.2 (c) 2100–2800 kcal. Healthy adults require 20–25 kcal per kilogram of body weight to satisfy daily caloric requirements. With the stress of disease or surgery, this need increases to 30–40 kcal per kilogram per day.

15.3 (c) In 1–7 days. TPN should be initiated in 1–7 days in patients requiring TPN who are catabolic and/or malnourished.

Chapter 16

16.1 (c) Evaluation of suspected perforated duodenal ulcer. Endoscopy is contraindicated in the setting of any gastrointestinal perforation.

16.2 (b) Coumadin should be held for 5–7 days prior to the procedure and low molecular weight heparin should be administered until the night prior to the scheduled procedure. The patient is undergoing endoscopy for evaluation and management of solid food dysphagia with the potential of having a dilation performed. A dilation is considered a high-risk procedure for potential bleeding; therefore, anticoagulation with coumadin should be held 5–7 days prior to the scheduled procedure. Bridge therapy with low molecular weight heparin should be administered while the coumadin is being held because a mechanical valve in the mitral position is considered a high-risk condition for a thromboembolic event.

Chapter 17

17.1 (c) Gastroesophageal acid reflux. High-amplitude contractions (>180 mmHg) were proposed as a common etiology of noncardiac chest pain; however, this finding is common among asymptomatic persons and poorly correlated with symptoms of chest pain. Diffuse esophageal spasm and achalasia, which are characterized by aperistalsis of the esophageal body, can be associated with pain but more commonly present with dysphagia. Gastroesophageal reflux disease is the most common etiology of noncardiac chest pain and should be empirically treated or evaluated.

17.2 (b) Achalasia is defined by the lack of peristalsis of the esophageal body. This does not mean that there is an absence of contractions but rather that the contractions are simultaneous and nonpropulsive. The lower esophageal sphincter generally does not relax or relaxes incompletely, but this finding may be absent early in the disease course.

17.3 (a) Oropharyngeal dysphagia is most often the result of cerebrovascular accidents. The other etiologies can cause oropharyngeal dysphagia but are much less common.

Chapter 18

18.1 (b) Esophageal impedance. Upper gastrointestinal endoscopy is able to detect complications of GERD including erosions, ulcers and Barrett esophagus; however, it is insensitive for the diagnosis of GERD. Esophageal pH monitoring is effective in detecting acid reflux but is unable to detect nonacid reflux. Manometry can detect motility disorders but not necessarily GERD. Impedance can detect acidic and nonacidic reflux events.

18.2 (e) Increased heartburn upon discontinuation of PPI. Heartburn has been shown to occur after discontinuation of PPIs, presumably due to gastrin-induced hypertrophy of parietal cells. While associations have been noted between PPI use and *C. difficile* infection, pneumonia, bone fracture and hypomagnesemia, these associations, if true, are very rare.

18.3 (c) Endoscopic therapy. Currrent guidelines recommend endoscopic therapy including radiofrequency ablation, endoscopic mucosal resection or photodynamic therapy for patients with Barrett esophagus and high-grade dysplasia. Patients refusing endoscopic therapy may undergo surveillance. Esophagectomy is generally reserved for patients with cancer. Chemoprevention with COX-2-selective inhibitors has been shown in epidemiological studies to be associated with reduced cancer incidence; however, a randomized trial comparing celecoxib to placebo among patients with Barrett esophagus and dysplasia failed to demonstrate protection against high-grade dysplasia or cancer.

18.4 (b) Functional heartburn. Excessive acid production is extremely rare and is associated with gastrin-producing tumors (gastrinoma). Nonacid reflux can be diagnosed by impedance measurement but is the cause of symptoms in a minority of patients nonresponsive to PPIs. Alkaline reflux occurs after surgery that allows reflux of duodenal contents into the stomach and esophagus (Bilroth II anastomosis) but is not as common a cause of refractory heartburn as functional disease.

18.5 (a) Normal. This is the most common endoscopic finding, even among patients with documented GERD. A minority of symptomatic patients has erosive disease, and 5–15% of patients with heartburn have Barrett esophagus. Strictures occur but in a small minority of patients.

Chapter 19

19.1 (d) Intestinal metaplasia (Barrett esophagus). Esophageal adenocarcinoma is significantly more common among individuals with the following characteristics: white race, male sex, advanced age, GERD, and Barrett esophagus. Alcohol is not a risk factor and while smoking is associated with cancer, it is not as strong a predictor as the other variables.

19.2 (c) National society guidelines recommend endoscopic therapy for patients with Barrett esophagus and high-grade dysplasia. Previous guidelines recommended either endoscopic surveillance every 3 months with biopsies in four quadrants every 1 cm, or esophagectomy; however, the efficacy of endoscopic therapy coupled with the morbidity and mortality associated with esophagectomy have placed endoscopic therapy into the optimal position. Visible lesions such as ulcers, nodules or masses should be treated via endoscopic mucosal resection to remove the lesion and confirm high-grade dysplasia without invasive cancer. Flat regions of high-grade dysplasia as well as the nondysplastic regions of Barrett esophagus should be treated with endoscopic radiofrequency ablation, photodynamic therapy or endoscopic mucosal resection.

19.3 (c) Alcohol. The primary risk factors for ESCC include African-American race, alcohol, smoking, and male sex. These factors are different from those associated with esophageal adenocarcinoma (see question 19.1).

Chapter 20

20.1 (b) Venting gastrostomy and feeding jejunostomy. This intervention has been illustrated to provide adequate symptom relief for patients with gastroparesis refractory to medical therapy. Gastric pacing (low-frequency, high-energy pulses) is rarely effective in improving gastric emptying or symptoms. Total parenteral nutrition is an option but should be reserved for patients in whom all other alternative have been examined due to the severe adverse events associated with this intervention. Total gastrectomy and other surgical options have had generally disappointing results.

20.2 (c) Octreotide delays gastric emptying and prevents the accelerated emptying seen in dumping syndrome. In addition, octreotide inhibits release of many of the enteric hormones and insulin secretion that play a role in symptom development.

20.3 (d) The 4-h assessment of gastric emptying after ingestion of a solid radiolabeled meal is most accurate for diagnosing gastroparesis.

Chapter 21

21.1 (b) Acid suppression. The most common etiology of elevated gastrin among patients presenting with recurrent peptic ulcer disease is acid suppression, usually due to proton pump inhibitor therapy. Acid is the most potent suppressor of gastrin production and in the face of PPI therapy, gastrin elevations are common. Gastrinoma produces hypergastrinemia but this is a rare tumor. Gastric atrophy associated with pernicious anemia is also associated with gastrin elevations but this is not common in young patients.

21.2 (c) Gastric pH. pH testing of gastric secretions is the most expeditious method of ruling out gastrinoma. Gastric pH will be acid (low) if hypergastrinemia is due to gastrinoma; however, causes of elevated gastrin due to hypochlorhydria (PPI use, atrophic gastritis) will reveal a relatively neutral pH. Secretin stimulation and acid output testing are useful to confirm the diagnosis of gastrinoma but require specialized equipment not as readily available as pH paper. Serum chromogranin A is a diagnostic test for gastrinoma but is not as expeditious as simply checking the gastric acidity.

21.3 (b) Bismuth, metronidazole, and amoxicillin. The issue is antibiotic resistance, especially with the clarithromycin regimens. While sequential therapy has excellent results, these are somewhat geographically disparate and US trials have not observed the same rates of eradication as non-US studies. Clarithromycin and metronidazole plus PPI has excellent eradication results but in treatment failures it is recommended to change clarithromycin to another agent. Quadruple therapy consisting of four times daily bismuth, metronidazole, and amoxicillin with twice-daily PPI is an effective salvage regimen after failure of triple therapy.

21.4 (c) CT scan of the abdomen. The most likely diagnosis is upper gastrointestinal hemorrhage due to peptic ulcer. At this point, there is no evidence of continued gastrointestinal hemorrhage; therefore, endoscopy is not emergent. The abdominal rebound tenderness with elevated WBC is worrisome for perforation, which can be detected by CT scan and would be a contraindication for endoscopy. *H. pylori* serology treatment is useful for prevention of recurrent ulceration but has no role in the acute management of complicated ulcer disease.

Chapter 22

22.1 (a) Proton pump inhibitor. Proton pump inhibitors treat functional dyspepsia, ulcer disease, and gastroesophageal reflux disease. In the absence of advanced age or alarm symptoms, an empirical trial of acid-reducing medication is acceptable. *H. pylori* eradication is indicated only if testing is performed and positive. Upper endoscopy is not necessary in this case due to the low risk of malignancy or other serious organic disease. CT scans are rarely diagnostic in dyspepsia without alarm features, especially with normal laboratory test.

22.2 (d) Normal. The most likely diagnosis is functional dyspepsia; therefore, a normal examination is likely. Duodenal and gastric ulcers are generally associated with *H. pylori* infection and/or NSAIDs; therefore, they are of low probability in this patient. Erosive esophagitis is possible but unlikely if proton pump inhibitors fail to alleviate symptoms.

22.3 (d) Reassurance. This patient has functional dyspepsia. Further evaluation is highly unlikely to identify a structural etiology for her symptoms. Reassurance and a supportive therapeutic relationship will be essential for improved quality of life.

22.4 (d) Tricyclic antidepressant. Of the strategies listed, TCA is the option that has the best evidence supporting effectiveness in functional dyspepsia. Amitriptyline, using a starting dose of 25–50 mg at bedtime, increasing to 75–100 mg over the course of several weeks, has been shown to reduce symptoms. Since *H. pylori* is not present, eradiction is not indicated.

High-dose proton pump inhibitor therapy has not been shown to improve symptoms more than standard dose therapy. Metoclopramide can be used to accelerate gastric emptying but this patient has not been assessed for this condition and the adverse event profile is more extensive than for TCAs.

Chapter 23

23.1 (c) Tumor with mucosal ulceration and GI bleeding. GISTs often present clinically with GI bleeding and are found to have an overlying ulcer on EGD. The presence of an ulcer is generally associated with a larger tumor; however, the presence of an ulcer with GI bleeding is not necessarily a high-risk feature. Biopsy of the ulcer base should be performed if active bleeding is not present as it often will result in sufficient diagnostic tissue.

23.2 (c) CT. A CT scan should be performed once the diagnosis of gastric cancer is made to evaluate for metastatic disease. If metastatic disease is identified on CT scan, an EUS is not necessary since local/regional staging will not have an impact on overall stage of the disease (stage IV disease). If there is no evidence of metastatic disease on CT scan then an EUS should be performed for local/regional staging.

Chapter 24

24.1 (c) Oats. Oats appear to be safe for most patients with celiac disease. Other safe grains include amaranth, buckwheat, corn, millet, quinoa, sorghum, and teff. Toxic grains include wheat, rye, and barley (including malt).

24.2 (d) Antigliadin antibodies. As shown in Figure 24.1, the initial evaluation of suspected celiac disease includes serological testing for anti-tTG IgA and IgG, and/or antiendomysial antibodies, followed by confirmatory testing with small bowel biopsies. Total IgA may be assessed because 2–3% of celiac patients may be IgA deficient, leading to a false-negative IgA test. However, antigliadin antibodies have lower sensitivity and specificity compared to tTG and antiendomysial antibodies and are no longer recommended.

24.3 (c) While symptomatic improvement after initiation of a gluten-free diet may be reported as soon as 48 h after it is initiated, recovery of normal intestinal histological features often takes much longer (i.e. months), and abnormalities persist in 50% of patients, despite strict adherence to the diet.

Chapter 25

25.1 (a) Calcium oxalate. Hyperoxaluria is due to increased absorption of dietary oxalate, particularly in the colon. Steatorrhea causes an increase in luminal fatty acids, which preferentially bind to calcium, leaving oxalate that is readily absorbed in the colon.

25.2 (d) D-lactic acidemia. D-lactic acid is derived from malabsorbed fermentable carbohydrates that are metabolized by colonic lactobacilli to D-lactic acid. The clinical syndrome consists of encephalopathy, D-lactic acidosis with compensatory hyperventilation.

25.3 (c) Antibiotics. D-lactic acidemia is caused by colonic fermentation of malabsorbed carbohydrates by lactobacilli. Treatment with antibiotics will reduce the D-lactate load. Reduction in dietary carbohydrates, and perhaps probiotic administration, will also reduce symptoms.

25.4 (b) Medium-chain triglycerides. Medium-chain triglycerides are absorbed in the absence of bile salts and do not require resynthesis in the enterocyte. Both short- and long-chain triglycerides require micelle formation that is facilitated by bile salts.

Chapter 26

26.1 (c) Side-viewing upper endoscopy. Patients with FAP are at increased risk for developing ampullary adenomas/adenocarcinomas. Therefore, side-viewing upper endoscopy should be performed every 1–2 years to examine the major papilla and duodenum for the development of adenomas. Double balloon enteroscopy and CT scans are not recommended for surveillance purposes. Standard upper endoscopy may also be performed for careful evaluation of the stomach; however, adequate visualization of the major papilla can be difficult with a forward-viewing endoscope.

26.2 (c) Urinary 5-HIAA. Carcinoid tumors produce and release serotonin, which is then metabolized to 5-HIAA. Carcinoid syndrome typically occurs in patients who have metastatic disease to the liver; therefore, a liver function panel (AST, ALT, alkaline phosphatase, bilirubin) should be ordered. However, abnormal liver enzymes alone will not support the diagnosis of carcinoid syndrome.

Chapter 27

27.1 (a) Approximately half of diverticular hemorrhage emanates from the right colon.

27.2 Although the majority of diverticula are found in the sigmoid colon, half of diverticular hemorrhages emanate from a right colonic source. There is no evidence to support the notion that seeds, corn or nuts may precipitate diverticulitis. Actually, there is some evidence to support an inverse association (i.e. possibly protective effect). Approximately 70% of individuals with diverticulosis remain asymptomatic. Barium enema is not recommended during an acute diverticulitis episode. However, a CT scan can be very helpful for clarifying the diagnosis and evaluating for complications.

27.3 (b) Abscess formation. A diverticular abscess should initially be managed percutaneously. If that fails, then surgery is indicated. Recurrent diverticulitis is an indication for surgical management. Research has shown that patients under age 50 are more likely to have recurrent attacks. Therefore, some advocate surgery on the basis of age along. Other indications for surgery include obstruction, inability to exclude carcinoma, and intractable symptoms.

27.4 (b) False. Most patients with diverticulosis are asymptomatic. There is some controversy as to whether or not uncomplicated diverticulosis can cause symptoms. Some patients have mild, intermittent abdominal pain, bloating, flatulence, and altered defecation, although coexistence of irritable bowel syndrome is possible.

Chapter 28

28.1 (a) Lubiprostone. Lubiprostone is a choloride channel activator that increases intestinal fluid secretion and facilitates intestinal transit. Dicyclomine is an antispasmodic. Alosetron is used in women with diarrhea-predominant IBS. Tricyclic antidepressants can modulate pain perception and may be most beneficial in patients with diarrhea. Atropine with diphenoxylate is an antidiarrheal.

28.2 (d) Association with ischemic colitis. The 5-HT$_3$ receptor antagonist alosetron is a potent treatment for refractory diarrhea-predominant IBS. Because this agent increases the risks of severe constipation and ischemic colitis, it is prescribed only through a restricted program. Because it has not been adequately studied in men, it is only approved for women with severe diarrhea-predominant IBS.

28.3 (d) Tricyclic antidepressant. Tricyclic antidepressants exhibit significant potency in patients with significant pain. Tricyclics may also reduce symptoms in those with prominent diarrhea. Polyethylene glycol solution, tegaserod, and lubiprostone are effective at treating constipation. Tegaserod was withdrawn from the US market due to risk of ischemic colitis.

Chapter 29

29.1 (c) Stool examination for *C. difficile*. The incidence of *C. difficile*-associated disease is elevated in IBD compared to non-IBD controls, and can manifest in the absence of antibiotic use. Evaluation to rule out this infection is mandatory prior to initiation of immunosuppressive therapy.

29.2 (d) Surgical intervention. While IV steroids, infliximab, and cyclosporine are used in severe ulcerative colitis, the presentation of toxic megacolon with peritoneal signs warrants immediate surgical evaluation.

29.3 (d) Calcium oxalate. Small intestinal malabsorption of fat increases fatty acid binding to calcium, which in turn increases colonic absorption of oxalate. Malabsorption in the small intestine also increases bile salt exposure to the colon, increasing permeability to oxalate.

Chapter 30

30.1 (e) Colonoscopy. This presentation is concerning for colorectal cancer. Colonoscopy is the diagnostic test of choice in this setting. If the colonoscopy is negative, EGD would be appropriate as the next step for evaluating iron deficiency anemia. In many centers, these two exams would be scheduled concurrently to avoid the need for additional exposure to sedation and the inconvenience to the patient. A fecal occult blood test should be used only for screening for colon cancer. This patient requires a diagnostic test. If colorectal cancer is found, a staging abdominal and pelvic CT scan would be indicated.

30.2 (d) Colonoscopy now with referral for genetics counseling. This patient's family history meets the Amsterdam II criteria for the diagnosis of HNPCC because he has three relatives with HNPCC-associated cancers (colorectal and ureteral), involving at least two successive generations and at least one cancer was diagnosed before age 50. Ideally, genetic testing of his affected relatives could be done to identify which mismatch repair gene is affected, and if the patient does carry the mutation, then he would require annual colonoscopy. Annual FOBT and colonoscopy every 10 years are appropriate for average-risk individuals. CT colonography every 5 years is also recommended by some for average-risk individuals.

30.3 (e) None of the above. The US Preventive Services Task Force recommends against routine screening in individuals aged 76–85. If this patient was in good overall health, particularly if she had not been previously screened, then screening may be appropriate. However, given her negative colonoscopy 10 years ago, her risk for colorectal cancer is below average. In addition, she has significant comorbidity that limits the relative benefits of screening.

Chapter 31

31.1 (b) Second-degree hemorrhoids prolapse and require digital reduction. Actually, second-degree hemorrhoids prolapse with defecation but spontaneously reduce. First-degree hemorrhoids do not protrude from the anus. Third-degree hemorrhoids prolapse and require digital reduction, and fourth-degree hemorrhoids cannot be reduced and are at risk of strangulation.

31.2 (d) Anal fissure. A thrombosed external hemorrhoid can also present with severe pain and scant bleeding, though these two conditions are readily distinguished on physical exam.

31.3 (b) Anal fissure. When conservative therapy with a high-fiber diet, stool softener and warm sitz baths fails, topical nitroglycerin or calcium channel blockers, or intramuscular injection of botulinum toxin may promote fissure healing.

Chapter 32

32.1 (a) Immediate-release enzymes (nonenteric coated) have been shown to be effective in the treatment of chronic pancreatitis pain in a randomized controlled trial. However, immediate-release enzymes were recently taken off the market by the FDA and are currently not available in the US.

32.2 (b) Once the prediction of severe acute pancreatitis is made. Early initiation of enteral feeding in patients with severe acute pancreatitis has been demonstrated to decrease the risk of infection and decrease hospital stay, with a trend towards improving mortality.

32.3 (c) Higher concentration of CCK and secretin-secreting cells in the duodenum. Since there is a higher concentration of CCK and secretin-secreting cells in the duodenum, there is a theoretical advantage of bypassing this segment of bowel for enteral nutrition since feeding into the duodenum would stimulate release of CCK and secretin, resulting in increased stimulation of the pancreas.

32.4 (b) Shortly after presentation for mild acute pancreatitis, delayed days to weeks after presentation for severe acute pancreatitis. The guidelines for performing surgery in patients with acute biliary pancreatitis depend on the severity. For mild gallstone pancreatitis, laparoscopic cholecystectomy should be performed as soon as the patient has recovered and during the same hospital admission. In patients with severe gallstone pancreatitis, cholecystectomy should be delayed until there is a sufficient resolution of the inflammatory response and clinical recovery.

32.5 (a) Pseudocyst size greater than 6 cm. Size alone is not a sufficient reason to perform pseudocyst drainage. The decision to perform pseudocyst drainage should be based on symptoms or evidence of infection.

Chapter 33

33.1 (d) EUS FNA. EUS FNA is the best method for obtaining tissue for diagnosis of pancreatic cancer. CA 19-9 can be useful for following response to therapy if elevated at the time of diagnosis; however, it should not be used to establish the diagnosis.

33.2 (d) 70%.

33.3 (b) Mucinous cystadenoma. The findings of an elevated CEA >200 ng/ dL, low amylase, and no duct abnormalities on EUS examination suggest the diagnosis of mucinous cystadenoma. Theses lesions do have potential for malignant transformation and should either be resected or monitored closely.

Chapter 34

34.1 (b) Klatskin tumor

34.2 (d) Celiac sprue. Refer to Table 24.1.

34.3 (e) Type V. Type V cysts are characterized by one or more cystic dilations of the intrahepatic ducts, without extrahepatic duct dilation. If multiple cystic dilations are present then the disease is known as Caroli disease.

Chapter 35

35.1 (c) Hypotension. The Charcot triad consists of RUQ abdominal pain, fever, and jaundice and is suggestive for cholangitis. Hypotension and confusion in addition to the Charcot triad make up the Reynolds pentad, which is suggestive of a more fulminant course.

35.2 (c) Type III. Type III SOD consists of biliary-type pain with normal liver tests and normal-caliber common bile duct.

Chapter 36

36.1 (d) CT scan is the imaging test of choice for suspected intra-abdominal abscess with a sensitivity of approximately 90%.

36.2 (c) Infliximab IV. Antitumor necrosis factor agents, including infliximab, have been demonstrated in randomized controlled trials to reduce the number of draining fistula by up to 68% and to completely close all fistulae in up to 55% of patients.

36.3 (b) The hernia of Bochdalek is a posterolateral diaphragmatic hernia through the lumbosacral area and can cause respiratory insufficiency, failure to thrive, and intestinal strangulation.

Chapter 37

37.1 False. A vigorous immune response is responsible for an aggressive clinical hepatitis, but also is more likely to result in clearance of the virus.

37.2 (c) Core antibody, regardless of class, is present with acute, chronic, and resolved hepatitis B. The persistence of HBsAg beyond 6 months is considered an indication of chronic infection.

37.3 (d) Hepatitis E virus, which typically causes a self-limited infection after fecal–oral exposure, is associated with a high rate (15–25%) of fulminant hepatitis in women during the third trimester of pregnancy.

Chapter 38

38.1 (b) It is estimated that 20% of NASH patients may progress to advanced fibrosis/cirrhosis. The peak onset of Wilson disease is in the second decade of life. Kayser–Fleischer rings are not always present in Wilson disease, although are uniformly present in the setting of neurological involvement. A hepatic iron index >1.9 is consistent with hemochromatosis.

38.2 (d) Penicillamine and trientine are chelators of copper. Zinc inhibits copper absorption from the gut, and therefore is not used to manage pre-existing copper overload but rather for maintenance after copper depletion. There is no role for ursodiol in the treatment of Wilson disease.

38.3 (d) The characteristic histological features of NASH are steatosis, hepatocyte ballooning degeneration, lobular inflammation, pericellular fibrosis and Mallory hyaline, with unremarkable bile ducts.

Chapter 39

39.1 (d) HELLP syndrome and acute fatty liver of pregnancy are two severe illnesses that can present with cholestasis during the third trimester. Cholestasis of pregnancy and placental release of alkaline phosphatase follow a benign course.

39.2 (c) Positive AMA and elevated IgM levels are the classic serological findings in PBC. The classic histological findings of PBC are small bile duct destruction with florid duct lesions, and often with noncaseating granulomas. Imaging studies are not expected to show biliary dilation in PBC.

39.3 (b) The appropriate dose of ursodiol in PBC is approximately 15 mg/kg, not 5 mg/kg. PBC patients are likely to be deficient in fat-soluble vitamins and to have reduced bone density so the routine use of calcium and vitamin D supplementation is appropriate.

Chapter 40

40.1 (c) The typical pattern in alcoholic hepatitis is AST>ALT, with values under 300 IU/L.

40.2 (b) The inflammation on liver biopsy in alcoholic hepatitis is predominantly neutrophilic.

40.3 (c) Patients with alcoholic hepatitis benefit from alcohol cessation, regardless of disease severity.

Chapter 41

41.1 (a) Liver biopsy plays a very important role in confirming the diagnosis of AIH. Patients with type 2 AIH are unlikely (<5%) to have a positive ANA. The absence of viral hepatitis and the presence of IgG elevation increase the likelihood of the diagnosis of AIH, with additional points provided in the diagnostic scoring systems.

41.2 (c) Excess iron is not an expected finding on the liver biopsy of a patient with AIH. The histological findings are not specific, and can overlap with those seen in viral and drug-induced liver disease. Bridging necrosis is not uncommon in those with severe hepatitis on presentation. The inflammatory cells typically seen on biopsy in AIH are lymphocytes and plasma cells.

Chapter 42

42.1 (c) Type 1 hepatorenal syndrome is the more severe form of HRS and is typically irreversible without liver transplantation. It is associated with intrarenal vasoconstriction. Above an HVPG of 12, higher values do not correlate well with additional bleeding risk. Portopulmonary hypertension is due to pulmonary vascular vasoconstriction, while hepatopulmonary syndrome is related to intrapulmonary shunting.

42.2 (c) Recommendations are for the use of a nonselective β-blocker, such as propranolol, carvedilol or nadolol.

Chapter 43

43.1 (b) Hepatocellular carcinoma affects men more than women, with a ratio of greater than 2/1.

43.2 (b) HCCs typically show "washout" of contrast on portal and delayed images, resulting in a hypodense appearance.

43.3 (c) Patients with HCC within "Milan Criteria" (up to three lesions <3 cm or single lesion <5 cm) receive priority for liver transplant with MELD exception points. Only a minority of HCCs are resectable (5–20%), and the 5-year recurrence rates are approximately 50%. TACE can precipitate worsening liver function in patients with advanced liver disease, including those with high bilirubin.

Chapter 44

44.1 (b) Stool culture is not able to distinguish between toxigenic and non-pathogenic strains of *C. difficile*, and therefore cannot differentiate asymptomatic carriers from patients with colitis. While endoscopic evaluation is usually not necessary in the diagnosis and evaluation of *C. difficile* infection, findings of pseudomembranes are suggestive of the infection.

44.2 (d) Antibiotics are not recommended for this infection because they do not diminish the duration of symptoms or prevent complications, and may increase the risk of developing hemolytic uremic syndrome.

44.3 (b) While it can be challenging to do so, *C. jejuni* can be isolated from stool culture.

Chapter 45

45.1 (a) Ulcerated lesion with a pigmented protuberance. This is consistent with an ulcer and not a Dieulafoy lesion.

45.2 (c) Transjugular intrahepatic portosystemic shunt (TIPS). Although GAVE can be seen in the setting of portal hypertension, TIPS is generally not effective in managing bleeding due to GAVE.

Index

Yamada's Handbook of Gastroenterology, Third Edition. Edited by Tadataka Yamada
and John M. Inadomi.
© 2013 John Wiley & Sons, Ltd. Published 2013 by John Wiley & Sons, Ltd.